THE SHOPPER'S GUIDE TO ECONOMY, ECOLOGY, AND GOOD EATING

The Supermarket Handbook names names, national brands, ingredients, additives, nutritional values, and costs. It pinpoints manufacturer's deceptions and evasions, including those of some so-called natural foods, provides easy, low-cost ways of preparing convenient substitutes for many supermarket items, and offers a bibliography and recommended reading list. It is a very good book to have and to use.

"The label-reading authors know their way around the shelves . . . a good guide!"
—*Chicago Tribune*

"Highly recommended as an extremely useful, practical guide for wise food choices."
—*Organic Gardening and Farming*

"Invaluable."
—*Vogue*

"Supplies and prices being what they are, we've got to do better. And a good place to start is to take a look at *The Supermarket Handbook.*"
—Howard K. Smith, ABC-TV

About the Authors

Nikki and David Goldbeck have teamed up their professional as well as personal lives to write and lecture about the basics of food, nutrition, and ecology. Their traditional approach to these subjects caused *The New York Times* to accuse them of trying to "reinvent the wheel."

Nikki Goldbeck received a B.S. in food and nutrition from Cornell University, then began her food career doing product development, recipe testing, and publicity for a Madison Avenue public relations firm. Appalled by how the "big business" of food was fed to the public, she left to devote herself to the natural foods field as a writer and food consultant. She is a regular contributor to *Organic Gardening and Farming* and author of *Cooking What Comes Naturally*, a vegetarian cookbook.

David Goldbeck received a B.A. in economics from Queens College and an L.L.B. from Brooklyn Law School. A former elementary school teacher and attorney, he left the practice of law in 1971 to work with Nikki. In addition to *The Supermarket Handbook*, together they have written *The Good Breakfast Book* and *The Dieter's Companion*.

The Goldbecks live in Woodstock, New York, in a house that resembles a log cabin which they renovated themselves.

THE SUPERMARKET HANDBOOK

Access to Whole Foods

Nikki and David Goldbeck

Drawings by Ellen Weiss

REVISED AND
EXPANDED EDITION

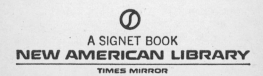

A SIGNET BOOK
NEW AMERICAN LIBRARY
TIMES MIRROR

*To the Preservation
of the Family Farm*

NAL BOOKS ARE ALSO AVAILABLE AT DISCOUNTS
IN BULK QUANTITY FOR INDUSTRIAL OR
SALES-PROMOTIONAL USE. FOR DETAILS, WRITE TO
PREMIUM MARKETING DIVISION, NEW AMERICAN LIBRARY, INC.,
1301 AVENUE OF THE AMERICAS, NEW YORK, NEW YORK 10019.

Originally appeared in paperback as a Plume edition
published by The New American Library, Inc.

A hardcover edition was published in the United States by
Harper & Row, and simultaneously in Canada by
Fitzhenry & Whiteside Limited, Toronto.

Library of Congress Catalog Card Number: 73-4084

 SIGNET TRADEMARK REG. U.S. PAT. OFF. AND FOREIGN COUNTRIES
REGISTERED TRADEMARK—MARCA REGISTRADA
HECHO EN CHICAGO, U.S.A.

SIGNET, SIGNET CLASSICS, MENTOR, PLUME AND MERIDIAN BOOKS
*are published by The New American Library, Inc.,
1301 Avenue of the Americas, New York, New York 10019*

FIRST SIGNET PRINTING, NOVEMBER, 1976

3 4 5 6 7 8 9

PRINTED IN THE UNITED STATES OF AMERICA

Contents

Acknowledgments

We wish to thank the many readers who have taken the time to write and share with us their ideas and suggestions, all of which encouraged us to update and expand *The Supermarket Handbook*.

The object of all unprincipled modern manufacturers seems to be the sparing of their time and labour as much as possible, and to increase the quantity of the articles they produce without regard to their quality. The ingenuity and perseverance of self-interest is proof against prohibitions and contrivances to elude the vigilance of the most active government.

—Frederick Accum, *A Treatise on Adulteration of
Food and Culinary Poisons, etc.,* London (1820)

Preface to the First Edition

How much do you really know about the foods you buy?

Why is it, we wonder, that in America, land of overstocked supermarkets, rapid communication and mass education, that improper diet and poor nutrition prevail?

America has been characterized as a "nation of nutritional illiterates" who know very little about what foods to buy or how to go about preparing them. But why should it be otherwise when so many of the available foods are pre-prepared packages intended for human consumption, yet generally devoid of a complete list of ingredients or otherwise useful information—anonymous foods?

Unless you've had some particular interest in food and nutrition, your education is probably limited to a public school home-economics class at best. Moreover, the policies of secrecy maintained by both government agencies and food processors make it almost impossible for even the knowledgeable and concerned consumer to really determine the quality of the food he or she ingests.

Although all the foods we need to live healthy, satisfied lives already exist in nature, the food industry would have us believe that "new," "improved" products are necessary—foods built around a framework of synthetics of questionable food value and potential physical harm.

The result of using even nontoxic additives is a product that replaces fresh top-grade ingredients with lower quality raw materials enhanced and alchemized to *appear* like the real thing. Less real food is needed when artificial ingredients intensify a taste or duplicate a texture. With the use of chemicals, foods that have outlasted their natural life span can appear "unstale." The question of whether these foods are still nutritionally alive is answered by industry with the use of synthetic nutrients to "revive" their creations. Much of the profit of food processing comes from this ability to use less food matter and to take chemical short cuts, otherwise known as "skimping on the recipe."

While many exposés tell us what *not* to buy and why, no one has taken the time to educate us as to what good choices we can make and how to go about preparing them. Because so much money is spent on promoting concocted foods, the real foods they imitate or replace are becoming unknown to us. But these basic foods do still exist.

A new food consciousness is in order to help us select and substitute whole, unprocessed foods for the bulk of the junk on the food market.

In our personal concern to succeed in developing this new food awareness, we investigated and lived with many different alternatives. We eventually learned to prepare meals without convenience foods in the same convenient amount of time. We found that eating unprocessed and unadulterated foodstuffs, closest to their natural state—what we refer to as whole foods—need not be expensive; in all truth our food bills are measurably reduced and we are able to do most of our shopping in our neighborhood supermarket.

We know that many other men and women still find cooking an enjoyable part of their lives and would gladly forgo the chemicals and extra expense of packaged, processed goods if they knew how to secure healthful raw materials among the supermarket stock; particularly if they knew that in doing so they could reduce calories, chemical consumption and food costs.

The Supermarket Handbook is designed to guide you past the nonnutritive, chemically laden nonfoods in the supermarket to the whole, healthy items that are still available. It will help you to understand labels and select foods with a discerning eye; it will teach you to prepare whole foods and use them to replace processed ones. *The Supermarket Handbook* aims to minimize chemical ingestion and maximize eating pleasure. We hope it will also encourage the food industry to provide more and more whole foods on the market, protecting the American farmer from extinction, so that we can once again get in touch with the basic elements of the food we eat.

Nikki and David Goldbeck

Woodstock, New York

Preface to the Revised Edition: Journey Through the Food Spectrum

We left a trail of half-full grocery carts and curious grocery clerks from coast to coast. We got to know intimately the aisles of local Ralphs, Krogers, A&P's, and K-marts. We hunted down Safeways, Waldbaums, even the Berkeley Coop. Our biggest find was a quiet, all-night supermarket.

For more than two months we traveled America in search of the best that regional supermarkets had to offer. Our aim was to broaden the recommendations of *whole foods* that appear at the end of each chapter, so that this second edition of *The Supermarket Handbook* would be useful to people in every section of the United States. These recommendations include the brand names of items available in supermarkets that meet our test of *wholeness*—that is, foods "free of chemical additives, colorants, or artificial flavoring, left in the whole, unrefined state or processed as little as possible to render them suitable for eating."

We are happy to report that our research proved successful; we have found hundreds of supermarket products that merit your attention. Dozens of whole grain breads, crackers, and flours; canned fruits without added sugar and juices without sugar or salt; untainted dairy products and peanut butter; pure mayonnaise, oil, and margarine; plus brown rice, dried fruit, nuts, wheat germ, molasses, honey, and more.

What amazed us, though, was to find how different the food supply is from one part of this country to the next. For example, while on the East Coast we see a choice of dairy products—yogurts, cottage cheeses, and sour creams—that are free of chemical adulturants, in the rest of the country there is rarely one acceptable brand. While the West offers an abundance of high-quality whole grain baked goods, most of the country has only two or three acceptable breads to choose from; in the Middle West we rarely encountered any additive-free whole grain breads at all. (This last observation was reinforced by a customer in a New York supermarket who was in the process of buying fifteen loaves of whole grain bread to send to a friend in Nebraska.)

This crazy-quilt pattern continues. Additive-free canned beans, offering convenient, inexpensive protein, are readily available in the Southwest, yet are generally nonexistent in the West. Unadulterated ice cream, taken for granted on the East and West Coasts, is a rarity elsewhere. Nutritious alternatives to the "American style" breakfast cereals are found mostly in the East and West. Pure oils, with the exception of peanut and olive oils, are also largely confined to the coastal states.

The most encouraging discovery of our trip, however, was the realization that for every staple food there is at least one brand available, and more often several, that meets the standards of a whole food. While the supermarket shopper will probably not find acceptable choices in all food categories in just one store, our research proves that such foods can, and do, exist.*

An interest in diet and nutrition can be both a selfish and a selfless concern, for the modern techniques that are supposed to supply food for mankind now seem to be linked to many of our personal, social, and economic problems.

Consider modern feed-lot techniques which fatten animals in less time but produce meat that contains residues of feed additives (particularly the highly suspect hormone DES), and meat so fatty that it is increasingly thought of as a contributor to obesity, heart disease, and cancer.

Consider white flour, pasta, bread, rice, and over-processed vegetables and fruits; while these foods have been suspected for a long time as being poor sources of nutrition, they are now viewed with increased concern because of their lack of fiber, a potential cause of digestive illnesses ranging from simple constipation to cancer of the bowel.

Consider a food supply containing artificial flavors, colors, sweeteners, preservatives, and the like, whose safety is constantly in doubt and whose use allows manufacturers to employ inferior raw ingredients.

Consider the FDA and the USDA, the two federal agencies we have entrusted with the tough job of protecting and policing our food

*Note that the Exemplary Brands listed, while extensive, are not and never will be a complete list of all whole foods available in the United States. Because of the size of this country and the ever changing nature of our food supply, products come and go and ingredients are subject to change. Moreover, food processors have been generally uncooperative in filling the gaps in our research. So in the end, it is up to each shopper to compile his own list of exemplary brands.

supply; both are so corrupted by the interests they were intended to oversee that the regulators are now controlled by those who were to be regulated.

Consider the "Green Revolution," industrial farming techniques which use so much energy that our homes, factories, and cars must now compete with our stomachs for fuel. This agricultural situation is due largely to our dependence on artificial fertilizers—chemicals that require vast amounts of fuel for their manufacture. It is understandable that chemical fertilizers are needed to supplement the available natural ones, but at present we ignore 1.6 billion tons of animal wastes and an equal amount of human waste—enough waste, once treated, to fertilize at least half of America's farmland. "Farming uses more petroleum than any other industry," state two Cornell researchers writing in *Science* magazine.

Consider the separation of suppliers, growers, processors, warehouses, wholesalers, retailers, and consumers, which adds an enormous surcharge to food costs and a needless drain on our limited fossil fuels. Several studies have shown transportation to be the second largest energy user in our food production system.

Because energy-intensive farming techniques were developed for large-scale farming, government farm policies favor the factory-farm. With lack of federal and academic support, more than 2,000 farms have been closing down each week since the 1940's; farms that provide employment and high-quality local produce with minimum energy input. As one observer has put it, ". . . the small farmer is no longer an agricultural problem; he is a welfare problem." Although a few states, including North Dakota, Kansas, and Minnesota, have laws that prohibit or curtail corporate farming, lack of public interest has kept a Federal Family Farm Anti-Trust Act in congressional committee.

In much the same way, our national encouragement of a diet high in meat has brought about inefficient use of our remaining farmland. Much of the valuable crops produced on the land, like soy and grain, are fed not to people but to cattle. Professor Georg Borgstrom of the University of Michigan estimates that the developed world, which makes up only 28 percent of the world's population, consumes three fourths of the world's fish supply and two thirds of the world's grain —not as human food, but indirectly, through the meat we eat.

One reason why we eat what we eat, is the tantalizing packaging that surrounds factory foods, nine tenths of which you throw away when you get home. It is estimated that merely cutting packaging in half would save 200,000 barrels of oil each day.

America's food advertising, which uses high-powered media techniques, exposes children to an average of twenty TV commercials an hour, eighteen of which sell edibles on the basis of their "sweetened, sugared, or crisped quality." The billions of dollars spent each year on public relations and advertising have so perverted our eating habits that many people now prefer the taste of factory-made foods to their real counterparts. As Dr. Ross Hume Hall has written in his excellent book *Food for Nought/The Decline in Nutrition:*

> When food technologists began to separate nutrition from palatability, they also undermined the ability of the human senses to assess the quality of the food. Texture, color, odor, taste, and feel of natural food are all human guides, not only to the nutritional value of food, but also to its sagely. At one time, one could use one's own senses to determine accurately the freshness of food, but man's senses no longer guide him in his choice of food items.

A U.S. Senate Report (1973) established that there were more than 12 million malnourished people in this country, spanning all economic sectors. This malnutrition can be directly linked to one of America's most tragic faces, that of the retarded child. Because of improper diet during pregnancy and infancy, the national incidence of learning disabilities, social maladjustment, and neurologic disorders is increasing rather than diminishing.

And, saddest of all, we are now in the business of exporting food technology, so that American cola drinks are available even in remote villages; improperly prepared infant formula is replacing mother's milk in underdeveloped countries; and, in an attempt to emulate the American life-style, many nations are forsaking their traditional diet and are encouraging in its place a fatty meat regimen.

We feel that by learning to feed ourselves and others whole foods, we can minimize the possible cause of many serious illnesses, including birth defects, diabetes, cancer, and heart disease. By encouraging small farmers and purchasing locally grown, minimally packaged foodstuffs, we can generate enormous energy savings while we simultaneously employ people. Lastly, by learning to use and appreciate all protein sources, we can help make sufficient protein available to all people.

We are convinced it is within our power as consumers to make whole foods available in our own areas; hopefully the information that the lists of Exemplary Brands provides can serve as a catalyst for improving the available food supply for all of us. By selecting the unrefined, unchemicalized foods in the supermarket, you show the store manager and manufacturer your preference. By asking for those items you do not find, you encourage the store to order them. And, as Majorie Mohr of the *Farmington New Hampshire News* suggested in her review of the first edition of *The Supermarket Handbook,* we hope that this book will inspire supermarket owners so that "they may develop a sense of responsibility to make a positive contribution to the health of the citizens they serve."

In addition to the expanded Recommendations, this second edition of *The Supermarket Handbook* contains a bibliography, reading list, and a number of updated footnotes.

David and Nikki Goldbeck
Woodstock, New York
July, 1976

A Key to the Book

In the forthcoming chapters we hope to acquaint you with the best choices you can make in the supermarket to bring flavorful, nutritious, and wholesome foods into your home. As you travel with us through the aisles of the supermarket we will point out which foods can add the most to your diet and how you can go about selecting the best of them. From many of the shelves you will be able to choose freely and confidently; from many you will not be able to buy at all. In between these two extremes we will come upon many products that offer some brands which are excellent along with some that we prefer to leave exactly where they are. In those cases we will try to help you evaluate the contents so that you will always be able to make a wise purchase.

In researching and preparing this book we naturally had to set certain standards. Our main consideration for each food item in question was, "Is it as unadulterated or unprocessed as possible?" With few exceptions we blanketly reject any product that contains any uncalled-for chemical additives or highly processed ingredients such as white sugar and white flour. What we are left with are foods that we call "whole"—foods which have undergone only enough processing to render them tasty without destroying their inherent value; foods which do not depend on highly processed ingredients in their manufacture and foods free of artificial flavoring, artificial coloring, chemical preservatives, or other synthetic additions. In general these foods are not "organic," although we personally think organic foods are best.

At the end of each chapter in Part I, "A Shopping Tour," we have prepared for your convenience a summary of what we feel we can recommend in each particular category. This list of "Recommendations" lays out a general rule of purchase and, where possible, suggests exemplary brands or items. Once you have read through the book and are ready to tackle your local supermarket you can simply refer back to these summaries in making up your shopping list, or take the book with you on your shopping rounds.

Many of the brands in your supermarket may be unknown to us;

this does not mean they do not offer a perfectly sound choice. Here we can only counsel you to read the label, keeping in mind the suggestions we have given as to what to look for in that particular product. If the list of ingredients does not violate any of our warnings, by all means buy.

Even after you've gotten your shopping down to a system where you know at a glance what you will and will not buy, go back to checking the labels on occasion. This way you'll know when anything new has been added—either to the product or the available choices.

Our choices are not without mistakes in either direction. We are sure items may be included here which, if we had had more information, would have been excluded. And as we said, we know that there are many more items we would have liked to recommend that were not made known to us. These shortcomings are partially the result of our own human handicaps, but in large part they are due to the secrecy of industry and the policies of our government.

The federal standards of identity leave many loopholes open to the manufacturer and at the same time remove many labeling requirements. This, and the deceit and chicanery often practiced by the food industry, have combined to keep us ignorant of the food we eat. By researching the federal food laws and other appropriate materials, by making in-the-supermarket investigations, and by querying many food processors by letter and telephone we have attempted to bring you the information *you are entitled to.* At the back of the book you will find "A Glossary of Terms," which will enhance your understanding of some of the words used in the text that may be foreign to you. Perhaps you will find things less of a mystery if you give these definitions a quick glance before you begin.

In addition, to help you resist the temptation of buying where no suitable selection can be made, Part II, "In Your Kitchen," will provide you with some easy ways you can cook the high-quality foods you've brought home. Homecooking doesn't have to be complicated or lengthy; it only has to be good, and we hope to show you how to make all your future meals live up to that high expectation.

We know this book will be helpful in many ways and to many people. We hope that it will not only help people who already eat well to eat better but will also assist those who now, through poverty or ignorance, eat poorly.

A KEY TO THE BRAND NAME RECOMMENDATIONS

To facilitate finding the "Exemplary Brands" in your supermarket, certain foods which are not generally distributed nationwide—dairy products, breads, peanut butter, for example—have been classified by their distribution areas as follows:

East—all states east of the Mississippi

Middle—all states situated between the Mississippi and the Rockies

West—all states west of the Rockies

Where distribution is more widespread, or where a product is marketed nationwide, food items may be broken down by variety, i.e., by the specific type of bean, flour, cereal, beverage, oil, etc.

Within each grouping, brands are listed alphabetically by trade name.

When requesting brands from your supermarket, keep in mind that most items from other "distribution areas," particularly the one nearest you, can probably be made available in your area too.

JOIN US

The Supermarket Handbook is a living, growing volume and we welcome your advice to help keep it that way. Have you discovered a noteworthy item in your supermarket that we've neglected to mention? Has something new been added to the picture that should be included in these pages? Have we erred in any of our recommendations?

If you have any information you feel would be helpful to your fellow supermarket shoppers we would be happy to receive it, check it out, and include it in future editions of this book. Make sure you include full particulars concerning your recommendation: brand name, product type, ingredient list, price, and address of manufacturer (or just send us the label).

We regret we can no longer offer free books for usable recommendations, nor can we acknowledge letters unless a stamped, self-addressed envelope is enclosed.

Our mailing address is R.D. 1, Box 452, Woodstock, N.Y. 12498.

Part 1

A Shopping Tour

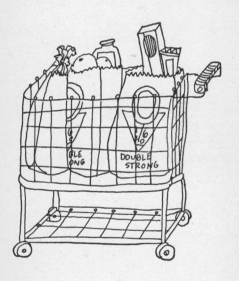

The Good Egg

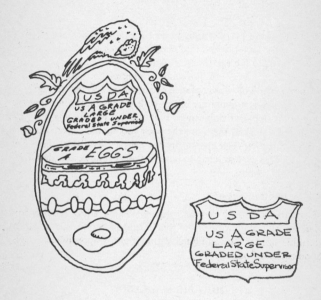

When it comes to nutrition, eggs are at the top of the list of the most highly regarded foods. It is the egg, not milk, that should have been popularized as nature's most nearly perfect food, for, with the exception of vitamin C, the egg is a balanced source of all the important vitamins and minerals; at the same time each egg boasts 6 grams of high-quality protein. Although there's been a lot of adverse publicity linking the egg and cholesterol, the egg is actually only a partial contributor to dietary cholesterol. If you are concerned, you'd be better off paying closer attention to your intake of animal fat in the form of meat, milk, butter, cheese, and other whole-milk dairy products instead of eliminating eggs from your diet. We're not, however, suggesting you ignore the advice of your doctor (although most doctors know surprisingly little about nutrition) or go on an egg binge. Too much of even a good thing is bad.

Do make good use of this nutritionally rich food, and while you're cutting down on your meat intake, build some of your meals around egg dishes.

BUYING EGGS

Fresh eggs are by no means perfect on the chemical score since traces of the antibiotics and feed chemicals given to laying hens may be transferred to the egg (See "Making the Best of Birds"). Because free-running chickens are becoming a thing of the past, most hens have never made the acquaintance of a rooster. Too bad though, for a fertilized egg is a living organism, with the vital enzymes that are present only in once living things. If eggs from free-running hens are sold in your market, these are the ones you should choose. If eggs from grain- rather than chemically fed hens are available, these will be richer in flavor, less likely to have chemical residue and should be your priority choice.

Grading and Inspection

Eggs are graded by size and quality. The grading requirement differs for each state with a legal weight range for a dozen eggs set to determine size labeling and quality grades set by appearance. Size is no indication of quality.

HOW BIG IS AN EGG?

Size	Weight
Extra Large	27 to 30 ounces per dozen
Large	24 to 27 ounces per dozen
Medium	21 to 24 ounces per dozen
Small	18 to 21 ounces per dozen

There is a voluntary government inspection program for eggs as well. The three grade marks, shown in an official government seal, are U.S. Grade AA (or Fancy Fresh Quality), U.S. Grade A, and U.S. Grade B. Many state grade standards are the same as the U.S. grades. When grade is marked on the carton, select U.S. Fancy Fresh Quality (Grade AA) or your state equivalent. Sometimes lightly cracked eggs are offered for sale; if there is a grading system these are the lowest

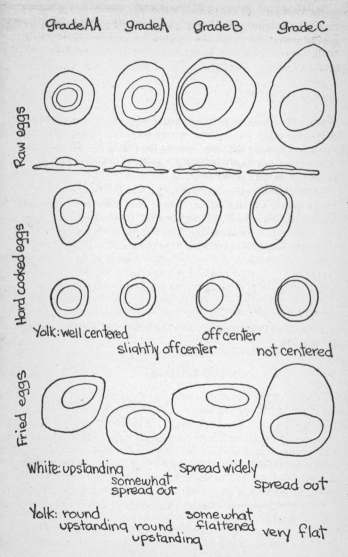

Grade AA Grade A Grade B Grade C

Raw eggs

Hard cooked eggs

Yolk: well centered

slightly off center

off center

not centered

Fried eggs

White: upstanding

somewhat spread out

spread widely

spread out

Yolk: round upstanding

round upstanding

somewhat flattened

very flat

5

grade. They may contain bacteria which can easily seep through the crack and penetrate the internal membrane. Unless the egg is *well cooked* you're taking a big chance when you use cracked eggs. High-quality grade eggs have better flavor, are fresher (at least when graded), and most lower grade eggs are destined for commercial use anyway.

Freshness

Modern technology has intervened in egg marketing to the benefit of the consumer. Eggs on the market today are fresher than ever, sometimes arriving within one to two days of laying. Whether your supermarket puts them out for sale immediately is a matter of chance, dependent on their turnover.

Many states have a dating code on eggs which indicates the last day the carton should be sold. Let this be your guide in selecting the freshest eggs available in your supermarket. If only the date of inspection is given, your purchase date should be within ten days. (For more information, see "Interpreting Food-Dating Codes: Blind Dates.")

Temperature is a key factor in egg deterioration. At room temperature an egg loses more quality in one day than it will if held one week under refrigeration. Make sure you buy from a refrigerated case.

Color Is Only Shell Deep

It shouldn't surprise you to learn that brown and white eggs are the same inside.

DOING YOUR OWN EGG GRADING

As an egg ages, the inner air pocket grows larger. A truly fresh egg will float; an old egg will sink.

When you break a really fresh egg the area it covers is small. The yolk remains round and upstanding and the thick white stands plentiful and firm around the yolk. Surrounding this thick white will be a smaller area of thin white albumen. As the egg ages, the white begins to spread and the yolk begins to flatten. The amount of thick white becomes smaller and smaller until finally the yolk is flat and breaks easily and a large, thin white area surrounds it. This is an old, low-quality egg.

You can detect aging in a hard-cooked egg when the yolk is far off center and the air pocket is large.

LIQUID EGGS AND FROZEN OMELETS

The frozen omelet mixes in our supermarket are all pasteurized. This is optional in liquid eggs, the only requirement being that the proportion of yolk and white be a natural one. Unpasteurized egg products are a possible source of Salmonella, a nasty bacteria that causes food poisoning. If this type of egg is not heated sufficiently when cooked at home the bacteria will not die. On the other hand, the process of destroying the Salmonella by pasteurization destroys some of the native vitamins and enzymes. You're caught in the middle and the only way out is to crack your own eggs, beat them with a fork, and presto—you've liquefied your eggs at home.

Although the brands of frozen omelets we've encountered thus far don't have added chemicals, monosodium phosphate and monopotassium phosphate may be added to preserve the color. The label will indicate whether these unnecessary, but relatively harmless chemicals are included.

DRIED EGGS

Other processed egg products include dried whole eggs, dried egg yolks, and dried egg whites. In all cases this involves spraying the liquid egg into heated air. Sometimes the glucose is reduced by adding a yeast preparation or an enzyme preparation in a hydrochloric acid solution. These products will say "stabilized" or "glucose removed." An anticaking agent may be added as well, and the whites may have an added whipping agent.

Dried eggs are not usually available on the consumer level, so many of us assume we needn't be concerned here . . . except that dried egg products are added to commercial breads, cakes, cookies, pasta, and all conceivable egg-containing foods. If you wouldn't personally consider using powdered eggs in your home, why bring them in in this disguised form? Watch the label of egg-containing foods and stick to those prepared with fresh eggs, just as you'd do in your own kitchen.

EGG SUBSTITUTES

There are several egg replacers on the market designed to serve those people on a restricted cholesterol diet. Essentially they are egg-white preparations with added starch, nonfat dry milk, and vitamin enrichment which are available in dried and liquid form. The addition of noxious chemical additives is left to the discretion of the manufacturer and will always be revealed on the label.

Our biggest beef with the "no cholesterol" eggs is the manner in which they are promoted. Egg substitutes (which approximate rather than duplicate the "nutrition of farm-fresh eggs" as one manufacturer implies) are a valuable dietary aid for those with a cholesterol problem, much in the same way that artificially sweetened jams were developed for diabetics. But that is all they are, and the precise balance of nutrients in a real egg preserves its status as "nature's most nearly perfect food" for all unafflicted consumers.

PUT ALL YOUR EGGS IN ONE (COVERED) BASKET

Keep eggs in the refrigerator, and although they will not spoil for several weeks, try to use them within one week. If you don't use eggs frequently, buy a half dozen at a time rather than hold them at home. The shell of the egg doesn't offer total protection. There are tiny holes which make it porous, and outside odors and flavors are easily absorbed. Keeping them in a covered egg box will cut down this invasion. Eggs should never be washed before storage. Washing enhances germ penetration.

Once cracked, eggs can be stored two to three days in a covered container in the refrigerator (with a small loss of quality and nutrients).

Extra egg white can be stored in a tightly covered container in the refrigerator for a week. For longer storage (up to six months), place the container in the freezer. Yolks are best kept under a covering of cold water in a closed container. They can be held in the refrigerator only two to three days, and freezing is not recommended because of their high fat content.

COOKING EGGS

Time and temperature are the focal points of egg cookery, as for all protein foods. People have their own opinion or family method of how an egg should be cooked. All experts, however, agree that the key to the most nutritious, tender, and flavorful egg is *gentle cooking*.

If your hard-cooked eggs have tough, rubbery whites and the yolks have a strong flavor or a dark ring around the outside, it's because the eggs were "hard boiled" instead of "hard cooked," as they should be. This is how we make "hard-cooked" eggs and it works just fine:

Place eggs in large saucepan and add water to completely cover them. Place over moderate heat and bring water to a boil. Immediately cover the pot and remove from heat. Let eggs remain in the covered pot for 20 minutes. If you're cooking more than six eggs in one pot let them stand 5 minutes longer. Remove eggs and immediately rinse under cold water until they are cooled. This stops further cooking. Refrigerate the eggs until you're ready to peel them.

Soft-cooked eggs can be made in the same way, this time letting them stand in the covered pot 1 to 3 minutes, depending on how soft you like them. Again, rinse under cold water to prevent further cooking and serve immediately.

If you are plagued with eggs that crack when they are cooked in the shell, try poking a tiny pin hole in the large end of the egg before cooking.

The Shell Game

We wish we had an easy method to offer for peeling eggs, but we don't. Maybe you'll find it encouraging to know that most egg experts insist newly laid eggs are the hardest to peel, so you can take comfort in the fact that your eggs are fresh as you struggle with the shell.

Frozen Omelets and Fresh Omelets

The latest item in our supermarket is frozen omelets, ready to thaw, shake, and pour into the frying pan. The label boasts three seasoned omelets, ready-mixed, pasteurized, and frozen for only 89¢. We make omelets regularly with those old-fashioned eggs in the shell. Instead of anonymous "seasonings" we add salt and freshly ground pepper; bits of leftover vegetables or cheese replace the bits of onion, mushroom, or bacon they've frozen into the mix. The leftovers don't cost us anything and at 59¢ a dozen a two-egg omelet costs 10¢. As for convenience—it takes less than a minute to crack and beat the eggs, and while the omelet sets on the heat you can chop up the filling. It takes longer than that to thaw the prepared variety.

EGGSPERTISE

To encourage you to do more cooking from scratch and take advantage of the versatility of the egg, here are a few tips to help you avoid some common egg crises:

●All beaten egg dishes (for scrambling or omelets) should be cooked in a hot pan with enough butter or oil to keep the eggs from sticking. Once the eggs are in the pan, the heat should be lowered for gentle cooking.

●Separate eggs when they are cold. The yolk is firmest in a chilled egg and this way there is less chance of it running into the white portion. Never attempt to separate an egg over a bowl of egg whites. If you miss, your whites will never beat to maximum volume.

●Egg whites whip better at room temperature, so after the eggs have been separated you'll get more volume if you let them stand out a bit. (This doesn't mean several hours . . . quality is still better than quantity.) Make sure there are no traces of yolk mixed in and that your beaters are completely clean. Any foreign particles, especially fat, inhibit the incorporation of air which is what makes egg whites an excellent leavening agent and produces those feather-light dishes.

●If you're using eggs to thicken soups, sauces, or puddings and are having trouble getting a smooth consistency or maximum thickening power, it's probably because your egg is curdling on contact with the hot liquid. To solve that problem, add a bit of the hot mixture to the egg first and beat it well to bring the egg gradually to the higher temperature. This is known as "tempering." Now you can fearlessly add the egg back to the hot pan. When reheating the mixture, don't let it boil or you'll have scrambled eggs.

RECOMMENDATIONS

General Rule of Purchase: Buy eggs from free-running, grain-fed hens, if available. Buy only from refrigerated case and check the last day of recommended sale.

EXEMPLARY BUYS:
U.S. Grade AA, or state equivalent

Milk and Its Many Forms

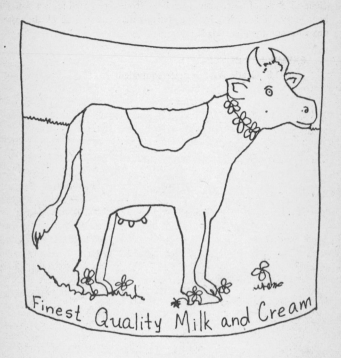

Finest Quality Milk and Cream

Even a simple food like milk is available in so many forms today it's dizzying. But before we begin investigating the varieties, let's look into "milk" in general. Is it really nature's most perfect food? Many highly regarded medical people say no. There are two schools of thought here. One contends that milk is meant for babies only, and that only in America and certain western European countries do grown-ups consume milk. The second group of anti-milk theorists feels that it's not milk, but mother's milk that is the ideal food, and that cow's milk is meant for calves. In part, these theories have held up. As many people grow older they find they have a reduced capacity to tolerate milk; cramps, diarrhea, and bloating are the resulting symptoms after drinking milk or milk products. Blacks and Orientals are more frequently plagued with this problem. Whole milk is also the biggest contributor to high cholesterol in the diet, and suspicion is high that milk fat may impair clot-dissolving enzymes in the blood vessels, leading to clogging. Finally, milk is linked to many intestinal disorders which lead to nutritional depletion.

WHOLE AND SKIM MILK

Despite all this, many people can handle milk with no trouble at all, and for them milk is a highly nutritious food. Milk is an excellent source of protein, calcium, and phosphorus and, except for low-fat milk, offers a good source of vitamins A and D. Nowadays, most skim milk and nonfat dry milk have A and D added.

Almost all the milk available in the supermarket is pasteurized. In a country where so much milk is produced daily this is necessary to destroy harmful bacteria. But despite the dairy industry's proclamations to the contrary, the heat of pasteurization *does* lower the quality of milk. Thiamine, one of the B vitamins, is reduced after pasteurization, and the native enzymes and any natural vitamin C are completely destroyed. In a few areas certified raw (unpasteurized) milk is available. Certified means it has been government-inspected and meets rigid sanitary regulations. On occasion we have been lucky enough to buy raw milk, and we think it's much more flavorful. The *Alta Dena* Dairy in California offers raw milk and raw milk products to supermarket consumers.

Most milk today is homogenized as well, so that the fat particles are evenly distributed throughout the liquid. Supposedly this milk has more body and a creamier flavor. Personally, we like to skim off the fat for cream and find the remaining milk much more refreshing. If you have the choice, at least try the nonhomogenized type.

Standards for the composition of whole milk vary from state to state, but 3.25 percent milk fat and 8.25 percent milk solids are usually the minimum requirements for it to meet the "whole milk" specification. As the percentage of fat is reduced it becomes known as "partially skimmed" and then "skimmed" milk. Although protein, mineral and B vitamin contents remain unaltered, a reduction in fat also means the loss of some fat soluble vitamins. Since most milk does have added vitamins A and D, switching from whole to skim milk is an advisable way to cut down animal-fat consumption. Milk fat, however, does contain vitamins E and D, and although no specific requirements have been established for these vitamins they are vital to your health; so at least an occasional supplement of whole milk is a good idea.

HANDLING FRESH MILK

Fresh and skim milk are sold in bottles and plasticized containers. In most metropolitan areas bottled milk is hard to come by, but worth a trip to the supermarket that offers it. Milk in containers is never quite as cold or quite as fresh-tasting. The soft containers never really seal the milk off from the outside environment once they've been opened, so the milk picks up funny odors in the refrigerator. Also, milk bottles are recyclable (some milk companies are now offering their product in biodegradable cartons). It is true, though, that exposure to light causes vitamin loss in milk, so that clear glass is not the ideal container by any means.

Here are some hints to preserve the freshness and high-quality food value of your milk:

●Milk perishes; not all at once, but gradually. Every minute out of the refrigerator shortens the life of your milk, so keep the container out just long enough to pour what you need.

●Light, as we said, is destructive to milk, and particularly to the B vitamin riboflavin, which is another reason milk shouldn't be kept out too long. Tinted bottles on the bottler's part would help cut down on lost riboflavin too.

●If you've poured more milk than you can use, don't pour it back into the container. Store it separately in a jar. Don't mix it with other stored milk either.

●Use milk within three to five days of purchase. Milk dating is totally unstandardized, but if open dating does exist in your city, the milk will state right on the carton "not to be sold after" a certain date. Heed the warning.

FLAVORING MILK

If your family insists on flavored milk there are many alternatives to chocolate. One reason milk is so highly regarded is that it is a rich source of calcium. Chocolate inhibits calcium absorption, so you're defeating your own purpose when you drink chocolate milk. Try these simple flavoring ideas instead:

Taffy Milk: Add 1 tablespoon of molasses per 8-ounce glass of milk. Instead of detracting from the value, you'll be adding calcium, iron, and B vitamins. To turn it into *Banana Taffy Milk,* beat in ½ ripe banana and, if desired, sprinkle with nutmeg.

Peanut Milk: Mix 1/3 cup of peanut butter, 2 tablespoons of honey, and 1 quart of milk with rotary beater until smooth. Mix or shake again before serving.

Vanilla Milk: Combine 8 ounces of milk, ¼ teaspoon of pure vanilla extract, and 1 teaspoon of honey.

Fruit Shakes: Combine 3/4 cup of milk, 1 to 2 teaspoons of honey, and fruit of your choice in blender container. Fruit can include 1 peach, 1 orange, ½ banana, ½ cup of diced cantaloupe, ½ cup of berries, or some combination of these. Blend at high speed until smooth, then add two ice cubes, one at a time through the feeder cap while machine is running, and process until ice is liquefied. Pour into a tall glass and garnish with nutmeg or cinnamon if you like. To fortify these shakes you can add 1 tablespoon of wheat germ and/or nonfat dry milk powder to the container before blending.

Other suggestions for enhancing a glass of milk are found in the chapter "Breakfasts: Unseating the Sugar-Frosted Fortified Fakes."

COOKING HINTS

When you cook with milk, keep the heat low and pay attention. Milk curdles easily. Acid also curdles milk, so if your milk is going to be added to a vegetable mixture (as in a cream of vegetable soup), heat the milk part first, add the acid food gradually, reheat, and serve as soon as possible. Even if the milk does begin to separate, it will taste fine.

BUTTERMILK

Buttermilk is produced in commercial dairies and is no longer, as it once was, the liquid that remains after butter has been churned, but a bacteria "culture" of milk with added butter granules. Usually fluid skim milk is the basis of buttermilk, although it may also be made with whole, concentrated, and nonfat dry milk. Much of it is reclaimed, stale, pasteurized milk. Produced in this manner, buttermilk undergoes a lot of handling and altering of its natural properties so we really don't include it in the list of "natural" milks in the same way we do fresh or skim milk. Real buttermilk, not the "cultured" kind, is a fine, wholesome food.

CREAM

Cream and half-and-half are both milk derivatives. They differ from each other only in the percent of fat. To prepare these products, the fatty portion is separated from the milk, and milk (whole or skim, fresh or dry) is added back to the fat to meet the fat percentage required for the specific product (heavy cream, light cream, half-and-half etc.) in your locale.

Imitation cream, on the other hand, is a chemical substance made in the image of cream. Some of these products contain animal fats, while others are completely nondairy. Nondairy does not mean nonfat. Many people use imitation cream and coffee whiteners because they have been told that butter fat is high in saturated fat; what they don't know is that coconut oil and palm oil, the vegetable fats used as the base for imitation dairy products, are highly saturated fats as well. At the same time they are ingesting chemical stabilizers, emulsifiers, corn syrup, and artificial flavoring. Our conclusion is that if you are going to use cream, you should make it the real thing.

Whipped Cream

When it comes to whipped cream, buy heavy cream and whip it yourself. Fresh whipped cream is highly unstable and should be made within an hour of use. After that it will begin to wilt. The reason the aerosol cans of whipped cream stay so nice and fluffy is the added chemical thickeners and stabilizers. Cream is highly perishable—buy it fresh; don't let it stand around already whipped in the supermarket waiting for you (not you!) to buy it.

When you want to whip cream:

1. Place fresh cream in a chilled bowl.
2. Beat with an electric or rotary beater until soft peaks form.
3. To sweeten: fold in 2 tablespoons of honey or maple syrup and ½ teaspoon of vanilla extract for each 2 cups of whipped cream.
   Yield: 1 cup of heavy cream makes 2 cups when whipped.

16

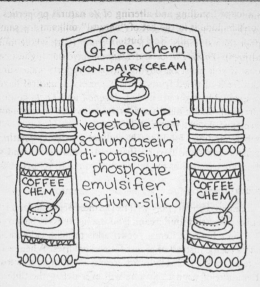

Coffee-chem
NON-DAIRY CREAM

corn syrup
vegetable fat
sodium casein
di-potassium
phosphate
emulsifier
sodium-silico

COFFEE
CHEM

COFFEE
CHEM

For a low-fat, low-calorie whipped topping, see the recipe given in the discussion of nonfat dry milk.

YOGURT

Yogurt is the result of the interaction of milk and special bacterial cultures. The long life of people in Bulgaria and many eastern countries is often attributed to the huge quantities of yogurt in their diet. Whether this is true or not is subject to speculation; however, there is no doubt this is a highly valuable food. All the nutritional benefits of milk are carried over into the yogurt, and in the process a change occurs that makes yogurt tolerable to many who cannot digest regular milk. In addition, the yogurt culture acts in the intestine as a cleanser and has the ability to destroy many harmful bacteria.

Yogurt is available nationwide, plain (unflavored) and in a variety of flavors. Many of the flavored brands rely on imitation flavoring, coloring, and other chemical additives. All contain refined sugar. Buy plain yogurt and do the flavoring yourself with honey, fresh or dried fruits, jam, or fresh vegetables (diced cucumber, tomato, garlic), and

17

herbs (mint, dill). You can top it with nuts and wheat germ.

Among the unflavored brands, *Colombo* (which is made from whole rather than skimmed milk), *Continental* (both whole milk and lowfat cultures), *Yami, Lacto,* and *Dannon* have our highest recommendations. If you insist on buying flavored yogurt, make sure that nothing but fresh or dried fruits or fruit preserves, natural flavoring, and the unavoidable sugar are added. *Dannon* and *Lacto* conform to this requirement. *Lacto* also has a brand new line of fruit-flavored, honey-sweetened yogurt worth sampling.

Remember, modified food starch, sodium caseinate, gelatin, corn syrup, artificial color and flavor, citric acid, tartaric acid, and potassium sorbate are extraneous matter when it comes to yogurt-making.*

Cooking with Yogurt

Plain, unflavored yogurt may well be the most versatile food in your kitchen. Like sweet and sour cream, it adds a lightness to baked goods. But unlike these high-fat items, yogurt adds protein, calcium and B vitamins to a recipe instead of excess fat and calories. Whenever your bread, cake or cookie recipe calls for cream, sweet or sour, substitute an equal amount of yogurt. No one will ever detect the difference.

In the same manner yogurt can replace cream or even milk in quiche, Hungarian stews, salad dressing, pureed vegetables, sauces, custards, etc., for added nutrients and a curiously fresh taste. Weight watchers and people on a restricted fat diet will particularly appreciate this idea:

FRESH MASHED POTATOES

Allow 1 to 1½ potatoes per serving. Boil or bake the potatoes, unpeeled, until tender. Puree in a food mill, skin and all. Beat in 1 tablespoon yogurt or more per potato until light and fluffy. Season with salt and pepper to taste.

SOUR CREAM

Like buttermilk, today's sour cream is not much like the kind your grandmother might have made. Old World sour cream was nothing more than heavy sweet cream allowed to sour in the warmth of the back of an old coal stove. This sour cream was rather thin, and varied from mildly tart to quite acid. The sour cream you buy today has

---

*We regret not having included an explanation of the ease with which yogurt can be made at home, but refer you to page 47 of our *Good Breakfast Book* (Links Books).

licked the problem of inconsistency of flavor. Dairy technology has created another "cultured" product in which a special bacteria culture is added to the cream, and through a series of exposures to extreme heat and pressure a thick, taste-controlled product is created. The original cream to which the culture was added didn't have much nutritional significance to begin with so, after the multiple heat treatments used in its creation, sour cream cannot be depended upon to add anything but calories to your food intake. It can, however, add variety of taste and texture to many dishes, so if there is a brand in your supermarket without added thickeners, you may want to select it. The preceding section on Cooking with Yogurt will, it is hoped, convince you to forgo this purchase, though, and use the less expensive, nutrient-rich yogurt in its place.

NONREFRIGERATED MILKS

Nonfat Dry Milk

Nonfat dry milk powder is a very useful form of milk, but shouldn't be used exclusively to replace fluid milk. Like liquid skim milk it is missing the fat-soluble vitamins, A, D, E, and K. Government regulations allow for synthetic replacement of A and D. The label will tell you if the brand you've selected is so enriched. What the label won't tell you, though, is how the milk has been processed.

There are presently two methods for drying milk: spray-drying, a low-heat process which apparently does not significantly change the nutritional makeup, and hot roller- or drum-drying, which requires two drying periods and subjects the milk to temperatures extreme enough to denature one of the essential amino acids, reducing the protein quality and destroying vitamins in the product. Our recent research indicates that all nonfat dry milk currently packaged uses the spray-dry process.

Always buy dried milk that has the U.S. Extra Grade mark in a shield. This means the milk comes from a government-inspected plant and is your safeguard against Salmonella, a common milk contaminant.

The idea behind nonfat dry milk is to create a product with a long shelf life. This does not mean it lasts forever. Once the package is opened, air and moisture can enter and the Salmonella problem crops up again. To avoid bacterial growth, the opened package of nonfat dry milk powder should be stored in an airtight container in a cool place. Reconstituted dry milk should be handled the same way as fresh fluid milk.

Using Nonfat Dry Milk So That Everyone Enjoys It

The taste of reconstituted dry milk is not as tempting as the fresh milk it came from. There are several ways to overcome this. One way to stretch the milk money and come up with a flavorful product is to mix equal amounts of reconstituted dry milk and fresh fluid milk. Another way to mask the taste, but guard the nutrition, is to use nonfat dry milk to replace fluid milk when it is to be mixed with other ingredients, as for cream soups, sauces, shakes, and the other flavored milks described in the section on Flavoring Milk.

Nonfat dry milk is an inexpensive replacement for fresh milk when making homemade yogurt and is the substance of the following low-calorie whipped topping.

LO-CAL WHIPPED TOPPING

Combine ½ cup of nonfat dry milk powder and ½ cup of ice water in a chilled bowl. Beat with an electric or rotary beater until soft peaks form, approximately 5 minutes. Add 2 tablespoons of orange juice, 2 tablespoons of honey, maple syrup, or raw sugar, and continue beating until fluffy, about 5 minutes. Keep refrigerated until needed and use within 2 hours.

Some companies have tried to overcome the public's resistance to nonfat dry milk by introducing flavored dry milk powders. The artificial sweetener they add and the imitation flavoring make them a less, rather than more desirable product in the end.

CANNED MILK

Evaporated Milk

Evaporated milk is produced by the removal of water from fresh, whole milk—pasteurized, homogenized, and usually vitamin D fortified. It is sealed in cans and heat-sterilized so no refrigeration is necessary. So far so good. Unfortunately, a variety of chemical stabilizers may be added, and only one of them, carrageenan, must be indicated on the label. So you're taking a chance of bringing home several unwanted chemicals when you buy evaporated milk.

The carrageenan, for example, added for "body," is a seaweed derivative and although formerly considered safe, new processing techniques have greatly altered this additive. Today carrageenan is bleached with sulfur dioxide and cleaned with harsh alkali. It has been linked to colitis, among other disorders, in animals.

Sweetened Condensed Milk

Sweetened condensed milk is no more than evaporated milk (both unfortified and chemical-free at least) plus 40 percent sweetener in the form of sucrose, dextrose, or corn syrup. If you plan on adding refined sugar to whatever you are using the sweetened condensed milk for, you might as well keep this product on your shopping list, but if you turn to the chapter "Sweet Things" you'll find out why we've crossed it off ours.

FILLED MILK

Filled milk looks, smells, and tastes like evaporated milk but is actually skim milk to which vegetable fat has been added. When soybean oil replaces the original butterfat, such milk is lower in saturated fats and cholesterol and may be desirable for those pursuing a low cholesterol diet.

Although filled milk has been on the market for the past fifty years its sale is banned in at least eighteen states based on an archaic law which the White House Conference on Food, Nutrition and Health termed "a major impediment to nutritional progress."

We have not found filled milk in any markets, but if it is no more than soybean oil and skim milk (the label will tell you), it may indeed be a valuable milk substitute for low-saturated fat food plans.

IMITATION MILK

Last (and also least) is imitation milk, also prohibited from being sold in many states. The product is fully labeled and as you will see is no more than corn syrup, protein, vegetable fat (the saturated coconut oil kind), plus a lot of chemical emulsifiers, stabilizers and flavoring. This milk contains only a fraction of the calcium and phosphorus of natural milk.

MILK IN ITS MANY FORMS

1 cup	calories	protein (grams)	fat (grams)
whole milk	160	9	9
partially skim milk	145	10	5
skim milk	90	9	trace
half & half	325	8	28
light cream	505	7	49
heavy cream	840	5	90
sour cream	485	7	47
yogurt, from partially skim milk	125	8	4

RECOMMENDATIONS

FRESH MILK

General Rule of Purchase: Most milk available is pasteurized, homogenized, and fortified with vitamins D and/or A. Some milks have added nonfat dry milk solids as noted on the container. If "certified raw milk" is offered, try it.

> EXEMPLARY BRANDS:
> *Alta Dena* raw milk
> *Gates Farms* raw milk
> *Mathis Dairy* raw milk

CREAM

General Rule of Purchase: Purchase fresh cream; avoid imitation cream and coffee whiteners. Purchase fresh heavy cream for whipping. Note: Sterilized or ultra-pasteurized products will not whip.

YOGURT

General Rule of Purchase: Select plain, unflavored yogurt. Undesirable additives appear on the label and include modified food starch, sodium citrate, gelatin, corn syrup, artificial color and flavor, citric acid, tartaric acid, and potassium sorbate. When buying flavored yogurts, look for those with preserves, fruit plus sugar or honey, and other natural flavorings only.

EXEMPLARY BRANDS:
East—*Breakstone's* Stay 'n' Shape
Breyers
Colombo (plain only)
Dannon
Lacto
Shop Rite (plain only)
Yoplait
Middle—*Breyers*
West—*Continental*
Golden Creme (plain only)
Knudsen (plain only)
Milk and Honey

SOUR CREAM

General Rule of Purchase: The natural thickening of the cream during the souring process is what gives sour cream its consistency, not locust bean gum, carrageenan, or mono- and diglycerides.

EXEMPLARY BRANDS:
East—*Axelrod*
Breakstone
Crowley
Michigan Old Fashioned
Penn Maid
Sealtest
Shop Rite
Waldbaum's
Weis
White Star Dairy
Middle—*Food Club*
Raskas

> West—*Anderson*
> *Arden*
> *Carnation*
> *Dari-Valley*
> *Knudson* Hampshire
> *Lucerne* (additive-free in West only)
> *Model Dairy*
> *Valley Gold*

NONFAT DRY MILK

General Rule of Purchase: Buy freely with U.S. Extra Grade the preferred choice. When processing is indicated, choose milk that has been spray-dried rather than hot roller- or drum-dried.

ADDITIONAL CHOICES:
  Darigold Powdered Cultured Buttermilk

CANNED MILK

General Rule of Purchase: Of the many additives possible in canned milk, carrageenan is the one most likely to appear on the label and should be avoided. Although free of chemicals, sweetened condensed milk is highly sugared.

EXEMPLARY BRANDS:
  Acme Louella Evaporated Skimmed Milk
  Miracle Brand Evaporated Goat Milk
  Pet Evaporated Skimmed Milk
  Real-Fresh California Whole Milk

Cheese: Why the Mouse Roared

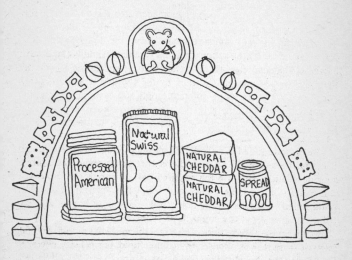

Cheese dishes are featured domestically and internationally on almost every menu. The fact that cheeses are delicious and easily adaptable to so many recipes certainly doesn't hurt their popularity, but more suited to our discussion is their nutritional significance.

Cheese is a concentrated source of many of the nutrients found in milk. The protein you get from cheese is of equal quality to meat protein and at a much lower cost, and because of the relative surplus of the amino acid lysine, it is valuable for increasing the protein quality of foods deficient in this amino acid, like grains. In addition, you get calcium, phosphorus, vitamin A, and much of the riboflavin and thiamine from the original milk. Although rich in nutrients, cheese is relatively sparse where calories are concerned. As a rough guide, one ounce of cheese (1 medium slice) furnishes about 100 calories. If you are counting calories, you are even better off with cottage cheese, pot cheese, farmer and ricotta cheese, containing about one third the calories of most other cheese.

WHAT IS CHEESE?

Cheese is a man-made food phenomenon stemming from a highly developed art form centuries old. Cheese-making is basically a process of separating the milk solids (the curd) from the liquid portion (the whey) facilitated by the action of the enzyme rennin and/or lactic acid bacteria. The characteristic flavor and body are produced by varying the milk source (cow, goat, sheep), by the addition of salt and other added seasonings, by using different molds and bacteria for ripening the cheese, and by changing the time, temperature, and ripening climate. The result is hundreds of different tastes, textures, and varieties of cheese.

The bacteria added to milk during cheese production are lactic acid bacteria; these are the same bacteria that bring about the normal souring of milk. Because the required pasteurization has destroyed this bacteria there is no choice but to put this "starter" back. The rennin used to accelerate the liquid-solid separation is a natural enzyme obtained from the stomach of young calves.

Because these constituents of cheese—the milk, the rennin, and the bacteria—are real, as opposed to manufactured, ingredients, cheese is included in the classification of whole or natural foods. Not all cheese, however, is unadulterated.

The composition of cheese is regulated by a government standard of identity which specifies the ingredients that may be used, the maximum moisture content and minimum fat content, and sets requirements for pasteurizing or holding the milk to remove the chance of harmful bacterial growth. Many chemical additives are also permitted in this government standard, with some exempt from labeling; we will delve into them shortly.

Since there are so many possibilities when it comes to cheese buying, we'd best first evaluate the different cheese-making processes to eliminate those not fit for a whole foods kitchen. The labels of all cheeses, with the exception of natural cheese, will indicate by which process they were made.

NATURAL CHEESE

In this case "natural" refers to a cheese made directly from the milk solids (and sometimes the whey) by separating the curds and whey, heating, stirring, and pressing the solids until the desired cheese characteristic is obtained. The milk itself may come from a cow, a goat, or a sheep, and is usually whole milk, although certain cheeses include skim milk, cream, and whey. Salt is added to almost every cheese.

In this country, unfortunately, certain unnatural steps may enter the process, like the addition of calcium salts and acidifying agents along with the bacteria, rennet, or clotting enzymes, the use of artificial coloring agents, and the use of potassium or sodium sorbate as preservative. Where preservatives are used, the law requires a statement on the label, but as to other chemical intervention, it is most often in the form of hidden (unlabeled) ingredients. In our description of specific natural cheeses we will give you some clues as to what to watch for, both on the label and off, so you can make the best choice.

UNNATURAL CHEESES

Those cheeses that are not "natural" are known as "process" cheeses and must be so labeled. During the "processing" they are heated to halt ripening and keep the flavor and texture constant. An assortment of emulsifiers and stabilizers are added to guarantee their consistency. Their supposed advantage over natural cheese is that they melt and spread easily and smoothly and are thus considered more convenient. The flavor, however, never approaches the richness of natural cheese, the controlled texture is dull, and a large part of the price goes toward the purchase of chemicals.

Pasteurized Process Cheese

This cheese is always described with the adjectives "pasteurized process" on the label (although you might have to read the fine print to locate it). It is made by grinding and blending one or more natural cheeses which are then heated and mixed with water and emulsifier, which may be any combination of thirteen different chemicals not appearing on the label, and some optional acids, artificial coloring, and flavoring ingredients in an effort to create a smooth, homogeneous, "plastic" mass. Some of the more popular forms of pasteurized processed cheese are American cheese (from Cheddar or colby), pasteurized process Swiss, sweet munchee, and brick.

Unlike natural cheese, which continues to develop flavor with age, the flavor of a pasteurized process cheese is controlled. These cheeses are often enhanced with bits of fruit, vegetables, or meat. Most varie-- ties are packed with preservatives but listing is mandatory on the label.

Blended Cheese

A blended cheese is made by combining one or more natural cheeses and differs from the pasteurized process cheese in that cream cheese or Neufchatel cheese may be included. Blended cheeses usually contain added bits of fruits, vegetables, or meat. Added coloring must be stated on the label, but many other chemicals used in these spreadable cheeses do not have to be given. Do not despair. Further on, suggestions for your own cheese blends are given. These cost less and have a much more lively taste.

Pasteurized Process Cheese Food

This cheese is almost the same as the pasteurized process cheese except that it contains less cheese with a dairy product (milk, nonfat dry milk, cream, or whey) plus water used as a replacement. The resulting cheese has a lower fat content and more moisture. It is mild in flavor, melts easily, and is chock full of chemicals.

The only advantage of the process cheese food over the process cheese is that all the optional ingredients (color, salt, acidifying agents, flavoring, preservatives) must appear on the label; don't waste your time reading it.

Pasteurized Process Cheese Spread

Just another version of the pasteurized process cheese, only this time the moisture content is even higher in order to produce a food that is spreadable at 70°F (as specified in the government standard). This necessitates yet another chemical, a stabilizer, to prevent the separation of the ingredients. This item is usually packaged in jars or loaves and often has added pimientos, fruits, vegetables, or meat. *Velveeta* and *Cheese Whiz* are among those commonly known.

All ingredients are listed on the label and there are always a number of undesirable ones.

Cold Pack (Club, Comminuted) Cheese

The only difference between these and the pasteurized process cheeses is the absence of heat in the processing; the chemicals remain the same, and sweetening agents like sugar or corn syrup may be added. Leave them on the shelf along with the pasteurized process variations. You can identify them by the term "cold pack, club, or comminuted" on the label. In the case of cold-pack American, the word "American" may appear alone on the label, but the undesirable processing is still there. There is no such thing as natural American cheese, so don't be deceived by the lack of descriptive adjectives here.

Smoked Cheeses

Smoke from hardwood sawdust is used to impart a "smoked flavor" to many cheeses. Compounds known as hydrocarbons enter the picture here, and since hydrocarbons have been inconclusively investigated in connection with cancer, we suggest selecting unsmoked varieties. The label will always indicate when a cheese has been "smoked."

CHOOSING PROCESS CHEESES

Don't!

CHOOSING NATURAL CHEESES

Almost every country has its cheese specialties and an acquaintance with some of these will greatly expand your food choices and cooking repertoire. Modern supermarkets are well stocked with natural cheeses from around the world and you can begin your cheese venture by checking out the varieties available in your locale and learning about them in the forthcoming section. This way you'll know what to expect from your purchase and how to introduce it to your family table.

Since all natural cheeses are not exactly "natural," let's take a look at some of the varieties to root out the offenders. Keep in mind that imported cheeses are less likely to contain some of these undesirable additives. Abroad, cheese is a treasured food item and very few nations want to risk changing that feeling.

UNRIPENED NATURAL CHEESE

Soft Unripened

An unripened cheese is one that is not aged, but is made to be eaten soon after manufacture. Soft unripened cheeses have a high moisture content and are highly perishable. They include:

COTTAGE CHEESE

This unripened cheese is made from skim milk, either fresh or dried, plus salt and a lactic bacteria which brings about the curdling. Some manufacturers use acid, however (like phosphoric or hydrochloric), to bring about the separation of the milk, a method unsuited to a natural foods kitchen. Those brands that employ acid say "directly set" or "curd set by acidification" on the label and should be left, in preference for the more natural ones.

Except for the special diet brands and low-fat cottage cheese, most cottage cheese is "creamed" which means the addition of cream or cream plus milk along with the possibility of a whole load of additives. Some cannot be detected by reading the label but those that can be include: the stabilizers in the form of vegetable gum, carrageenan salts, lecithin, furcelleran, to name a few, and these are in combination with several other additives which need not be mentioned; lactic, citric, or phosphoric acid (acid set); artificial flavor. A rich-tasting superior product can be made without these additives. Fine examples come from *Hood, Friendship, Breakstone, Axelrod, Jerseymaid, Carnation, Arden, Tuttle. Crowley's* makes one variety which contains neither cream nor salt.

CREAM CHEESE

Cow's cream, and possibly fresh, dry, or concentrated milk plus water are the basis of this soft, spreadable cheese. What you want to look out for here is the addition of propylene glycol alginate which appears on the label and is used in conjunction with another chemical not made known to you. Never buy cream cheese which contains this additive. Other added ingredients may include gelatin and more commonly vegetable gum, both of which are added to thicken the cheese and impart a "rubbery" texture. Again, their presence is indicated on the label and although both are natural, rather than chemical substances, they are not natural to dairy products. If you can, avoid them. Neufchatel cheese is practically identical to cream cheese, with a slightly lower fat content. Unlike most other cheeses, cream cheese does not contribute much in the way of protein.

POT CHEESE

Similar to cottage cheese, but drier, never creamed, made without salt and free of the undesirable additives. Acceptable choices are made by *Friendship, Breakstone.*

FARMER CHEESE

Farmer cheese is also much like cottage cheese and pot cheese, only it is pressed into block forms. Potassium sorbate preservative may be added; look for it on the label. *Crowley* and *Breakstone's* Farmer Cheese is free of preservatives. Although the small packages of *Friendship* Farmer Cheese include this additive, the bulk packages distributed to the delicatessen counter don't, so you're better off buying your pot cheese at the delicatessen counter than from the cheese case if *Friendship* is available in your area.

RICOTTA CHEESE

Another cheese which resembles cottage cheese, but with a finer, lighter texture. It is excellent for baking and filling Italian noodles. Lightly sweetened and mixed with chopped dried fruits, nuts, and grated chocolate, it makes a heavenly dessert. The milk whey used in this cheese may be from whole or partly skimmed milk, as indicated on the label, with or without added milk solids. A starter and salt may also be added; any other ingredients mentioned on the label, like locust bean gum, carrageenan, mono- and diglyceride, dextrose, and citric acid are quite unnecessary, so do not buy these brands. *Polly-O* is a favorite of Italian-Americans and is available both whole and partially skimmed. *Hood* and *Brunetto* also offer unadulterated choices.

31

FETA

A fresh curd cheese set in a concentrated salt solution. Feta may be domestic or imported, and made from either goat's or sheep's milk. This is a sharp, salty cheese excellent for topping salads. All brands are chemical-free.

Firm Unripened

Firm unripened cheeses differ from the soft in that they contain less moisture, making them firmer and less perishable.

MOZZARELLA

Mozzarella is the best-known cheese in this category and, while purchased fresh rather than aged, it is not as perishable as the soft ripened cheeses. The cow's milk used may be whole or skim (indicated on the label), and there are no undesirable elements used here, either on the label or off. In special "low-moisture" varieties, however, preservatives may be added. If so, it will be indicated. Use this cheese for melted cheese sandwiches and topping lasagna, pizza, and casseroles. Also delicious uncooked with crackers and jam for dessert.

RIPENED CHEESES

A ripened cheese is one that is aged under conditions favorable to the growth of certain molds or bacteria on the surface which produce the characteristic flavor and texture. The rate of this "curing" varies with the moisture content and temperature and is carefully controlled in each variety to produce the highly cherished flavor. The longer the cheese ages the more pungent it becomes, and you will notice, if you eat part of a ripened cheese soon after it is purchased and go to have another piece several days later, that the flavor may be quite different. Storing cheese in the refrigerator slows the curing process. The softer the cheese, the higher the moisture content and the quicker this flavor change will take place.

Soft Ripened

The soft ripened cheeses are all free of artificial coloring and preservatives and include: Brie (mild or strong in flavor), Camembert (mild to strong), and Limburger (always strong and smelly). Soft ripened cheeses are best served for an appetizer or as dessert with crackers and fruit.

Semisoft Ripened

Less moisture makes the semisoft ripened cheeses somewhat firmer than the soft varieties. They are all well suited to appetizer and dessert service like their softer sisters, but may be used for cooking with excellent results too. They start out quite mellow but some develop a fuller flavor with age. Included here are Bel Paese, Munster (which stays mellow), Monterrey Jack (similar to Munster but saltier and good for Mexican dishes and baked combinations), and Port du Salut. The only additives to watch for here are preservatives which must be indicated on the label.

Firm Ripened

Firm ripened cheeses are excellent eaten plain or used in cooking for toasted cheese sandwiches, casseroles, and sauces. As you'll see from the descriptions which follow, some may be subject to a bit of chemical tampering.

CHEDDAR

Cheddar comes in varieties of mild, medium, and sharp. Artificial color may be added, but not stated. It is often found in the yellow-orange varieties. To be on the safe side choose white (Vermont) cheddar. If mold inhibitors are added, it will say so on the label.

EDAM

This cheese originates in the Netherlands and is made with partially skimmed milk, giving it a lower fat content. Imported varieties are free of artificial color, domestic ones may not be. The surface of the cheese is coated with a red paraffin that is usually artificially colored, but is not too crucial since you discard it. The presence of preservatives must be stated on the label, but no other clues as to what's inside need be given. *Maybud,* of Wisconsin origin, gives a pledge of purity ("natural ingredients, no preservatives added") on the package.

GOUDA

Almost identical in mellow flavor and handling to Edam. The only difference between the two is that Gouda is made with whole milk and so has a higher fat content.

PROVOLONE

This cheese comes from Italy and is highly salted and often smoked. If smoked, the label will inform you. Provolone may have coloring added, but not stated, and may be made from bleached milk, which means some vitamin destruction. The label will state if the milk has been bleached. Again, preservatives are allowed but are subject to the mandatory labeling requirement.

SWISS (EMMANTHALER)

The milk used to prepare Swiss cheese (usually partially skimmed) may be bleached first to give it that pale yellow color. There are a number of chemicals that can be employed in this process, and as a result the vitamin content of the milk is diminished. When the milk is bleached, synthetic vitamin A is added. The label must tell you if the milk has been treated, and it is advisable to buy a brand that is not. Unfortunately, unbleached cheeses may have added color, and there is no sure way of telling since it isn't on the label. Mold inhibitors may be added to Swiss cheese or the packaging, but the label must reveal this. Without preservatives the cheese will last several weeks with proper handling. The holes, by the way, come from the gas produced by harmless bacteria which penetrate the interior to ripen this type of cheese.

GRUYERE

Gruyère is a variation of Swiss and the flavor is slightly altered (somewhat sweeter), due to the addition of natural flavoring enzymes. No coloring or bleached milk may be used in this cheese, making it an excellent choice. The milk may be whole or partially skimmed. Mold inhibitors may be added, and this information is given on the label.

Hard Ripened

Hard ripened cheeses are used extensively for grating and tend to be sharp-flavored. Because of the low moisture content, these keep without much change in flavor or running the risk of mold growth for many weeks, but for some reason the standard of identity permits the addition of preservatives anyway. As with all cheeses, this is revealed on the label.

PARMESAN

Parmesan cheese is made from partially skimmed cow's milk which may be bleached. If so, it will be stated on the label. No coloring may be added to the cheese itself, but the rind may be waxed or colored without your knowing it. Check the label for preservatives—they are common in domestic varieties, less so in the imported ones.

This cheese is easy to grate in the blender or a hand grater. It can be purchased already grated but lacks the freshness of home-grated cheeses and many pre-grated brands include a sorbate preservative and an anticaking agent. If you do buy grated Parmesan, *Progresso*, for one, is free of additives.

ROMANO

Not too different from Parmesan but made with whole milk so it has more milk fat. Blue or green coloring matter may be used in this cheese (not stated) and again, bleached milk may be the basis of this product (stated). Look for preservatives on the label. The Italian imported varieties are made with sheep's milk (as stated on the label) and are quite tasty and unlikely to contain any undesirable matter.

Mold Ripened

Mold ripened cheeses are characterized by the blue veins that run through them. They depend on mold to grow in the interior during the curing time to impart the tangy flavor and the characteristic blue-green veins. All are semisoft and may be pasty or crumbly in consistency. Best used in salads and salad dressings, dips, and spread on crackers or vegetables.

BLUE (BLEU)

The spelling "Bleu" is an indication of the French imported version, "Blue" is domestic. Blue or green coloring may be added (unstated), the milk bleached (stated), and it may have preservatives (stated).

GORGONZOLA

The main difference between this and "Blue" is its homeland, Italy. Also, Gorgonzola may be made from goat's or cow's milk or a mixture of the two. If goat's milk is used, the label will advise you. Coloring, bleaching, and preserving are the same as for Blue.

ROQUEFORT

This form of Blue cheese is made with sheep's milk and is free of all unwanted additives. It is the preferred choice among the blue-veined cheeses.

THE GREAT DANES

Because the Danish cheeses are so good-tasting and the least likely to have any undesirable added ingredients, look for some of these in your store and give them a try: Samsoe, similar to Swiss in taste and texture; Danish Saint Paulin, a somewhat sharper cheese; Fontina, delicate, just right for sandwiches; Danish Blue; and Crema Danica, Danish Camembert, and Brie, all excellent dessert selections.

CHEESE CHECKPOINTS

Here's a quick summary of what to look for on the cheese label before you buy:

• If the cheese is "natural," the name appears alone, such as "Cheddar Cheese," "Swiss Cheese," or is preceded by the word "natural." If the cheese is otherwise processed, the words "pasteurized process," "pasteurized process cheese food," or "pasteurized process cheese spread" will appear, with the name of the variety or varieties of cheese included. Cold pack cheese will be labeled as such or as "club" or "comminuted." American cheese is the one exception; the descriptive adjective may be missing, but it is never a natural cheese.

On the label of natural cheese look for:
- Added preservatives
- Bleached milk

You can also discover from the label:

• Where present, the degree of curing, such as mild or mellow, aged or sharp.

• The animal the milk came from. If not stated, the milk is cow's milk. Other possibilities include sheep and goat's milk. Many people prefer these cheeses since sheep and goat's milk are less likely to contain high levels of DDT.

Most domestic cheese is made with pasteurized milk; otherwise it is cured for a specified period of time to insure its safety. Only pasteurized-milk cheese may be imported by law.

STORING CHEESE

All unripened cheeses are perishable and must be stored in the refrigerator. The soft unripened cheeses are often dated with the last recommended day of usage, and, if not dated, should be used within ten days of purchase.

All other cheeses should be kept in the refrigerator for long-term storage, but if cheese moves quickly in your house you can follow the European example and have a special cheese drawer or box left out at room temperature—the temperature at which cheese should be served. Cheese not refrigerated will become stronger sooner.

The rind or wax coating on cheese will protect unexposed surfaces. By buttering exposed edges you can keep the cheese moist and preserve the consistency. An alternate method for keeping the cut surface of cheese from drying out is to store it in a plastic wrapper, preferably a reusable plastic bag.

Smelly cheeses should be tightly covered so their odor doesn't penetrate other foods.

Cheese will not turn rancid but will become stronger and stronger with age until you will no longer enjoy the flavor or the odor. Then it's time to get rid of it. In its last days it can be used in dishes that call for melting. Mold on the outside of cheese is not harmful but should be cut or scraped off before using. This is a sign that the

cheese has passed its prime, so use the remainder in the near future.
Save dried-out ends of cheese for grating.

SERVING CHEESE

Except for the unripened cheeses, cheese is best served at room
temperature. This is the only way the full flavor and proper texture
can be achieved and savored. Remove the cheese from the refrigerator
at least thirty minutes before serving whenever possible.

"Cheese Closes the Stomach"

David's mother has a saying: "Cheese closes the stomach," an
expression that summarizes the ease with which cheese satisfies hunger pains. Because of its high protein and high fat content a small
piece of cheese can curb a large hunger.

USING CHEESE

Because cheese is so nutritious it is wise to incorporate it into the
menu often. With such a variety to choose from there is surely a
cheese to suit every member of your household.

Whenever you cook with cheese be sure to keep the heat low. High
temperatures cause the protein in cheese to become tough and stringy.

One-fourth pound of cheese, when grated, will make one cup.
Some of the many ways of incorporating cheese into your daily
meal routine include:

•Main dishes, in the form of fondues, soufflés, omelets, pizza, or
baked casseroles with potatoes, pasta, grains, or vegetables.

•Salads and salad dressings.

•Cheese wedges with fruit, nuts, or crackers for appetizer, dessert,
or anytime snack.

•Spreads and dips.

•Grated into soups, sauces, and as a topping for stews and casseroles.

•Sliced cold or melted on sandwiches.

•For topping fresh fruit pies; in cheese cakes and pies; in bread and
biscuit batter.

Stuffing, Spreading, and Dipping

For appetizers or parties, stuff raw vegetables with your own, not store-bought, spreads. Cream cheese, pot cheese, and cottage cheese are ideal for this purpose. Combine them with chopped scallions, green pepper, chopped olives, radishes, garlic, herbs, chopped nuts, and chopped dried fruits for a variety of spreads and fillings. Any of these mixtures can be thinned or smoothed with a spoonful of milk.

If you'd like to make some homemade cheese spreads for entertaining friends these two are quite impressive.

HOMEMADE BOURSIN SPREAD

¼ cup cottage cheese
1 tablespoon butter
2 tablespoons chopped parsley
2 cloves garlic
1 teaspoon sea salt

Drain all liquid from cheese and work in butter to form a smooth paste. Pound together parsley, garlic, and salt, and work into cheese paste. Shape into a flat round on an oiled board using oiled hands. Serve with crackers or toast.

To store, wrap in foil and chill. *Yield:* 1 small ball.

POTTED CHEDDAR SPREAD

2 cups grated Cheddar, about ½ pound before grating
1 tablespoon yogurt
½ teaspoon nutmeg
Pinch of cayenne
¼ cup apple juice

Mash all ingredients together with a fork to make a stiff paste. Pack into custard cups or small, wide-mouthed glasses, cover with foil, and refrigerate. Spread on crackers or use to fill vegetables. *Yield:* about 1 cup.

Dips for crackers or raw vegetables can be made with a cottage cheese base that's creamed in the blender instead of the more traditional sour cream. Cottage cheese is high in protein; sour cream is high in fat. Try this Roquefort Vegetable Dip and vary it by replacing the Roquefort with fresh herbs and caraway seeds.

ROQUEFORT VEGETABLE DIP

1   pound (2 cups) cottage cheese
¼   cup milk, skim or regular
1   teaspoon sea salt
1   tablespoon chopped chives
1   tomato, chopped
2   ounces (½ cup) crumbled Roquefort cheese

Puree cottage cheese and milk together in blender or food mill until smooth. Fold in remaining ingredients. *Yield:* about 2 cups.

RECOMMENDATIONS

General Rule of Purchase: Buy "natural cheese" only; if otherwise processed, the label will state "pasteurized process" or "cold pack." Although most ingredients are not listed on the label, if preservatives are added, it will be so stated. Imported cheeses, particularly from Denmark, are the least tainted. For specifics, see the descriptions in this chapter.

Soft cheeses like cottage cheese and ricotta should not have any thickening or stabilizing agents like carrageenan, vegetable gums, or mono- and diglycerides added. Nor should they have preservatives. All pot cheeses are chemical-free.

EXEMPLARY BRANDS:
  Cottage Cheese
    East—*Axelrod*
        Breakstone
        Crowley
        Friendship
        Hood
        Lawson
        Michigan Old Fashioned
    Middle—*Anderson Erickson* (large, small, and dry curd)
        Hy-Vee (4 percent fat varieties)
    West—*Anderson*
        Arden

      Carnation
      Cream 'O Weber
      Janet Lee
      Jerseymaid
      Knudsen (contains vegetable color)
      Lady Lee
      Lucerne Dry Curd
      Model Dairy
      Ralphs
      Tuttle
      Valley Gold

Ricotta
    East—*Axelrod*
          Breakstone
          Brunetto
          Falbo
          Hood
          LaMagna
          Maggio
          Micelis
          Polly-O
          Shop-Rite
          Sorrento
    Middle—*Micelis*
    West—*Gardenia*

Cream Cheese
    West—*Arden* (no vegetable gum)

Butter vs. Margarine:
The "Higher Priced" Spread Wins Again

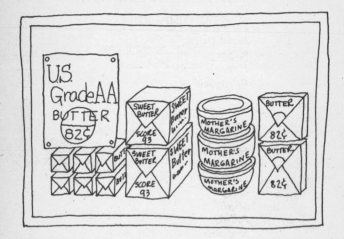

The substitution of margarine for butter is a common practice in many American households. Although margarine is less expensive than butter, economy is rarely the motivating force behind the switch. Unsaturated fat is the big selling point for margarine these days, and those concerned with heart disease consider margarine to be the miracle food of the century. We seriously question the validity of their sentiments.

The standard of identity for margarine defines it as a "plastic food" and, believe us, that's just what it is. There is hardly anything real in it! Let's analyze the contents.

MARGARINE AND FATTY ACIDS

Fat makes up 80 percent of both butter and margarine.

Where does the fat in margarine come from? There are three choices. One type of margarine is made exclusively from the fat rendered from animals, that is cattle, sheep, goat, or swine. Like the milk fat that butter is made from, these animal fats are saturated. The second type of margarine is primarily vegetable fat, or oils, which contain varying amounts of unsaturated fats (fatty acids). The third combines the animal and vegetable fat into one product.

A FAT COMPARISON

Source	Total Fat	Saturated Fat[1]	Unsaturated Fat[2] linoleic acid
(per 100 grams)	(grams)	(grams)	(grams)
Corn oil	100	10	53
Cottonseed oil	100	25	50
Olive oil	100	11	7
Peanut oil	100	18	29
Safflower oil	100	8	72
Sesame oil	100	14	42
Soy oil	100	15	52
Margarine hydrogenated or saturated oil first ingredient on label	81	18	14
liquid oil first ingredient on label	81	19	29
Butter	81	46	2

1. A saturated fat is one in which all possible locations for hydrogen atoms have been filled. Saturated fats are thought to accumulate in the cells of the heart and blood vessels, blocking the passageway and bringing about thickening and hardening of the arteries. Saturated fats may also increase the level of blood cholesterol.

2. Unsaturated fats have one or more possible sites available for hydrogen atoms. They do not contribute to bodily cholesterol and are the preferred form of fat consumption. Linoleic acid is only one of many unsaturated fats, but it is the most important. It is necessary for proper functioning of the nerves, brain, hormones, digestive system and general upkeep of the body. Linoleic acid cannot be synthesized by the body and therefore must be supplied by food. It is found primarily in fats of vegetable origin.

As far as saturated and unsaturated fats are concerned, the margarine which employs animal fat obviously offers no benefit over butter. Now if you look at the advertising promotion closely, you'll notice certain vegetable oils used in margarines are billed as "high in polyunsaturates." Perhaps the original vegetable oil was a rich source of many polyunsaturated fatty acids, but in order to obtain a butterlike consistency, vegetable oil must be at least partially hydrogenated (which means saturated). So all the manufacturer has succeeded in doing is creating a saturated fat from a previously highly unsaturated one. Bravo!

A small clue to the extent of saturation of fats in the resulting margarine appears on the label. Margarine ingredients are listed in order of decreasing amounts; for example:

• If the only fat listed is "hydrogenated or hardened oil," then the oil has been completely saturated.

• If the label states "liquid soybean oil, partially hardened safflower oil" then you have more unsaturated than saturated fats present.

• If the order is reversed and the partially hydrogenated oil appears before the liquid, then the saturated fat predominates.

The source of the oil is less important here than what has been done to the oil. One hundred percent corn oil margarine in which a large percent of the oil is hydrogenated has no greater health benefits than any other conventional margarine. If you are looking for a margarine with fewer saturated fats, the "soft" margarines are somewhat better.

The Type of Oil—Fit for Human Consumption?

There is, however, another reason for considering the oil used in the margarine, and we find most brands undesirable for yet another reason—one of the oils they employ is cottonseed oil.

As we've said in other sections of this book, cotton is not considered a food crop and therefore receives more than its share of chemical sprays. Food products derived from cotton are not fit for human consumption. Cottonseed oil is present in all "pure vegetable oil" margarines. This is your reason for selecting pure corn oil or safflower oil margarine over the pure vegetable oil variety.

The Other 20 Percent

The liquid portion of margarine comes from cream, milk (and both of these contain saturated fat), skim milk, buttermilk, nonfat dry milk, just plain water (and maybe some ground soybeans), or a combination of these.

What about the other ingredients in margarine? These include phony color and artificial butter flavor; emulsifiers and plasticizers (lecithin, monoglyceride); synthetic vitamins; salt (not too compatible with the low-sodium diets of many heart-conscious consumers); carotene (a natural source of vitamin A and color), and seven different "permissible" preservatives (including the sorbates, isopropyl citrate and disodium EDTA). Your only consolation is the fact that it's all there on the label for you to see and reject. Personally we wouldn't bring any of them into our kitchen but if you are still not convinced, you may be lucky enough to find one of the few brands on the market that contain neither cottonseed oil nor preservatives.

Among those we recommend are:

Autumn 100% Natural (free from all chemicals, including artificial flavoring)
Shedd's Willow Run (no chemicals or animal products)
Fleischman's Unsalted Corn Oil (in the freezer case)
Nu-Maid
Royal Scott
Sweet Rose
Golden Maid

The last three, all made by the Miami Margarine Company, are made entirely from partially hardened soy oil, or palm oil, a largely saturated oil.

Do not be misled by margarine that is labeled "Danish Flavor," leading you to believe it is of higher quality, as most Danish dairy products are. "Danish Flavor" margarine is 100 percent American and is made primarily from coconut and palm oil, both more highly saturated than animal fat, cream, plus the usual long list of chemicals.

A Final Note

All margarine must be refrigerated. Despite the fact that the tub it comes in says "Refrigerate" prominently, our supermarket insists on displaying one brand of soft margarine in a large cardboard bin. If your store follows this practice, make sure you bypass the bin.

BUTTER

In most cases, oil can be substituted for margarine or butter in cooking. (See "Salad Dressing, Oil and Vinegar.") Where it can't, as for spreading on bread, why not use butter, but sparingly? If you're going to eat saturated fats you might as well stick to those that are naturally saturated. Used sparingly, butter will be less detrimental to your health than margarine, for at least the additives are held to a minimum. The best butter you can buy bears the statement "made from sweet cream" on the label. Other butters are made from stale or soured milk or cream with a lot of salt added to inhibit mold growth and an alkaline salt added to neutralize the salty taste. U.S. grades of butter are determined first by flavor, then body, color, and salt. The only one you should concern yourself with is "U.S. Grade AA" or "U.S. 93 Score." Any other type exhibits a variety of off-flavors from slight flatness (a lack of natural butter flavor), aging (a lack of freshness), and smothering (an indication the cream was improperly cooled) to "musty, weedy, woody, barny" (all flavors associated with the animal it came from) and a plain old stale taste. The lesser grades also show body defects. All these off-flavors and poor textures are the result of mishandling of the cream during processing.

Once you've selected your U.S. Grade AA sweet cream butter, make sure it's unsalted. Salt is added to butter to mask any off-flavors (and off-quality). Salt also helps preserve butter, so salted butter can be more easily mishandled. Greater care is taken with unsalted butter to insure its safe arrival at the supermarket.

Now the only additive you have to concern yourself with is the added color, which may be natural or synthetic and can be added without your ever knowing it. This is unavoidable in purchasing commercial butter.

Despite all your care, butter may be held by the supermarket in cold storage for several months. Make sure you select a package that is well wrapped, and if you detect any off-flavor or odor, return it to the store. Rancid fats destroy fat-soluble vitamins in the digestive tract, literally

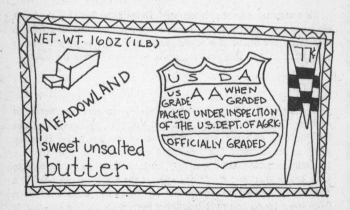

robbing your system. If it looks or tastes funny, don't think you're oversensitive. Return it.

"Whipped butter" is made by incorporating air or gas into regular butter. If you want it whipped, you can save the money by whipping it in your blender.

ONE MORE ALTERNATIVE

As we said before, most of your cooking can be done with oil in place of butter or margarine. If you seriously want to cut down on the use of saturated fats and butter why not spread your bread with something else altogether.

Here are a few suggestions for spreadable substitutes:

- Cottage cheese moistened with skim milk
- Ricotta cheese
- Homemade oil and vinegar dressing
- Yogurt
- Tahina (sesame butter)
- Mashed avocado

RECOMMENDATIONS

BUTTER

General Rule of Purchase: The label generally gives no ingredients. Buy sweet cream, unsalted butter and season it yourself. U.S. Grade AA or Score 93 is of highest quality.

> EXEMPLARY BRANDS:
>> East—*Breakstone (Sugar Creek)* Unsalted
>> *Dairy Maid* Whipped, unsalted
>> *Land O Lakes,* unsalted
>> *Lucerne* Sweet Cream
>> Sunnyfield Unsalted
>> *Waldbaums,* unsalted
>> *Weis* Sweet Cream, unsalted ·

      Middle—*Breakstone (Sugar Creek)* unsalted
          Lucerne Sweet Cream
          Roberts Sweet Cream Unsalted
          Select Brand Unsalted
      West—*Challenge,* unsalted
          Creamland Unsalted
          Daisy Whipped, unsalted
          Darigold AA-Grade Unsalted
          Knudsens Sweet Cream, unsalted
          Lucerne Sweet Cream
          Select Brand Unsalted

N.B. Many local dairies offer additional choices.

MARGARINE

General Rule of Purchase: All ingredients are on the label. Margarine is never highly recommended, but look for those free of cottonseed oil and with the least amount of hydrogenated or hardened oils and additives.

EXEMPLARY BRANDS:
    Autumn™ 100% Natural
    Fleischman's Unsalted Corn Oil (frozen)
    Hy-Vee
    Nu-Maid
    Shedd's Willow Run Soybean
    Staff

The following brands are also relatively additive-free but contain partially hardened oils only and are therefore more saturated.
    Albertson's
    Pomco
    Red and White
    Royal Scott
    Staff Corn Oil
    Sweet Rose (Golden Maid)

Meeting the Challenge of Meat

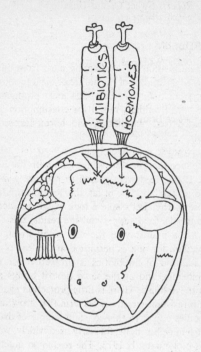

Is meat a natural food? This may seem like a silly question, but so many chemicals are ingested and injected into our livestock it's hard to say how much is real animal and how much is chemically induced. We don't eat meat anymore, but we aren't saying everyone else must do the same. There's no question, though: Americans should consume less meat. All over the world meat is considered a luxury, except in our country where it's assumed to be a necessity.

If you are eating a well-balanced diet of whole foods, which this manual will help you to do, reducing your meat intake offers physical and monetary benefits worthy of your consideration. These are outlined for you in the chapter "Meatless Main Dishes and Nutrition."

As you read the following chapter on meat, seriously weigh what you learn and perhaps you too will join the movement toward less meat in the American diet.

THE REAL PROBLEM

The original motivation for eliminating meat from our diet came with our increased awareness of the nature of meat production in this country. Right from their very inception meat products meet with food pollution—most animals raised for consumption grow up on chemically treated feed, antibiotics, and hormones, so they grow faster and fatter.

By feeding livestock scientifically mixed feed the cattle rancher manages to produce the greatest weight gain with the least amount of actual feed. If this feed were geared to produce a more healthy animal, high in protein and low in fat, this feed manipulation would indeed be praiseworthy. Let's take a look at what is actually being added to the animal's food supply and the results this diet has.

Antibiotics are a mainstay in the diet of all livestock bred for slaughter. Penicillin, for one, is permitted in the feed of all animals. The random addition of antibiotics is protection for the rancher against any epidemic, and at the same time it brings about faster weight gain in the animals. There is little protection against residues in the meat and resistant strains of bacteria that grow in the animal once his antibodies adjust to this constant supply of drugs.

Stilbestrol, a female hormone, formerly used widely, was banned in animal feed as of January 1, 1973. The reason so much concern is centered on this chemical hormone is its extreme potency in altering sex characteristics. It has also been implicated in cervical cancer in women. Although banned in feed, beef and lamb may still be implanted with pellets of the hormone under the new regulations. Stilbestrol is used to make the animal more feminine, in other words, to bring about a gain of fat and water.*

To keep the animals quiet and attentive to their eating, tranquilizers

---

*The first edition of this book contained a footnote in this space indicating that DES had also been removed from animal implants; however, this ban was overturned in 1974, so that DES is now in full use. Even if DES was banned, there are many substitutes (also suspicious); thus our attitude that the *whole system* of food and feed additives must be questioned.

go into the feed and the lights are often left on continuously so the "hungry" stock can feed at night too. Another favorite hormone blocks the action of the thyroid gland, thus causing weight gains.

Perhaps none of this would be so alarming but for the biological similarity of the animal these chemicals are being given to, and the animal who will ultimately consume the treated flesh—YOU! It's not a pretty picture, and consequently more and more people are choosing to limit meat in their diets.

For those of you who are sticking with meat, there are, of course, some guidelines to help you shop wisely. Let's analyze some of the categories of meat products and see what we're left with.

FRANKFURTERS

Ever since the early days of food processing, the era of the "muck-rakers," Upton Sinclair and *The Jungle,* aspersions have been cast on that great American invention, the hot dog. There have always been rumors that "everything but the squeak" goes into its production. Today it would still be a guess as to whether these rumors are fact, but we can guarantee the presence of some equally repugnant nonfood items. For example, chemical coloring and preserving agents like sodium nitrate and nitrite, among the most potentially dangerous additives on the market, have found a home in this widely consumed in food, can disable hemoglobin, the molecule in red blood cells that transports life-giving oxygen. Both nitrates and nitrites can lead to the formation of cancer-causing chemicals.* The other scientific-sounding names you encounter on the label of frankfurters are antioxidants, added to prevent fading of the artificially induced pink color. You might watch for a new addition as well, sodium acid pyrophosphate, a unique ingredient which "will cut the manufacturing time down 25 to 40 percent." Who knows how long it will cut your time down?

As far as the food ingredients in this meat product go:

•The term "all meat" on the label does not mean the product is nothing but meat. According to the USDA such franks can contain 10 percent added water and 5 percent other ingredients (spices, flavoring, chemicals).

---

*The U.S.D.A. has proposed (1975) that nitrate preservatives be banned from all meat products except dry-cured and fermented sausage, and that the amounts of sodium nitrite be reduced in bacon, cooked sausage, canned cured products, dry-cured meats, and fermented sausage. No matter what action the U.S.D.A. takes, *you* can still ban nitrites from your table.

•Perhaps the label should say "all kinds of meat," for if you purchase "all-meat" frankfurters, you receive muscle tissues from cattle, pigs, and chickens with up to 30 percent of their natural amount of fat. Thus 45 percent of "all meat" frankfurters may be fat, water and additives.

•If they're "all beef," the difference is that the meat part will be derived from beef animals only.

•According to the USDA publication, *The Yearbook of Agriculture,* processed meat items use Utility, Cutter, Canner, and Cull grades of meat. This is a polite way of saying flesh of senile, fatty, tough, useless animals along with other unwanted parts.

•Corn syrup, a refined sugar extract, is present in all varieties.

You'd probably be better off with the simple "frankfurter" which extends the meat products with cereal, defatted wheat germ, and milk solids, contains only 2.5 percent less meat than "all meat" varieties, and is more nutritious in the long run.*

FRANK FACTS

1 pound frankfurters	calories	grams of protein
All meat	1343	59.4
with nonfat dry milk	1361	59.4
with cereal	1125	65.3
with cereal and nonfat dry milk	not available	64.4

OTHER PROCESSED MEAT

The picture doesn't improve for other processed meats.

Worried about cholesterol? Pork sausage and breakfast sausage may be as much as 50 percent fat. And in addition to the nitrate coloring agents in the "meat" itself, there are chemicals added to the synthetic casings to preserve the contents. Although you don't consume the casing of sausage, bologna, salami, etc., the meat sits in it for months.

We're far from the end of the adulteration of processed meats.

---

*As of July, 1976, what were formerly called "all meat" frankfurters will now be labeled "frankfurters," "weiners," or "hot dogs." If made only from one species, the label may say "beef" or "pork" as well. If meat other than muscle meat is used, the term "with byproducts" or "variety meats" must be included. The "frankfurter" that contains cereal or milk solids must now state these ingredients in the name, as "hot dogs with soy flour" or "nonfat dry milk added."

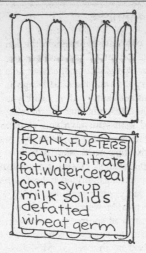

FRANKFURTERS
sodium nitrate
fat. water, cereal
corn syrup
milk solids
defatted
wheat germ

Curing is no longer the lengthy process of salting the meat and allowing it to hang to dry, but involves artificial incorporation of chemicals and sugars into the flesh for quick curing. To cure ham, a brine of salt, sugar, and nitrates may actually be injected into the arteries. If the total weight gain after this processing is up to 8 percent, the label will read "Ham, with Natural Juices." You'll notice on many labels it says "Water Added," which means an 8 to 10 percent weight gain, and as this goes up, the product is called "Imitation." As of February 1973 cured meats must carry a list of all ingredients used in the curing process. You may discover as many as ten different curing agents in your favorite corned beef sandwich or frank 'n beans dinner.

Additional processes are used to flavor, smoke, insure maximum juice retention, and further preserve these products. Reading the label gives few clues to any of this.

Included in this category are frankfurters, sausage, bologna, salami, corned beef, canned cured hams, picnic shoulders, bacon, pepperoni, and other smoked meats. Thus far we have found the following brands to be chemical free: *Jones* sausage, *Tobin's* Brown and Serve Sausage, *Taste Wright* Brand Pure Pork Sausage, plus several sausages which, unfortunately, include MSG. In any event, processed meats contain such high levels of fat that the best advice here is to choose something else instead.

CANNED MEAT PRODUCTS

Consider all those convenient dinners in the can that someone else has prepared for you, so that all you have to do is pay for it, take it home, and heat it up. One glance at the label tells you all the things that were used to prepare your meal (although it won't reveal how much of anything was used) and will reassure you that you're still a better cook than General Foods with all their experience.

You are concerned with your own and your family's health and growth. Producers of canned meat products are concerned with making money. Take a can of corned beef hash, one of those products given a formula to follow in the form of a government standard of identity. What you're actually buying is beef, which may be fresh, cured, or canned to begin with; potatoes, which are fresh or dehydrated and probably treated with chemicals to prevent darkening; curing agents in the form of sodium or potassium nitrate or nitrite; seasoning of salt, sugar, and spice extracts; and the optional extras of onion, garlic, water, beef broth, beef fat, MSG, and hydrolyzed plant protein. What you are getting is the cheapest, most undesirable parts of the animal doctored up with spices and chemicals.

Wouldn't it be much nicer to dice up some fresh onion and garlic, sauté until tender in oil, add pieces of boiled potato (leftovers are fine), throw in yesterday's meat scraps, season the mixture with salt and pepper, and cook until the potatoes are lightly browned and the meat is heated through? This way you know just what it is you're getting in your hash.

To further discourage you, here are some of the percentages the government requires food processors to include in their canned meat products:

Chili Con Carne with Beans—25 percent meat
Beef with Barbecue Sauce—50 percent meat
Deviled Ham—up to 35 percent fat
Meat Balls in Sauce—50 percent meat balls which contain 12 percent extenders, and if the label reads the other way around: Spaghetti Sauce with Meat Balls—the percentage of meat balls drops to 35

As for chemicals, as we've said, they're all there on the label, so check for yourself.

FROZEN MEAT PRODUCTS

We're having such a good time quoting percentages from canned meat, we thought you might like to hear about some of their sister products as well. So here goes:

> Veal Parmigiana—40 percent *breaded* meat
> Meat Pies—25 percent meat
> Lasagna—12 percent meat
> Entrees of meat, gravy, and one vegetable—30 percent meat
> Meat casseroles—25 percent uncooked meat or 18 percent cooked

When you consider the percentage of meat and its quality, you're paying a lot of money for a lot of additives, extenders, and packaging.

Go on to the next section and begin choosing your own fresh meat to be certain you're getting the best the supermarket has to offer.

BUY FRESH MEAT!

Let's look through the meat case together and determine what the best buy for your health is. You'll notice some of the meat is frozen or has a sign indicating that it has been frozen and defrosted. Meat that is frozen is not as fresh, has often gone through partial defrosting and refreezing, and is subject to more degradation and higher bacterial count than fresh meat cuts. If you want frozen meat, take home a fresh piece and freeze it yourself. It cannot be frozen indefinitely and this way you are sure its life isn't being overextended. Unless you have a zero degree freezer frozen foods will not be properly frozen. In the case of meat this can lead to considerable bacteria growth. If you do have a zero degree freezer consider buying a whole animal carcass, have it butchered and flash frozen. This is often the cheapest way to buy meat and provides plenty to share.

VEAL

The less fatty animals lead the recommended list. Veal, especially milk-fed veal, although becoming more and more costly, is your best bet. Firstly, this is the meat of a young calf, and since it is slaughtered at an early age it usually misses the hormone treatment. Secondly, as this is the leanest of meats, you not only do your heart a favor, but also your pocketbook, for there is very little waste and you can see just how much you're getting for your money. Veal cutlets, scallops, and chops are all versatile, tasty choices. Because there is so little fat, veal cutlets may be tougher than other meat products. To "tenderize" the meat, place it between two sheets of paper and pound it with a mallet or hammer. This will break the connective tissues as well as provide a great outlet for your aggressions.

LAMB

Lamb also comes from a young animal (it's mutton if it's fully grown) and so has had less mistreatment in its short life. Although breast and shoulder chops are more expensive, making them appear more desirable, leg of lamb is up to half as fatty.

Of all the foreign meat imported into the United States, New Zealand Spring Lamb is the most noteworthy. Raised, slaughtered, aged, cut, inspected and flash frozen in New Zealand, the meat is inspected again by the USDA before it is allowed to enter this country. One of the most significant facts about New Zealand lamb is that it is not chemically treated. The New Zealand Lamb Information Center tells us that "in New Zealand all sex hormones and 'tenderizers' are banned, and animal tranquilizers are not in use." Hygienic conditions in New Zealand are reportedly good, and this lamb, which is imported and distributed in the frozen state, is a good choice if your supermarket maintains good freezing techniques. Most supermarkets indicate when "Genuine Spring Lamb from New Zealand" is being offered.

Many people object to lamb, insisting that it has a "gamey" taste. You'll find if you don't overcook it, it has a very pleasing, delicate flavor.

BEEF

Beef is the most available, most popular, and most tainted of all meat products. This is also the meat that most often boasts a USDA grading shield, so we'll take a brief detour to explain the role of the government in meat sales.

Grading and Inspection

There are three different categories of meat-judging in this country. Most important is the inspection procedure, which is required by law for all meat sold across state lines. For meat sold within state lines, state inspection laws apply. What the inspectors check for are sanitary conditions in the slaughterhouse, proper labeling and packaging, and healthy animals. Although the sampling is only random, so that many animals with hormone and antibiotic residue are likely to get through, and although carcasses which are only partially affected by disease and drug residue are passed once the involved portions are removed (and it takes a very wise inspector to know for sure that all the cancer has been removed), you should always check for the round inspection stamp on any meat you consider buying.

Next is the government grading system, which is a voluntary service purchased by the slaughterhouse. This grading is not based on food value, but on appearance. Higher grade carcasses are more uniform in size, with a good intermingling of fat with lean and a thick, firm fat covering; this meat will be juicier and more tender. Lower

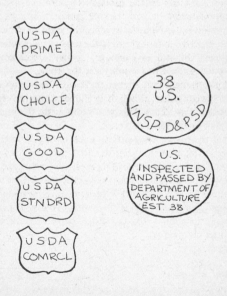

grades actually have more protein and vitamin value. Grades range from Prime, Choice, and Good for all animals to an additional five gradations for beef (Standard, Commercial, Utility, Cutter, and Canner), three for veal (Standard, Utility, and Cull), and two for lamb (Utility and Cull). Prime choices rarely go to the retail market and many stores only offer "Choice." A government grade is indicated by a shield with the letters USDA and the grade.

Many supermarkets buy ungraded meat to avoid the extra payment for grading, and many companies do their own grading based on their own standards. Beware of stickers similar to the official seal without the letters USDA.

If they're available in your area, there are two excellent reasons for choosing the lower grades of beef, that is, "Good" to "Commercial." Firstly, these cuts are less fatty, and although this may result in a less tender cut of meat, proper preparation (dealt with below) yields a highly desirable end product, and the reduced animal fat intake will be a boon to your health. One farmer suggests buying commercial grade beef as a remedy to the problem of hormone implantation, under the rationale that "a cow that has run on the range all of her life and grown fat on grass never reaches the good to choice grade." This is the second reason for bypassing the upper grades of beef. Don't worry, this meat will still have enough fat, but in competition with artificially induced fat it just won't meet the grade.

The final government grading system is called a Yield Grade and rarely affects the consumer, although an animal with a low-yield grade usually provides leaner cuts. This won't appear on the precut packages on display in the meat cooler.

It's difficult to let your eye be the guide to beef-buying these days. The chemicals available can doctor diseased, decaying, and just plain stale meat, and with all the misleading meat-case lights and layers of transparent wrapper all you can do is rely on the federal, state, or local inspector (and a friendly butcher). When you have the chance to view the meat, remember: fresh meat is cherry-red in color. The darker the meat, the older the animal. Texture should be velvety, not coarse; fat portions white, not yellow.

GROUND MEAT

Behind the sterile white showcase and the plastic see-through wrappers in the meat department of every supermarket there stands a butcher. Although he may be separated from you by a glass window, try to get to know him. If you intend to eat meat, his friendship can prove invaluable. Even supermarket butchers can grind meat to order. This is your only guarantee that the substance of your ground meat dish is not derived from old, undesirable or fatty parts, and that the luscious red color (usually an indication of freshness) doesn't come from a nearby jar of blood.

Chopped sirloin makes the leanest ground meat, followed by chuck. The label "hamburger" or "chopped meat" is a euphemism for a package which may contain pork, lamb, and veal trimmings, hearts, and other organs and is more than 25 percent fat. Since most ground meat is ground on the premises, it is not subject to federal regulations, which limit fat content to 30 percent. Although organ meats, an excellent source of vitamins, are often included in "hamburger," the high fat content of the trimmings used makes it a poor buy, except for your pet.

ORGAN MEATS

Meat is given the prime position it occupies in menu planning because it is so rich in protein, B vitamins, and minerals, particularly iron. The best source of these nutrients in the meat department is found in what are termed "variety meats." These include liver, tongue, brains, and heart, usually from steers, calves, and chickens.

Choose only fresh, not frozen, organ meats and never select a package that has been frozen and defrosted. Supermarkets often save the liver, kidney, etc., from large carcasses of whole birds in the freezer, accumulate enough to offer for sale and then defrost them so they appear fresh at first glance (although any ethical butcher will put out a sign: "frozen, defrosted"). Variety meats are more perishable than other cuts and by buying them in this manner you risk faulty freezing and defrosting and high bacterial growth. *Never* refreeze organ meats.

If you want your family to like liver, select calf rather than steer liver. Liver from the young animal is tender, with a delicate flavor, rather than tough and dry and "livery." Do not overcook liver. It is the overcooking, not the liver itself, that turns it into shoeleather (and destroys the high quality of the protein).

ORGAN MEAT AND MUSCLE MEATS COMPARED, 1 lb. BEEF

Cut	Calories	Protein (grams)	Fat (grams)	Calcium (grams)	Phosphorus (mg)	Iron (mg)	Vit. A (I.U.)	Thiamine (mg)	Riboflavin (mg)	Niacin (mg)	C (mg)
Chuck, boneless	1,166	84.8	88.9	42	720	10.7	150	.31	.64	17.2	–
T-bone, bone in	1,596	59.1	149.1	32	543	8.8	300	.25	.53	14.2	–
Hamburger	1,216	81.2	96.2	45	708	12.2	160	.35	.72	19.5	–
Brain	567	*47.2	39.0	45	1415	10.9	0	1.08	1.18	20.1	82
Heart	490	77.6	16.3	23	885	18.1	90	2.42	3.98	34.1	9
Kidney	590	69.9	30.4	50	993	33.6	3130	1.61	11.57	29.2	68
Liver	635	90.3	17.2	36	1597	29.5	199,130	1.16	14.79	61.6	140

PORK

Pork is a questionable buy. The tantalizing fresh pink color is an indication of nothing since it is usually induced by a tranquilizer injection into the animal before slaughter rather than by good health.

There is presently no requirement for inspection of pork, and trichinosis is a serious problem if the meat is not sufficiently cooked. Our supermarket has this sign next to the pork display: "All raw pork products must be thoroughly *heated* or *cooked* so that all portions thereof reach a temperature of *not less than 140°F to prevent trichinosis.*" If you're preparing pork, be sure the internal temperature reaches at least *170°,* and if the juice is pink, keep cooking.

There is also no grading standard for pork and the amount of fat is appalling. Tests have shown that 60 to 80 percent of bacon is often lost in the drippings! If you do choose to purchase pork products, these suggestions can help you.

•Irradiation, or exposure to X-rays, is employed in this country for pork preservation. It is illegal in Denmark, so better choose the imported product.

•Don't buy unrefrigerated canned hams. Canned ham must be refrigerated at all times, although many supermarkets ignore this fact.

PACKAGING

While we're at the meat counter we'd like to put in a word about packaging. This is an important consideration for your health and the health of the environment. Note the tray in which the meat is resting. Is it plastic? Plastic is a nondegradable product (see the chapter on "Ecology at Home") which remains in the environment forever. You and your butcher have a choice. Compressed paper containers, although not recommended for long-term storage, are made from recycled paper and as garbage they can be broken down and returned to the land. Victory Markets have recently introduced a nonplastic see-through meat tray that burns cleanly and decomposes completely. Discourage your store from using plastic.

A last warning: don't purchase any meat if its container is damaged in any way.

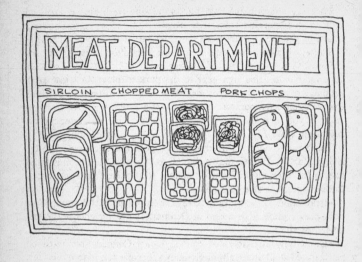

HANDLING AND STORAGE

Meat spoils quickly. It must be stored in the coldest section of your refrigerator, and then not for more than a few days. If you plan on using the meat within two days after it's bought, it can be refrigerated in the original (transparent) wrapper. If your supermarket sells meat in market paper, rewrap it before chilling. If you plan to hold the meat longer than two days, remove excess moisture and make sure it is wrapped loosely so that air can circulate. This will discourage bacterial growth.

Use fresh cuts within three to five days, fresh sausage, variety cuts, ground or stew meat in one to two days, and cured meats within one week.

If you intend to keep the meat longer, freeze it. Do not wash meat before freezing, but wipe the surface with a cloth to remove any surface bacteria. Make sure it's dry before you wrap it; the idea is to keep out all air and moisture. Rewrap so that it is air- and moisture-tight, label with both the cut and the date of freezing, and freeze as soon as possible after purchase—as meat ages, both flavor and food

Product	Storage Period	
	Refrigerator 35°-40°F Days	Freezer 0°F Months
Fresh meats		
Roasts (Beef and Lamb)	3-5	8-12
Roasts (Pork and veal)	3-5	4-8
Steaks (Beef)	3-5	8-12
Chops (Lamb and Pork)	3-5	3-4
Ground and Stew meats	1-2	2-3
Variety meats	1-2	3-4
Sausage (Pork)	1-2	1-2
Processed meats		
Frankfurters	7	½
Ham (whole)	7	1-2
Ham (half)	3-5	1-2
Ham (slices)	3	1-2
Luncheon meats	3-5	Freezing
Sausage (smoked)	7	not
Sausage (dry)	14-21	recommended
Cooked meats		
Cooked meats and meat dishes	1-2	2-3
Gravy and meat broth	1-2	2-3
Fresh poultry		
Chicken and turkey	1-2	12
Duck and goose	1-2	6
Giblets	1-2	3
Cooked poultry		
Pieces (covered with broth)	1-2	6
Pieces (not covered)	1-2	1
Cooked poultry dishes	1-2	6
Fried chicken	1-2	4

value begin to deteriorate. Although freezing will halt further alteration, it will not improve a product.

Properly frozen, lamb and beef for roasts and steaks will last twelve months; veal and pork roasts, eight months; chops, cutlets, and variety meat, four months; ground and stew meat, three months; and fresh sausage, two months. Don't freeze cured meats, as the combination of high fat content and seasonings accelerates rancidity. For the same reason it is better not to season chopped meat before you freeze it.

It is not necessary to thaw meat before cooking, and steaks, hamburgers, and other cuts which are to be broiled without a sauce will have a fresher flavor if they are cooked directly from the frozen state. Thaw meat, whenever necessary, in the refrigerator. Never soak frozen meat in hot water to thaw; you'll be creating a haven for microorganisms. Do not refreeze meat.

Meat is a fine breeding ground for bacteria. As trivial as it sounds, please be very sanitary in the kitchen when you handle any animal products. Discard any paper immediately which has been in contact with the meat and be sure to wipe the work area, any utensils which have touched the meat, and your hands thoroughly before you begin preparing any other food. Various forms of food poisoning, from mild, hardly traceable but definitely uncomfortable varieties to the severe, deadly kind, are not uncommon in this country.

PREPARATION

The cooking of meat is of vital importance, for it is this exposure to heat that kills the harmful bacteria. Don't encourage the eating of blood-red or raw meat (even though it's very tempting to nibble during preparation).

At the same time, protein foods are extremely heat-sensitive. Very high temperatures not only destroy the protein, but denature it in such a way that overcooked meat will be tough and dry.

Longer cooking at a lower temperature will give juicy, tender results, with a uniform color, less shrinkage, and the least nutritional loss. Adelle Davis, the popular nutritionist, does a wonderful demonstration where she cooks a chuck roast, one of the leanest, toughest cuts around, for twenty-four hours at 165° and when it's done she slices up a beautiful pink, buttersoft roast beef. If you want to try her method, here are the directions: Be sure to adhere to the initial one

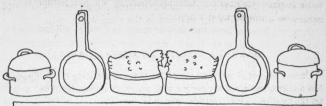

Product	Internal temperature when done °F
Fresh beef	
Rare	140
Medium	155
Well done	170
Fresh veal	170
Fresh lamb	
Medium	160
Well done	170
Fresh pork	
Loin	170
Other roasts	185
Cured pork (cook before eating)	
Ham	160
Shoulder	170
Canadian Bacon	160
Cured pork (fully cooked)	
Ham	130
Poultry	
Chicken	185
Turkey	180-185
Boneless roasts	170-175

hour at 300°; this heat is necessary to destroy the bacteria, which will otherwise multiply by the millions in the nice, warm oven.

MAKING A ROAST A LA ADELLE DAVIS

Choose any cut of meat you would like to roast, including the traditionally less tender ones. Brush the surface with oil, insert a meat thermometer, and set the meat on a rack in an open pan in an oven preheated to 300°. Let cook 1 hour to destroy surface bacteria. Now, lower the heat of your oven to the internal temperature that matches the desired degree of doneness for the choice you have made (see Doneness Temperatures below). Multiply your normal cooking time by three (not including the hour of preheating), and you'll have a pretty fair guide to how long to leave your roast in the oven. Following this method you can put a 4-pound chuck roast in the oven at 7:30 A.M. when you get up, give it the 1-hour sterilization, turn your oven down to 140° at 8:30 A.M., go out for the day and return home at about 6:30 to take a juicy, rare roast beef from the oven and sit down to dinner. (Based on an estimated 50 minute/pound cooking time for less tender cuts of beef.) Try it with veal and lamb as well as beef roasts.

Invest a dollar in a meat thermometer; you can purchase one in almost every supermarket, and if not in yours, the local hardware store or five-and-ten will have one. It takes the guesswork out of meat cookery. "Minutes per pound" is only a rough guide, and will vary with oven temperature (which is rarely the same as what you've set the dial at), thickness of the cut, bones, and fat content. The meat thermometer will let you check the temperature in the center of the meat. Make sure it isn't touching a bone.

Doneness Temperatures

If you want your roast beef rare, remove it from the oven when the thermometer reads 140°. Medium roasts come out at 155°, and the beef is well done when it reaches 170°–180°.

Veal should always be cooked well done, which is 170°.

Lamb is best when "medium," which again means an internal temperature of 160°–170°.

Never cheat with pork; let the heat reach at least 170°, and if the juice is still pink, put the roast back in the oven.

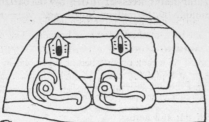

Place meat thermometer in the thickest part of the roast

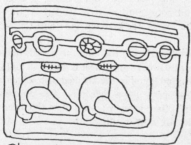

Place the thermometer in the center of the inner thigh of the turkey

Cooking Methods

Oven-roasting in an open pan gives the tenderest results even with the so-called tougher cuts, as you've discovered if you've tried the Adelle Davis method. This is by no means the only method of meat cookery though.

Braising

Large cuts can be potted, or more technically cooked with liquid in a covered pot by a method known as braising. The procedure is quite simple:

1. Place the meat on a rack or on a bed of vegetables in a large pot.
2. Add ½ inch of liquid for stews, ¼ inch for pot roasts. Choose water, vegetable broth, tomato juice, wine, etc. The more flavorful, the better.
3. Season with salt and herbs.
4. Cover, and you're ready to begin cooking.

Many people flour the meat first and brown it in a little oil. This is optional and actually causes shrinkage and toughens the outer layer; besides, it's more time-consuming and leaves another pot to wash.

Braising can be done on top of the range or in the oven.

5. For oven-cooking: place the covered casserole in an oven set from 250 to 350° and cook until meat is tender. Again, the lower the temperature the longer the cooking time and the more tender the product.
6. For range cookery: bring the liquid to a boil, reduce heat, cover and let simmer gently only until meat is done (45 minutes to 1 hour).

Be sure to use the liquid in the finished dish, either as is, or thickened with a flour paste for a rich gravy (see directions in "Do-It-Yourself Sauces"). Important vitamins from the meat and accompanying vegetables are now in this broth.

Broiling

Smaller cuts, such as steaks and chops, can be broiled or pan-broiled. Where broiler heat can be controlled, turn it to low and place meat on a rack about two inches from the heat. In an oven broiler, where heat cannot be varied, set the rack five to six inches from heat. Turn the meat halfway through cooking. Do not salt until serving time. Salt draws out the juices and will dry out your steak.

Pan-broiling should be done over low to medium heat in a heavy skillet. Do not grease the pan and do not cover. This method is best reserved for well-marbled steaks or cuts with a high fat content. While it is true that salting the pan first helps prevent sticking, this practice extracts flavorful, nutrient rich juices from the meat and should be avoided.

Pan-Frying

Meats with little fat, like veal, are good sautéed. This is done just like pan-broiling, but the pan is brushed with oil to keep the meat from sticking. Coating the meat with flour or crumbs first enhances the flavor and helps absorb the fat to enrich the taste and texture of the finished dish.

Leftovers

What you don't eat today makes a quick meal tomorrow. The addition of a sauce can completely change the taste of yesterday's meat and no one will ever know they're eating leftovers. Before we get too far ahead, take the freshly cooked extras (leftovers), place them in an airtight container and refrigerate them immediately. Letting meat stand warm creates a breeding ground for bacteria and is the worst thing you can do. Older cookbooks call for cooling meat (and gravy or broth) at room temperature before refrigerating. This was to compensate for the less-than-perfect refrigerator cooling systems of the day. With today's technology at work in the appliance area you can place hot food directly into your refrigerator with no risk of reducing the refrigerator's coldness. If you don't plan on using the leftover meat within two days, freeze it immediately. Gravy and broth should also be used within this two-day period. The high fat content of gravy makes it unsuitable for freezing; however, if you skim the fat from the broth you can freeze it as well.

Use Your Imagination: Now you're ready to change the character of the cooked meat. Although many cookbooks will supply you with numerous variations, we'd like to give you a few suggestions that can be prepared in minutes and require neither canned products nor a cookbook, only your imagination.

MEAT IN FRESH VEGETABLE SAUCE

1. Sauté a chopped onion in oil until it turns golden brown.
2. Add some chopped green pepper and cook for a minute or so.
3. Next, add a few diced tomatoes, salt, and pepper, and cook over moderate heat until the tomatoes become soft and release their juice. This will take about 10 minutes.

4. Now you can add the leftover meat, in slices or thin strips, and heat through.

When you add the green pepper, consider the other possibilities in your vegetable bin. Try adding some sliced mushrooms, leftover zucchini squash, green peas, or anything else that touches your fancy along with the pepper.

VARYING THE SAUCE

When you season the sauce with salt and pepper let your hand wander across the spice shelf. Basil, oregano, and marjoram will make your dish Italian; chili powder will give it a Mexican flavor; dill will make it taste like spring.

Make it sweet and sour with the addition of a tablespoon or two of wine vinegar and an equal amount of molasses or honey; then when you add the meat, toss in some raisins or diced dried apricots and plump them in the warm sauce.

SAUTÉED MEAT AND VEGETABLES

Quick-fried vegetables with strips of meat, a takeoff on Chinese cooking, is a good way to prepare a speedy meal and use the odds and ends in your refrigerator.

1. Heat a little oil in a skillet (or a wok if you have one) and quickly sauté any selected assortment of diced vegetables over high heat. Carrots, scallions, mushrooms, shredded greens, celery (almost anything except tomatoes will do).
2. Add the meat, cut in thin strips, a little broth or water, a spoonful of soy sauce (see recommendations for purchase in the chapter "Seasonings: Natural Food Enhancers"), cover and steam a few minutes over reduced heat.
3. For variety, top with chopped walnuts, slivered almonds, or toasted sesame seeds.

MEAT, RICE, AND VEGETABLES

The Chinese are experts at making a little bit of meat go a long way. Use leftover bits and pieces to make Chinese fried rice. Made with brown rice this dish will provide a hearty main course.

Leaving No Leftovers: The smallest scraps, even bones, can be reused. Keep a container in your freezer for these meat trimmings. Use them to season soups, dried beans, or to prepare a rich meat stock (see directions in "Homemade Soups" chapter).

WHILE WE'RE ON THE SUBJECT: MEAT TENDERIZERS

The essential ingredient in meat tenderizers is a natural enzyme from papaya known as papain. Papain has the ability to break down protein or partially digest your meat for you, thus making it softer, sometimes to the point of mushiness.

Where papayas are plentiful, the fresh fruit slices are often placed around meat before cooking to achieve this tenderizing effect. If you truly feel you need to "tenderize" your meat, fresh papayas are a much more sound method. In addition to the papain, commercial meat tenderizers include huge amounts of refined salt and sugar (and, as we mentioned before, salt draws the juices from meat, making it tougher and drier), spices, vegetable oil, and tricalcium phosphate—in other words, a variety of ingredients not suited to your meat dish.

If you follow the selection and preparation suggestions given here you can save the money you would have spent for this item and still have a tender, juicy product.

RECOMMENDATIONS

General Rule of Purchase: What you buy should be as fresh as possible, so check the date on the package. Fresh, unfrozen cuts are your best choice.

EXEMPLARY BUYS:
    Veal—always a good choice
    Lamb—particularly the leg; also, New Zealand Spring Lamb
    Beef—USDA "Good" grade your best choice
    Ground meat—have it ground for you
    Organ meats—particularly from young animals
    Rabbit—available frozen in some stores

N.B. A Special Word on Cured Meats:

Most cold cuts, frankfurters, bacon, sausage products, and other cured meats are undesirable on two counts: they contain many chemical additives, sodium nitrite in particular, and they have a high fat content. While high fat content is unavoidable in such foods, there are some brands of cured meat available that do not contain any chemical preservatives, although most include some form of sugar and are highly salted. Because of the paucity of choices in breakfast meats, we have included sausages containing MSG, but no nitrites. Keep an eye out for new and local brands of sausage, bacon, and frankfurters that avoid nitrite preservatives, propyl gallate, and BHT/BHA.

EXEMPLARY BRANDS:

East—*Ballard's* Honey B Farm Sausage (MSG)

    Bob Evans Farms Pork Sausage (MSG)

    Coleman's Country Style Sausage (MSG)

    Country Treat Whole Hog Pork Sausage (MSG)

    Crayton's Southern Brand Sausage (MSG); Country Cousin Brand Beef Sausage (MSG)

    Green Hill Country Sausage (MSG)

    Gunnoes Whole Hog Sausage (MSG)

    Gwaltney of Smithfield Pork Sausage

    Jake's Country Pork Sausage (MSG)

    Jamestown Pork Sausage

    Jimmy Dean Pure Pork Sausage (MSG)

    Jones Pork Sausage (no sweeteners, frozen)

    Lee Brand Fresh Sausage

    Odon's Tennessee Pride (MSG)

    Robbins Fresh Pork Sausage

    Rudy's Farm Country Sausage (MSG)

    S.M. Fortenberry Sausage

    Safeway Beef Breakfast Sausage (MSG); Pork Sausage (MSG in some varieties)

    Samuel Sandler Kosher Sausage (no sweeteners)

    Shiloh Farms Shiloh Dogs; Luncheon Meat; Beef Brown 'n Serve Sausage Links; Dinner Loaf (no sweeteners)

    Shop-Rite Country Style Pork Sausage

    Sinai 48 Kosher Beef Breakfast Sausage

    Smithfield Pork Sausage

    Tobin's First Prize Brown and Serve Sausage

    Wilson's Country Man Pork Sausage (MSG)

Middle and West—*Andy Griffith's* Whole Hog Sausage (MSG)

> *Bics* Pure Pork Sausage and Beef Breakfast Roll (MSG, but no sweeteners)
>
> *Bid Farm* Pork Sausage (MSG)
>
> *Carl's* Tasty Sausage (MSG)
>
> *Dubuque* Royal Buffet Iowa Sausage (beef)
>
> *Farm Pac* Brand Pork Sausage (MSG)
>
> *Food Club* Whole Hog Pork Sausage (MSG)
>
> *Hickory Hut* Italian Brand Sausage and Beef Breakfast Sausage
>
> *Iron Skillet* Brand (MSG)
>
> *Jimmy Dean* Pure Pork Sausage (MSG)
>
> *Jones* Pork Sausage (no sweetners, frozen)
>
> *Owen's* Country Style Sausage (MSG)
>
> *Prairie Maid* Pork Sausage
>
> *R.B. Rice's* Pork Sausage (MSG)
>
> *Safeway* Beef Breakfast Sausage (MSG); Pork Sausage (MSG in some varieties)
>
> *Shiloh Farms* Shiloh Dogs, Luncheon Meat; Beef Brown 'n Serve Sausage Links; Dinner Loaf (no sweeteners)
>
> *Taste Wright* Brand Pure Pork Sausage (no sweeteners)
>
> Wilson's Country Man Pork Sausage (MSG)

A Fishing Trip

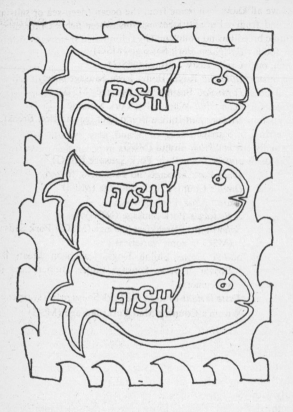

David grew up disliking fish. Or at least he thought he didn't like it. Fish is now one of his favorite meals. As it turns out, frozen fish is what he was scoffing at all those years.

The moral of this story is that frozen fish and fresh fish taste like two different animals. Moreover, fish, especially fresh fish, abounds in essential protein and minerals and, being a light food, is easily digested. As many supermarkets now have fresh fish sections, we strongly recommend you make use of them.

FISH THAT LIVE IN THE OCEAN

As we all know, fish come from the ocean (deep-sea or salt-water fish) and from lakes and streams (freshwater fish). Unfortunately, scientific breeding and pollution have eliminated freshwater fish from those foods that can be considered free of contaminants. Fortunately though, our vast oceans have thus far exhibited an amazing power to resist misuse, keeping deep-sea fish relatively safe. The following fish are all ocean varieties: bluefish, butterfish, cod, flounder, grouper, haddock (also known as baby scrod), hake, halibut, mackerel, mullet, ocean perch, pollack, pompano, porgie, red snapper, salmon, sea bass, sea herring, sole, striped bass, tuna, and, alas, swordfish.

Actually the pollution problem exists in ocean fish too, witnessed by the demise of swordfish on the market owing to high levels of mercury contamination. However, while mercury is a potentially dangerous element (and the methylated form found in fish is the most toxic) the mercury scare has proven less formidable than originally feared. Reports have shown that preserved samples of fish 300 to 2,000 years old contained mercury levels comparable to those in fish living today.

Although future developments may change the truth of this statement, fresh ocean fish presently seem to be the most untainted food product available in the nonorganic marketplace and offer an excellent source of relatively chemical-free sustenance.

CHOOSE FISH FOR FRESHNESS

Freshness is the *only* indication of quality in fish. Because of its delicate structure, fish meat spoils readily. A fresh fish never smells "fishy" or tastes "fishy." Its flesh is firm and springy; if you press it lightly with your finger, no indentation remains. The skin is firm and smooth. If you buy a whole fish, or have an opportunity to see the whole fish, make sure the eyes are bright and bulging, the gills intact, and the scales tight, bright, and shiny. Freezing masks all these visual signs and makes it impossible to determine how old the fish really is.

Fresh fish is usually packaged and shipped on ice and should be displayed this way.

Remember: if you suspect the fish was previously frozen, *do not buy it.* Once defrosted, fish deteriorates rapidly.

OTHER BUYING FACTORS

Fish, like most fresh foods, have a season, but with the exception of butterfish (April–December) and grouper (November–May), most ocean varieties are in season year-round. In addition, fish, like meat, vary in fat content. The fat contains important fat-soluble vitamins; it also contains calories and fatty acids. The following chart classifies ocean fish according to fat content. Personal preference should determine your selection where fat is concerned.

FISH	FAT OR LEAN
Bluefish	lean
Butterfish	fat
Cod	lean
Flounder	lean
Grouper	lean
Haddock	lean
Hake	lean
Halibut	lean
Mackerel	fat
Mullet	lean
Ocean Perch	lean
Pollack	lean
Pompano	fat
Porgie	fat
Red Snapper	lean
Salmon	fat
Sea Bass	lean
Sea Herring	fat
Sole	lean
Striped Bass	fat
Tuna	fat

CUTS OF FISH

Fish are sold in the forms described below, all of them ready to cook and eat.

Pan-Dressed: Scaled and freed from all viscera and blood. The head, tail, and fins are usually removed.

Fillet: The meaty sides of the fish, cut lengthwise away from the backbone. The skin, with the scales removed, may be left on one side.

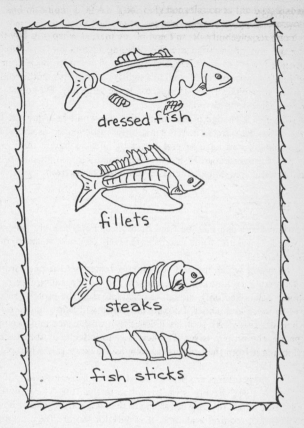

Steaks: Slices cut crosswise from the whole fish with skin and scales removed. These come from larger fish, weighing over 4 pounds.

Fish Sticks (not to be confused with frozen fish sticks): May also be available in your area. These are simply pieces cut from fillets or steaks into fingers 1 inch wide and 3 inches long.

As a buying guide, plan on ½ pound per serving if you buy pan-dressed fish and 1/3 pound per serving of fillets, steaks, or fish sticks.

STORAGE

Your responsibility doesn't end at the market when you buy fish. Storage and preparation are the deciding factors in your family's attitude toward seafood. Once you get the fish home, place it, in its original wrapper or transferred to a tightly covered dish, in the coldest part of your refrigerator. Plan to use it the same day. Do not keep it more than one to two days.

If there's a change in the menu and you won't be using the fish within two days, freeze it. Wrap in moistureproof paper, as you would meat, and if you have several steaks or fillets, separate them with pieces of freezer paper. Fish can be kept solidly frozen for one to two months. But remember, the taste will never be as fresh.

PREPARATION

Almost any fish may be fried or broiled. Fatty fish are generally favored for baking, while lean fish are lovely poached, steamed, or in chowders.

No matter which method you choose, remember the one cardinal rule: DON'T OVERCOOK. Overcooked fish is dry and tough. Fish should be cooked only enough to coagulate (set) the protein; then it will be moist and tender. Looking at the fish will help you determine when it's ready. As soon as it loses its translucence and becomes opaque, the protein is set. The best way to judge is by fork-testing, removing it from the heat just as soon as it flakes easily when poked with a fork.

Low temperatures are best for most fish cookery, especially if the pieces are thick. Frying is the exception to this rule. The important point is to adjust the time according to the temperature, and although cooking fish requires watching, it is only for ten or fifteen minutes.

Oven cooking requires the least watching and is simple to do and easy to clean up. To bake:

1. Season fish lightly with salt, pepper, and herbs of your choice and place in a greased baking dish.
2. Brush with a little oil or melted butter. A little lemon juice and grated onion mixed with the fat adds flavor.
3. Bake in a moderate oven (350°) about 20 to 25 minutes. Give it the fork test for doneness.

4. If a sauce is desired, vegetable broth, tomato sauce, or milk can be added to just cover the fish before baking.

Frying fish has several drawbacks. In general, frying is the least nutritious form of food preparation, adding unnecessary fats. It masks the delicate flavor of fish, is odorous, and isn't much fun to clean up afterwards. For those who long for the crisp crust and browned flavor of pan-fried fish, *oven-frying* is the answer. This requires much less fat and much less of your attention.

1. Dip the pieces of fish into seasoned milk, then roll in fine, dry bread crumbs. Flour, cornmeal, or cracker crumbs can be used, but these do not brown as well in the oven. Bread crumbs prepared from stale, whole wheat bread are preferable. To heighten the color add 1 teaspoon of paprika to each cup of bread crumbs.
2. Arrange the coated pieces side by side in a well-greased baking dish.
3. Drizzle a small amount of oil or melted fat over the fish, about 2 tablespoons per pound.
4. Place in a very hot oven, 500°, for 10 to 15 minutes.

Broiling is Nikki's favorite method of fish preparation, probably because that's what she grew up with. It's the quickest, simplest method we know.

1. Season fish as desired
2. Grease the broiler pan.
3. Place the fish directly on the broiler pan and brush with oil, butter, or homemade French dressing.
4. Insert the pan so the top of the fish is two to three inches from the heat and broil for 10 to 15 minutes. Thinner pieces may be done quickly and need not be turned. Thick pieces cook more evenly if turned halfway through cooking and will be delicately browned.

Poaching is a little more tricky. The first few times it's hard to handle the fish without breaking it, but this is the gourmet style of fish preparation. If you wrap the fish in a piece of cheesecloth, it will facilitate lifting it from the pot when it's done and minimize breaking.

1. Heat chosen poaching liquid in a deep skillet, using enough liquid to just cover fish. Milk, sea-salted water, vegetable bouillon, tomato juice, all work well.
2. Place whole fish fillets (tied in cheesecloth if you wish) in the liquid and adjust heat so the liquid is barely simmering.
3. Cover the skillet and cook until fish flakes easily with a fork, about 5 to 10 minutes.

4. Using a spatula, and great care, transfer the fish to a hot platter for serving. If you've wrapped it in cheesecloth, lift the bundle by hooking a long-handled fork into the gathered material on top.

Poached fish is best served with a sauce. Experiment with cream sauces (like cheese or mushroom), a flavorful herb sauce, lemon butter, or a fancy hollandaise. All fish is perked up with a few squirts of lemon, mayonnaise seasoned with chives, onion, dill, parsley, or just about any fresh herb. Sour cream is delectable on most fish steaks, especially salmon, and toasted slivered almonds add a nice crunchy topping. Be unconventional and try chopped walnuts and sunflower seeds as well. There are no rules when it comes to dressing up fish. Anything goes as long as it's not so strong it overpowers the delicate taste of the fish itself.

All fish can be prepared by any of the basic methods and varied in so many ways that if you don't like it one way, you're bound to like it another.

FROZEN FISH

As we've said, frozen fish is never as desirable as fresh. Fish is highly perishable, and in addition to the loss of flavor you can't be sure how the fish was handled between the packer (assuming it was at its peak of freshness when prepared) and the supermarket. Unless your store has a rapid turnover it's a good idea to stick with the fresh exclusively. If you insist on buying frozen fish, make sure it's solidly frozen and there are no tears in the wrapper. Have the clerk pack it in an ice cream bag. If it becomes soft on the way home, do not refreeze it, but change your menu to include fish that day.

There is no need to defrost the fish before cooking unless you plan to bread it or stuff it. Just add ten minutes or so to the cooking time. If you must thaw it, place the wrapped package on the refrigerator shelf for three to four hours. Thawing at room temperature is risky; if fish stands for any length of time once it's defrosted it will begin to decay. Cook the fish as soon as it's thawed. And remember, never expect frozen fish to be as juicy or delicate as the fresh kind.

PRECOOKED AND FROZEN FISH PRODUCTS

As a sales gimmick, fish is often completely seasoned and cooked for immediate eating. Unless the eating is immediate, however, which means just after cooking, the risk of getting harmful bacteria and food poisoning is extremely high. Unfrozen cooked fish that is offered for sale more than one day after preparation is not edible!

Frozen fish products are a story in themselves (a rather bad one), and after finding out how simple it is to cook fish from scratch you shouldn't even consider those prepared simulations. With the exception of frozen breaded shrimp, the bad news is on the package for you to read. You will be overpaying for "enriched flour, water, cornstarch, dextrose, salt, vegetable oil, dry yeast, malt, leavening, sugar, MSG, natural and artificial flavor, spice, dough conditioner, and caramel color." Artificial flavor is permitted in breaded fish, although not in shrimp batter.

SEAFOOD

Shellfish are a source of much controversy since they are taken from beds where the river empties into the sea, a place where much poisonous matter is deposited. They actually thrive in areas most likely to be contaminated with human waste. Although we personally consider shellfish a better source of protein than the tainted meat products, we recommend it only with reservation. Eat sparingly and apply the same precaution in selecting and handling as you would for fish. Although government inspection of fish is voluntary and not common in all places, this is one instance where government regulation is your only safeguard.

Lobster

If you purchase lobsters make sure they're alive when you buy them and use them within the next few hours. When you get the lobster home, place it on top of ice covered with several sheets of paper to keep it from suffocating as the ice melts. Cook the lobster while it is still alive. You can grasp it behind the claws; when you plunge it into boiling, salted water for cooking, the heat will do the rest.

Clams and Mussels

Clams and mussels should be alive when bought, too, which means the shells will be firmly sealed. They will open easily once they are cooked.

Scallops

Scallops are usually removed from the shell (or didn't you suspect that this animal lives between two shells just like the clam?). Bay scallops are the small pinkish variety, and are both rare and expensive. The sea scallop is the larger, meaty white version that is found in most markets. Frozen scallops are more common than fresh.

Shrimp

Shrimp are the most frequently chosen of the shellfish varieties, and here we say buy only the freshest. Frozen and old shrimp have an undesirable strong flavor and are always tough and chewy. Fresh shrimp are embarrassingly simple to fix.

1. Wash shrimp and place in enough boiling salted water to cover. Add herbs for flavor.
2. Cover pot and allow water to simmer (cook just below boiling) for 3 to 5 minutes, until the shells turn pink.
3. Drain and rinse. The shells can be removed easily now. Remove them and serve immediately, or clean and refrigerate the shrimp till serving time, or serve the shrimp in the shells and let everyone work on his own.

To keep cooked, peeled shrimp without losing its flavor, place on a bed of ice in the refrigerator. Do not keep longer than overnight.

Steer clear of frozen, raw, breaded shrimp. The recipe for this product is based on a government standard, a standard which allows the processor to include only 50 percent shrimp in the package. They might just as well call it "Shrimped Bread." Even the "Lightly Breaded" variety is only 65 percent shrimp.

CANNED FISH

The heat of canning is always destructive to protein, vitamins, and minerals. And the additives employed usually discourage us from buying any canned food we may have otherwise been considering. In the case of canned fish, however, we make an exception. Here are some of the suggestions we can offer in this area:

Anchovies

Anchovies are tiny fish of the herring family and are used almost exclusively in preserved form, salted or pickled and packed in oil.

They are very salty, but used with a light hand can add zip to salads, homemade pizza, sauces, and egg dishes. The best brands are imported from Spain and Portugal and feature the flat or rolled fillets in a bath of salt and olive oil.

Herring

The most common way you'll find herring in this country is salted, pickled, or smoked, and dressed with a sauce. Those pickled in vinegar or wine sauce like *Vita* Herring in Wine Sauce, Party Snacks, Sliced Lunch, and Bismarck Herring offer a chemical-free means of enlivening a meal. The pickled herring in sour cream that comes in a jar almost always has a sorbate preservative. If your supermarket has a delicatessen counter, chances are herring in cream sauce can be purchased there without the preservatives. Be sure to store the herring jar (or fresh salad) in the refrigerator.

Salmon

All popular brands of canned salmon are salted, but that's it (except for an occasional brand with salmon oil as well). The tiny bones left in soften into the fish and provide natural calcium enrichment in this food gem.

Sardines

The recommended variety of sardine—which isn't a kind of fish, but any very small ones—is labeled "natural." This means the tiny fish are packed in salted or unsalted brine, without sauce, oil, or any spices or flavoring. Several brands come packed in soybean or olive oil plus salt. These too are acceptable.

Tuna

There is a government standard of identity for tuna. The tuna can be packed in any one of a mixture of vegetable oils, olive oil, or water. Water and olive oil must be specifically stated on the label, while any other oils may simply be termed "vegetable oil."* All types are acceptable, except cottonseed oil (and if no specific oil is given, cottonseed oil is probably included). Various seasoning ingredients are also permissible, and, again, these will appear on the label. The only accepted

---

*New FDA ruling requires all fats and oils in foods to be identified by origin on the label beginning.

ones are salt, vegetable broth, and spices. The main thing to watch for on a can of tuna is a chemical used to inhibit crystal formation. Its official name is sodium acid pyrophosphate, but it may be simply pyrophosphate on the label. Many companies use it, but many house brands for some reason often seem to be free of this additive. So are *Progresso* Tonno (tonno means packed in olive oil), *Gill Netters Best*, *Bumble Bee* Chunk Light (packed in soybean oil), *Chicken of the Sea* Chunk Light, *Starkist* Chunk Light and Chunk White, *Carnation* Chunk Light (packed in water), *Geisha* Chunk Light and *S & W* Solid White Tuna.

The terms solid, chunk, white, light, etc., refer to the type and size of fish pieces and these differences cause a wide variety in tuna flavors.

●White tuna comes from the Albacore tuna only, considered the "choice" tuna and higher priced.

●Light tuna comes from the other five species and is just as nutritious and tasty.

●Solid tuna offers loins free of surface tissue with a few flakes.

●Chunk tuna includes pieces which still retain the muscle structure.

●Flake tuna still has the muscle structure but more than half the pieces are under ½ inch.

●Grated tuna is anything above a paste.

Quality is unrelated to these classifications, so choose according to taste, remembering the less expensive flake and grated are just as good for you and simplify preparation in dishes that call for ground, pureed, or flaked tuna.

RECOMMENDATIONS

FRESH FISH

General Rule of Purchase: Buy fresh, unfrozen fish, preferably saltwater varieties. Never buy prepared fish, either fresh or frozen. Check the date on the package and make sure it is only one to two days old. Follow the same rule for other seafood, and see that lobster, clams, and mussels are still alive at time of purchase.

CANNED FISH

General Rule of Purchase: When buying canned fish products, check the label to see that no chemicals have been added; all ingredients are given on the label. In particular check for pyrophosphate in tuna, preservatives and thickening agents in prepared herring and sardines, and aluminum sulfate and disodium EDTA in canned crab.

> EXEMPLARY BRANDS:
>> Anchovies—buy those packed in olive, rather than cotton-seed oil
>> Mackerel—contain salt and water only
>> Oysters—contain salt and water only
>> Salmon—contain salt and salmon oil only
>> Shrimp—contain salt, water, and sometimes citric acid
>> Crab—*Crown Prince* Snow Crab Meat
>>> *Roland* King Crab Meat
>> Sardines—"natural" or packed in olive, slid, or soybean oil
>>> *Crown Prince* Sardines in Tomato Sauce (as well as their other varieties)
>>> *Empress* Sardines in Tomato Sauce
>>> *Ocean Delight* Sardines in Tomato Sauce
>> Herring
>>> *Booth* Creamed Herring Fillets; Sliced Lunch Herring (sugar)
>>> *Empress* Kipper Snacks
>>> *Fancifood* Kipper Snacks
>>> *Marshalls* Scotch Herring in Tomato Sauce; Kippered Herring; Kipper Snacks
>>> *Noon Hour* Fillet Herring in Wine Sauce (sugar)
>>> *Sea Trader* Norway Kipper Snacks
>>> *Vita* Herring in Wine Sauce; Party Snacks; Sliced Lunch Herring; Bismarck Herring (sugar)
>> Fish Roe
>>> *Big Alpha* Tarama
>>> *Bumble Bee* Shad Roe
>>> *Marshalls* Cod Roe

Bonito

Clear Water Light Bonito Chunks

Eatwell Bonito Chunks

Giant Brand Portuguese White Bonito

Priority California Chunk Bonito

Sea Boy Light Bonito Chunks

Top Wave Bonito

Tuna

National Brands:

Argo Chunk Light

Bits O' Sea Grated Light

Brest O' Chicken Chunk Light in Corn Oil; in Vegetable Oil; in Water

Bumble Bee Chunk Light

Carnation Chunk Light in Oil; in Water

Chicken of the Sea Chunk Light; Solid Light; Diet Pack (in water, no salt)

Geisha Light in Oil; in Water

Gill Netters Best Chunk White

Lucky Strike Light Grated

Progresso Tonno

S & W Solid White

Starkist Chunk Light; Chunk White in Oil; Solid Light in Spring Water

Van Camps Grated Light

Many house brands also have acceptable varieties of tuna, particularly the light variety. For example:

Albertsons Chunk Light

Bluebrook Chunk Light

C.H.B. Chunk Light

Camelot Chunk Light

Coop

3 Diamonds Chunk Light

Empress Light in Water

Food Club Chunk Style Light

Gaylord Light, Chunk Style and Grated

Heritage House Chunk and Solid Light

Hy Vee Light Chunks

Iris Light Chunks

Kimbell Chunk Light

Kroger Chunk Light and Solid Light
Lady Lee Chunk and Solid Light
North Bay Grated
Scot Lad Chunk Light
Sea Trader Chunk Light
Shur Fine Chunk Light
Springfield Chunk Light
Staff Chunk Light
Top Wave Solid Light in Water
Weis Light
Western Valley Chunk Light

Other Fish Products

Art Brand Salt Codfish
Csardas Fish a la Paprika and Bakony; Fish Salad; Fish Soup

Making the Best of Birds

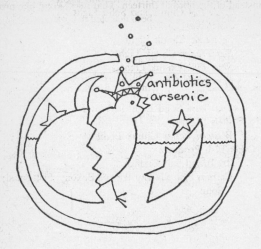

There are many common misconceptions about the nature of poultry production in this country. If you were to ask most people about how and where poultry is raised they would probably conjure up images of a cozy little farm, chickens running freely in the yard, and the farmer's wife feeding them grain from her apron. Nothing could be further from the truth.

Chickens in this country are raised in enormous coops, sometimes holding 10,000 or more birds. Each bird may be housed in an individual box which he never leaves. A "scientific blend" of feed and chemicals enters the "cell" through a tiny chute, and the light may be left on twenty-four hours a day so the chickens will eat continually.

Stilbestrol pellets formerly implanted in birds were only banned from animal feed as of January 1, 1973.* Antibiotics, though, are still very common in these animals, since not only are birds prone to infection, but the antibiotics, along with arsenic, vastly improve the efficiency of food utilization, speeding growth and weight gain. Thanks to modern science those plump little broiler-fryers, almost the

*See footnote page 50.

only variety of chicken available today, can now be turned out in nine weeks instead of the normal thirteen. That may sound like progress, but residues of chemicals have been detected in both the flesh and eggs of the birds.

Putting these drawbacks aside, chicken and turkey are both excellent sources of protein, less fatty and less costly than other meats. For those of you still interested, let's take a look at the available buys and see what you can spend your money on most wisely.

FRESH BIRDS: THROWING THE BIRD OUT WITH THE BATH

It's becoming increasingly rare to find fresh, unfrozen fowl on the market today. Most birds are frozen for shipping or shipped "on ice." Both these methods involve soaking the bird in a water bath. Conveniently, for the seller, the bird absorbs some of this water, adding excess weight. Most foreigners who eat poultry in this country for the first time are amazed at the lack of taste. One reason is that they are used to birds fed on grain. The primary reason for this obvious taste difference, though, comes from the water bath. Once the bird is thawed, this water seeps out, taking with it much of the natural flavor and vitamins. You're left with a soggy, tasteless bird. As one observer noted: "The only flavor they have is what will be absorbed from the cardboard and plastic wrappings they're presented in."

Often there will be a note in the chicken case indicating that frozen, defrosted chicken is being offered for sale. If you plan to use it in a day or two this saves you the trouble of thawing at home; however, if it means refreezing, select one that's still hard-frozen, make sure there are no tears in the protective wrapping, and take it home in an ice cream (freezer) bag, as you should all frozen foods. According to the *1969 Yearbook of Agriculture*, most poultry of the future will be frozen or processed in some way, so take advantage of fresh poultry while you still can if it is available in your supermarket.

Be wary; fowl, particularly turkeys, that are labeled "fresh" are often frozen, defrosted birds.

INSPECTION AND GRADING

To determine quality in poultry you'll have to rely pretty much on the government inspectors. All poultry must be inspected either by the

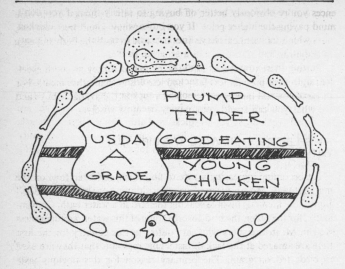

PLUMP
TENDER
USDA A GRADE
GOOD EATING
YOUNG CHICKEN

federal or state government. The round shield with the USDA stamp is your only guarantee that the processing plant was clean and the bird was properly processed and found to be "fit for eating." It is very important that the bird you eat has passed this inspection.

There is a grading system for poultry, done on a voluntary basis, but it is really not very significant since most poultry available in the supermarket is Grade A. This only means it is meaty, has a well-developed fat layer (even if it's chemically induced), and has no surface defects. Grade B and C chickens are usually sent to the processing plant to be turned into something else. Ungraded birds offered for sale in the supermarket are usually below Grade A.

CHICKEN CHECKPOINTS

Although physical appearance is scientifically induced in chicken, this is the only means you have of judging them. For tender meat, choose birds that are plump and show no surface skin defects.

Chickens are available intact, cut up, or in prepackaged parts so you can buy to suit your taste buds. Whole chickens are usually a better buy for the money, but if members of your family have preferences you're obviously better off buying to satisfy them if you don't mind paying the higher price. If you buy a whole chicken or chicken parts which include the giblets (neck, heart, liver, etc.), remove them immediately and refrigerate in a separate package.

Stewing hens are rarely found on the market today, most of them finding their way to the soup factory or other similar burial grounds for spent hens. If they are available in your area, they are satisfactory for soups or salads where texture is not the important factor. They are less expensive than the young chicks, and although the laying hen gets her share of chemicals to make her into an egg factory, the quantity and quality of these are less than that found in commercial eating varieties.

READY-TO-EAT CHICKEN

Many supermarkets are now offering ready-to-eat chicken in the meat showcase. We would caution you not to buy it. You have no way of knowing how fresh the bird was before it was cooked, how careful the cook was, or how the bird was handled after cooking. And if you don't plan to eat it immediately, the flavor will continue to degenerate and you'll end up with chicken texture and a cardboard taste.

Southern Fried Chicken

If your family insists on "Southern Fried Chicken," prepare it at home. Aside from the high price of a batter that's mostly water in both the fresh and frozen prepared fried dishes, chicken is one of the most easily mishandled products on the market. Compounding this is the low quality of frying oils which are used and reused in preparing precooked items. All you need for a "home fried" dinner is a paper bag, salt, pepper, any herbs you wish, flour, and, of course, the chicken.

HOME FRIED CHICKEN

Combine flour (sifted whole wheat or unbleached white) and seasonings in a paper bag. Plan on ½ cup flour, 1 teaspoon salt, ½ teaspoon of pepper, and ½ teaspoon of herbs per 3 pounds of chicken. Pat chicken pieces dry, add a few at a time, and shake to coat. Place the coated pieces in an inch or so of hot oil in a skillet. Cover and cook over medium heat until golden. Cooking time is from 45 minutes to 1 hour and the parts should be turned halfway through cooking.

"Shake and Bake"

If you haven't already realized it, this same method can be used to coat chicken for baking. For a crisp crust you can moisten the chicken with milk or water first and add fresh cracker crumbs to the paper bag mixture. Then bake as usual, in a greased shallow pan in a 350° oven for 45 minutes to 1 hour.

The packaged "shake and bake" mixes are a waste of money and an insult to your intelligence.

TURKEY

Butterball Turkeys

Butterball and self-basting turkeys are becoming more prevalent on the market. These birds have 3 percent injected fat (yes, literally injected), not necessarily butter as the name suggests, but more commonly coconut oil and water. While the turkey cooks, it "bastes itself" as the fat comes to the surface. This additional cost of 5 to 10¢ *per pound* saves you about two minutes, the time it takes to paint the bird yourself with melted butter or oil. By the way, coconut oil is a highly saturated fat and not on the recommended list of vegetable oils.

Turkey Roast

Another popular form of turkey is the turkey roast: boned turkey meat, rolled and ready to cook as is. Although a few products are no more than turkey meat, skin, and salt, most have such additional ingredients as "sodium tripolyphosphate, brown sugar, sodium hexametaphosphate, and sodium erythorbate (antioxidant to preserve freshness)." All have some sort of sauce added to the package which adds some more unwanted elements to this list.

DUCK

Since the demand for duck has not reached the proportions of either chicken or turkey, its production is still at a sane level. Long Island duckling is probably the best poultry buy in the supermarket.

HANDLING POULTRY

When you get your fresh poultry home, loosen any tight wrapping and place the bird in the coldest part of your refrigerator. The raw bird can remain in this state satisfactorily for one to two days.

For longer storage, freeze the bird. Chicken and turkey, wrapped for freezing (and, as with meat, don't wash the bird first but wipe with a clean cloth), can be frozen successfully for twelve months, duck for six months, and giblets up to three months. Any leftovers can be frozen for six months, but careful handling is essential and the taste will never be as good the second time around. We think you'll be a lot happier slicing the leftovers for sandwiches, dicing the meat for salads, or using it as you would leftover meat in a casserole or vegetable-grain dish.

GETTING THE BIRD READY

In general, poultry can be cooked directly from the frozen state or it can be thawed first. If you are adding other ingredients this thawing might be necessary to prevent excess water leakage into your sauce. Refrigerator thawing is the preferable way:

Place the frozen package in the refrigerator and let it stand one to two days. Turkeys over 18 pounds may take up to three days. If time is short, the bird can be placed in its watertight wrapper in cold water out of the refrigerator. Change the water often to hasten the process. Small birds will take about one hour, large turkeys six to eight hours by this method.

Poultry can also be thawed at room temperature, but if you resort to this method be sure the bird is away from the heat (and the cat) and is kept wrapped. There's going to be a lot of dripping, so set it someplace that can be cleaned up easily. To facilitate the clean-up, place the wrapped bird in a heavy-duty garbage bag. Leave it out only until it's just pliable.

STUFFING

As for prestuffed birds: why not stuff your own? Stuffing is often the favorite part of the dinner and when you make it yourself you have an opportunity to be creative, add some extra nutrients to your meal (as opposed to the pure starch stuffing the manufacturer puts in), and eliminate one potential source of food poisoning. Poultry stuffing is a good vehicle for leftover vegetables (dice them up for added flavor), dried fruits, and stale bread. When your bread gets hard, cube it and store it in an airtight container or in the freezer. This way you can make whole grain bread stuffing. Brown rice and other whole grain cereals also make tasty poultry stuffing.

Pack the dressing loosely into the bird (bacteria multiply rapidly in the nice, cozy environment, and when tightly stuffed, the heat cannot circulate properly to destroy them) and add an additional fifteen minutes cooking time per pound. If you insist on prestuffed poultry, follow the manufacturer's instructions and DO NOT THAW before cooking.

Immediately after cooking separate the stuffing and the bird (this goes for home or pre-stuffed specimens); never refrigerate leftover meat and stuffing together.

A CAVEAT

At the risk of sounding like scare-mongers: poultry is very easily contaminated! To avoid transferring bacteria to other foods, wash your hands and the work surface immediately before and after touching raw poultry and clean all equipment after you've finished with it.

Our final cautionary point—do not partially cook a bird one day and finish the cooking the following day. This practice only gives bacteria additional opportunity to grow. Cook the bird completely at one time; staphylococci are not your friends.

RECOMMENDATIONS

General Rule of Purchase: Buy birds fresh rather than frozen whenever possible, and never pre-prepared whether fresh or frozen.

The Grain Silo

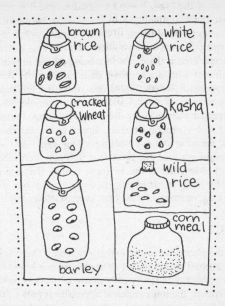

In other parts of the world some form of grain provides most people with their main source of protein. In India and Asia, people exist on rice and millet; in Africa and the Middle East they eat couscous (semolina) and cracked wheat; in North Africa and much of Europe, barley is the chief grain; in Eurasia, it's buckwheat groats, and in South America corn is the essential grain. In North America, rice is the only grain we pay much attention to, and if we had to depend on the white rice that is milled from it for anything other than carbohydrates we'd be in big trouble. White rice may look nice on the plate, it may fill you up, and it may make a perfect base for saucy foods, but it does little else.

How is it, then, that so much of the world exists so well on a diet that is primarily rice?

When rice is first harvested, the grain is surrounded by a harsh, indigestible hull. In more primitive countries a "paddy machine" is used to get rid of this coating, which removes the hull and some of the bran. Most of the bran, however, remains, and it is here and in the germ that the high-quality protein, along with calcium, phosphorus, iron, vitamin E, and most of the B vitamins, is found. Further debranning and polishing remove almost all of these nutrients and create white rice. That is the rice we are being offered in this country. Sometimes glucose and talc are even added to improve the appearance. To compensate for the nutritional loss, the polished rice is coated with a mixture of alcohol and zein (a protein derivative from corn), then treated with calcium and iron salts, dipped into the mix again, treated with synthetic vitamins, dipped again, and so on. With some brands, washing the rice before cooking removes the enrichment, so if you don't read the directions you may be washing your family's health down the drain. In those brands that are specially compounded for long-lasting effects, the enrichment is not affected by washing, cooking, or storage; it may not even be affected by digestion!

BROWN RICE

Why buy the phony when the real is available? There is hardly a supermarket around that does not offer at least one brand of brown (natural) rice, which, like the "paddy machine" variety, contains all the native nutrients. Even the enriched white rice is only a fair source of niacin and thiamine compared with the natural supply of B vitamins in the whole grain brown rice, plus protein, calcium, phosphorus, and iron, which are all plentiful before the grain is refined. We cannot overemphasize the nutritional gap the refining process creates.

Surprisingly enough, once brown rice is cooked, the color is only slightly different from "white" rice, a much more appealing creamy color. The taste—and come to think of it white rice really has no taste at all—is full and nutlike. Preparation is identical to white rice, except that brown rice requires longer cooking, and although cooking time is about forty-five minutes, there's no extra work involved on your part. Cooking instructions appear on the package of all brands of brown rice. Nikki's mother keeps complaining her rice comes out gummy; ours never does, so maybe you should follow our recipe.

N.B. With the growing popularity of brown rice, one of the major rice packagers has marketed a new brown rice product designed to be less "sticky or gummy." The heat steaming process this rice is subjected to is another example of unnecessary processing, reflected, of course, in the price. Save your money, prepare the rice like we do, and you'll have no problems.

HOW TO COOK BROWN RICE

Wash raw rice well and drain. Place in saucepan with enough room for rice to triple in volume. Add twice the amount of boiling water as you did rice and return to boil. Now cover and reduce heat to the lowest point possible, the lower the better. Let rice cook like this for 45 minutes. Do not stir; stirring makes rice pasty. Then remove from heat and let stand several minutes and it will steam and dry even more.

If I have an extra minute (while the water is coming to a boil), I stir the washed rice in a dry saucepan over medium heat until the grain is dry and lightly toasted. This enhances the nutty flavor.

Don't add salt until after the rice is cooked; it tends to harden the kernels.

Rice combined with beans or nuts provides all the essential amino acids; because brown rice is so rich we often sauté it with bits of diced vegetables, lots of scallions and cooked beans, bean sprouts and pine nuts, and have it as a main course. Season with soy sauce or a flavorful onion sauce (see "Do-It-Yourself Sauces") and you have a satisfying meal.

More Brown Rice Recipe Ideas

•*Brown Rice Pilaff:* Follow our directions for brown rice, only begin by sautéing a chopped onion (and some mushrooms if you like) and the washed grain in a tablespoon of oil. Cook, stirring often, until the onion is limp and the grain is dry. Now add the boiling water and proceed as usual.

•Instead of plain water you can add boiling meat or vegetable broth, or tomato juice, or add a tablespoon of curry powder to the water.

•Halfway through cooking add a handful of raisins, chopped figs, or a mixture of diced dried fruits, and some chopped nuts to the rice pot. Stir once, cover, and continue to cook until the rice is tender. A little cinnamon sprinkled on top after cooking will enhance the flavor of this rice dish.

CONVERTED, QUICK-COOKING AND SEASONED RICE MIXES

Sometimes rice is converted, or parboiled. This means that it is precooked and dried before polishing. The converting process forces much of the vitamin B into the grain before the bran is removed. This conserves some of the original nutritional value. As you will notice from the label, parboiled rice often contains the preservative BHT. Without this preservative rice will keep a minimum of three months, and we have kept brown rice, the most vulnerable type since the fat has not been removed, for a year and never had it turn bad.

All the quick-cooking varieties have chemicals added to reduce preparation time. Their nutritional contribution to the meal is barely significant and the texture of the rice is like damp cotton. Don't bother.

There are many pre-seasoned rice mixes on the shelf next to the plain, all replete with additives, as you'll see by the label, and all fantastically expensive. To enhance the flavor of rice, add your own seasonings, although with the natural richness of brown rice, all this jazzing up isn't even necessary.

CRACKED WHEAT

As long as you're up for adding variety to your meal, why not experiment with some of the other grains available in your supermarket. These are prepared in exactly the same manner as rice and complement meat and vegetable dishes just as nicely. Cracked wheat (made from the toasted grain with the bran and germ intact) is available in most supermarkets and takes only fifteen minutes to prepare. Do not buy the pre-seasoned brands, and where a spice packet is included (as in *Old World* Wheat Pilaff) add your own flavoring ingredients to avoid the chemical flavor intensifiers manufacturers add. This is our favorite way to prepare cracked wheat for four side-dish servings:

CRACKED WHEAT PILAFF

Chop 1 large onion. Heat 2 tablespoons of peanut oil in saucepan, add onion and 1 cup of cracked wheat. Sauté until wheat is glossy and onion begins to turn golden. Add 2 cups of boiling vegetable or meat broth or water. Reduce heat, cover, and cook until all liquid is absorbed, about 15 minutes. At this point we're ready to eat. Some people like to deepen the flavor, and bring about a drier roasted texture by transferring the cooked wheat to a covered casserole and baking for 30 to 45 minutes in a 350° oven. I'll admit it is particularly delicious that way, but I'm an impatient cook. To deepen the flavor, season with soy sauce.

Wheat pilaff is traditionally served with Mid-East food (like eggplant dishes), but it's fantastic with pot-roasted meat and gravy too.

KASHA

Kasha, or buckwheat groats as they are often called, is actually the fruit rather than the seed (as most grains are) of the buckwheat plant. It is a common supermarket item (*Wolffs* and *Pocono* being two widely distributed brands), and can be prepared just like the cracked wheat or according to the directions offered on the package. Serve it as a base for meat and vegetables or as a hot breakfast dish. In Jewish cuisine the cooked groats are baked with bow noodles for an accompaniment known as "Kasha Varenickas." Very tasty.

BARLEY

Barley, in the form of pearl, not egg, barley is another grain that can be purchased in your supermarket and combined with other foods for excellent eating. Most of us know barley as a common ingredient in soup. It can also be cooked with lentils to make a delicious meatless high-protein casserole.

LENTIL AND BARLEY BAKE

1 cup lentils
6 tablespoons barley
3½ cups water
1 onion, chopped
2 carrots, diced

½ teaspoon salt
1 bay leaf

Sauce: 3 tablespoons molasses
         2 tablespoons cider vinegar
         ⅓ cup reserved cooking liquid
         1 clove garlic
         1 teaspoon dry mustard powder
         ½ teaspoon salt

Wash lentils and barley in cold water and drain well. Combine lentils, barley, water, onion, carrots, ½ teaspoon salt and bay leaf in large saucepan. Bring to boil, cover, reduce heat and let simmer 45 minutes. Strain, reserving ⅓ cup of the liquid, and transfer cooked grain and vegetables to a 2-quart casserole. Prepare sauce by combining molasses, vinegar, reserved cooking liquid, garlic, dry mustard powder and ½ teaspoon salt. Pour over vegetables in casserole. Bake in 350°F oven until liquid is absorbed, about 20 minutes. *Yield:* 4 to 6 servings.

WILD RICE

Next on your list of supermarket grains is wild rice. On the East Coast only the rich gourmet can afford this costly product, but if you live in the Midwest you'll find the price of wild rice is much more reasonable. This delicacy is high in protein, phosphorus, and potassium, and provides some B vitamins as well. It is prepared in the same manner as brown rice; make sure to wash it several times before cooking to remove any foreign particles. Cooking time varies from thirty to forty-five minutes, and when it's done all the water will be absorbed and the rice tender. It can be used whenever you would use regular rice and we recommend it highly with poultry or delicate omelets.

CORNMEAL

Advice for buying cornmeal is given in the chapter, "Hot Cereals," but once you've learned what to buy you'll find it can substitute for both flour and grains on the menu. Use whole, unbolted cornmeal at dinnertime as well as for breakfast. The Cornmeal Polenta below makes an ideal base for any meal that has a tomato sauce and an Italian flavor. Use it instead of spaghetti—it's much more nourishing.

CORNMEAL POLENTA

1 cup yellow cornmeal
½ cup cold water
1½ teaspoons salt
2½ cups boiling water
¼ cup grated Parmesan cheese
A little butter or oil

Combine cornmeal, cold water, and salt in a saucepan and stir until smooth. This keeps the polenta from becoming lumpy. Stir in the boiling water, cover and cook over low heat about 20 minutes, until the water is absorbed and the cornmeal becomes thick. Stir occasionally. When done, spread polenta in a baking dish making a layer about 1 inch thick. Allow it to cool and thicken. Just before serving sprinkle on the cheese, dot with butter or brush with oil, and brown under the broiler. Cut into squares and place the cooked polenta under Italian stews. *Yield:* 4 servings.

Broiled without the cheese this cornmeal base can be served with meat and gravy. With Cheddar or Monterrey Jack cheese instead of Parmesan it complements Mexican-flavored dishes.

RECOMMENDATIONS

General Rule of Purchase: Buy whole, unseasoned grains including brown (unhulled) rice, cracked wheat (or bulgur), buckwheat groats (or kasha), barley, wild rice, and cornmeal (discussed in the chapter, "Hot Cereals"). The grain itself should be the only ingredient in the package.

EXEMPLARY BRANDS
Brown Rice
East—*Riceland* Natural
River Brand
S & W Natural Long Grain
Town House
Uncle Ben's

      Middle—*Comet* Natural
         Mahatma
         Riceland Natural
         S & W Natural Long Grain
         Town House
         Uncle Ben's
     West—*Christar*
         Co-op
         Diamond G Brand
         El Molino
         Evans
         Hime
         Port of Call
         Riceland Natural
         S & W Natural Long Grain
         Springfield
         Stone Buhr
         Town House
         Uncle Ben's
         Valley Farm Long Grain

Cracked Wheat
   Arrowhead Mills
   Catherine Clark's Brownberry Ovens
   Fancifood Wheat Pilaff
   Fisher Ala Bulgur
   Harrington's Hodgson Mill
   Jolly Joan Bulgur Wheat
   Old World Wheat Pilaff (remove the spice packet)
   Robinhood
   Stone Buhr
   Ziyad Brand

Buckwheat Groats
   Pocono
   Wolff's

Millet
   Datetree

Sifting Out the Flour

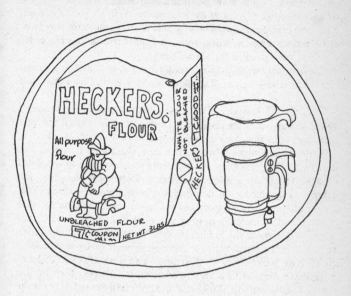

One of the most prevalent products on the market can be considered among the most unwholesome: white flour. What is put into the wheat, and what is taken out of it to create white flour, results in a product that adds nothing but calories to your diet and may actually do considerable harm.

THE STORY OF FLOUR

Once upon a time wheat was deserving of the title "the staff of life." The flour milled from this grain was rich in protein, calcium, iron, the B vitamins, thiamine, riboflavin and niacin, and vitamin E. This was known as graham or whole wheat flour. The flour was milled between two stones which ground the entire grain, bran, germ and endosperm, at a low temperature, into a fine powder and kept all the native nutrients intact. Then in the late 1880s modern science replaced the millstones with steel rollers and the process was refined to one of first cleaning and conditioning the wheat, then sorting out the bran and germ (the source of most of the vital nutrients) in a series of siftings. The large bran flakes could now be sold as bran, the germ was separated and marketed as wheat germ, and other siftings unsuitable for the flour were peddled for animal feed.

The flour that remained was creamy in color, although on standing it would become lighter. This flour is today known as unbleached flour.

Since the 1880s modern food processing has become big business, and time and money are involved in storing the flour while it ages and oxidizes. Aging improves the baking quality of flour, while oxidation lightens it (and turns it white, the false symbol of goodness and purity). So, a process known as bleaching was developed to speed this change. Today seven different methods of chemical bleaching and aging are available for the flour industry to whiten its product, sterilize it so it does not support insect life (or any other life for that matter), and incidentally destroy any of the vitamin B and E that might have escaped the milling process. The product that remains is known as white flour, but you should remember that you will see it on labels as "white flour," "wheat flour," and simply "flour." "Flour" is available today with a variety of modifiers. Durum flour, milled from a tougher variety of wheat, is used primarily in industry for the manufacture of pasta. Pastry flour (which is unbleached) and bread flour (which is somewhat higher in protein than all-purpose flour) are sold to bakers. All-purpose flour, which is high in nothing but carbohydrate, is sold to you. Cake flour and instantized flour are more highly processed versions of the already empty all-purpose flour. Self-rising flour, another white flour derivative, has sodium bicarbonate and acid-reacting salts added (a form of built-in baking powder).

The milling industry is well aware of the rape it has imposed on white flour. To "compensate," a standard of enrichment has been established for this flour . . . of the twenty-two nutrients removed at the mill three B vitamins are replaced and vitamin D, calcium and iron salts are added. This is "enriched flour"—*still lower* in all nutrients with the exception of riboflavin than the original whole wheat flour! You can tell by the label if your flour is enriched. Your flour may also have malted wheat or barley flour added to make up for any deficiency of natural enzymes, although you'll never know it.

According to government standards, certain "dough conditioners" or "improvers" can be added to flour to enhance the baking qualities. In this case the label will state that ascorbic acid has been added, or that the flour is "phosphated" or "bromated" (treated with phosphate or bromate salts).

BUYING REAL FLOUR

Your aim is to use primarily whole wheat flour, especially when it comes to bread-baking. You may also be fortunate enough to find whole wheat pastry flour in your supermarket, suitable for lighter baked products. You should *never* use anything less nutritious than unbleached white flour.

When you select whole wheat flour make sure the brand you choose is not "bromated" or "phosphated," which is permitted for this flour as well as the white and must appear on the label. In recent months many brands of whole wheat flour have become available to the supermarket shopper. Some of these brands like *El Molino* and

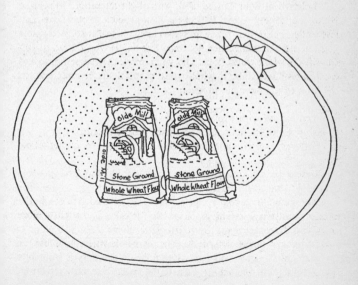

Elam's are ground from organically grown wheat and their distribution was formerly limited to natural foods stores. Many of these "health food" brands are now in the supermarket. In addition, many familiar flour manufacturers are offering whole wheat flour and other whole grain flours along with their traditional line of white flours. The list of brands which offer suitable choices appears at the end of the chapter under Exemplary Brands. For long-term storage, whole wheat flour should be kept in the refrigerator or some other cool place.

If you still insist on using white flour, make sure it is unbleached, choosing from the list at the end of the chapter. These flours, described by *Pillsbury* as "natural flours," are naturally aged and contain no chemical bleaches, preservatives, leavening or maturing agents. Keep in mind that unbleached white flour is only a minimal change from white flour as far as food value is concerned.

USING WHOLE WHEAT FLOUR

Unbleached flour is used exactly like bleached white flour and the results are hardly distinguishable.

Whole wheat flour can be used, with slight alteration, to replace white flour in any recipe. Expect the final product to be heavier and less tender, but tastier. If you find this change in texture objectionable you can use half unbleached flour and half whole wheat flour, or you can sift the whole wheat flour. This will remove the coarsest bran and create a product similar to whole wheat pastry flour. Be sure to return the bran to the flour bin to use in breads.

When baking with whole wheat flour:
- Do not sift the flour, but stir lightly before measuring.
- For every cup of white flour called for, use only ¾ cup of whole wheat flour.
- Reduce oil in baking with whole grain flour by using 2 tablespoons for every 3 called for in the recipe.
- More liquid than your recipe calls for may be needed to obtain the proper consistency; a tablespoon or two for cakes and slightly more for bread. Experience will be your best teacher.
- To thicken sauces with unbleached or whole wheat flour use the same amount as you would of white flour. When only a few tablespoons of flour are called for, cornstarch, potato starch or arrowroot

can be substituted. In this case use half the amount of corn or potato starch as the flour normally required.

OTHER FLOURS

For those who would like to try their hand at fancy bread-baking, rye and buckwheat flour are distributed to many supermarkets. These flours lack gluten, the protein which gives wheat flour its good baking quality, but by combining them with whole wheat flour you can turn out many fine products.

In some areas soy flour—a high protein, low starch flour—is offered. Use it to replace up to 1/5 the flour in a recipe to increase the protein value.

CORNSTARCH

Since it's called corn flour in Great Britain, this seems a logical place to mention the properties of cornstarch, a finely milled starch obtained from corn by removing the germ and grinding the remaining kernels. Similar to white flour in that the grain, minus the vitamin and mineral-rich germ, is the source of this product, it cannot be depended upon to contribute much in the way of nutrients. Unlike white flour, however, cornstarch is not treated with chemicals to alter its color or cooking properties. Therefore, its use as a thickening agent (in white sauces, puddings) can be recommended for home use. Do not, however, look too favorably upon manufactured soups and spaghetti sauces that rely on cornstarch. Used in this manner it is frequently a starchy substitute for high-quality ingredients.

There is no difference in brands when it comes to purchasing cornstarch.

POTATO STARCH

As its name implies, potato starch is the starch extract from potatoes. This fine white powder is used mainly as a thickener, like cornstarch, and it is free of additives. Use it to replace white flour in thickening white sauce, pudding and gravy. Do not use it, as the food industry does, as an inexpensive filler to replace beans, grains, meat or vegetables which give soups and sauces their thick, velvety consistency.

All brands of potato starch are the same.

GETTING AWAY FROM MIXES

Those who are dependent on white flour mixes, like pancake mix and biscuit mix, are getting a product whose basis is refined to nothingness, only to be mixed with unnecessary preservatives, artificial color, and other chemical additives. Do you have any idea how simple it is to make up a batch of whole wheat pancakes from scratch? Here's our recipe for a batter you can use immediately or store a few days in the refrigerator. The dry ingredients are a lot less costly than the prepared mix. The eggs and liquid you have to add either way.

WHOLE WHEAT PANCAKES

¾ cup whole wheat flour
2 teaspoons baking powder
½ teaspoon salt
1 tablespoon raw sugar or honey
1 cup milk (or water plus 4 tablespoons dry milk powder)
1 egg
1½ tablespoons oil

Combine all dry ingredients. Combine liquid ingredients and stir into dry ingredients only until moistened. Any lumps will cook out. If you like heavy pancakes add up to ¼ cup additional flour.

Cook as you would any pancakes: brush a skillet with a thin covering of oil and heat until a few drops of water sprinkled on the surface dance about. Spoon pancake batter onto hot skillet. When bubbles appear on the surface turn the pancakes and brown the other side. Oil the pan for the first batch only. *Yield:* 10 to 12 pancakes.

If you're still not convinced, you may find a box of *Fearn Soyo* Pancake Mix, *Krusteaz* Pancake Mix or *Stone Buhr* Pancake Mix in the natural foods aisle; they contain the pre-mixed dry ingredients (the flour will be whole wheat, buckwheat, soy or unbleached white) without those unnecessaries we mentioned.

If you find mixes an indispensable convenience, here is a basic biscuit mix you can keep on hand. Use it just as you would the commercial brands by adding milk or water, egg and any desired natural flavoring ingredients.

NIKKI'S HOMEMADE BISCUIT MIX

4½ cups whole wheat flour
1 cup nonfat dry milk powder
3 tablespoons baking powder
2 tablespoons raw sugar
½ teaspoon salt
¾ cup oil

Stir the flour, dry milk, baking powder, sugar, and salt together very well. Add the oil and mix together well with a fork or your fingers until the oil disappears. Store the·mix in a well-closed container in a cool place, and in the refrigerator during the summer. Use within one to two months. *Yield:* about 6 cups.

To measure, spoon lightly into measuring cup. When cup is full, level off with a knife. Do not pat the top to make it level.

BISCUIT MIX BISCUITS

3 cups Homemade Biscuit Mix
Scant 2/3 cup water

Measure biscuit mix into a bowl. Make a well in the center, add water and stir well to make a soft dough. Knead dough gently on an oilcloth or floured board about 15 times. Roll gently ½ inch thick and cut with a biscuit cutter or a glass with a 2-inch diameter. Put the biscuits on a baking sheet without sides and bake in a 400° oven until brown, about 15 to 20 minutes. *Yield:* 15 biscuits.

PECAN MUFFINS

2 cups Homemade Biscuit Mix
3 tablespoons honey
1 egg
6 tablespoons water
½ cup chopped pecans

Mix together honey, egg, and water, and add to biscuit mix. Stir only until moistened. The mixture should be lumpy. Fold in nuts. Fill greased muffin cups 2/3 full and bake in a 400° oven until golden, about 20 minutes. Diced fresh fruit can be used to replace the nuts. If you make this replacement, reduce water by 2 tablespoons. *Yield:* 8 muffins.

BLUEBERRY UPSIDE-DOWN CAKE

Glaze: ¼ cup butter
           1/3 cup honey
           1 cup fresh blueberries
           2 teaspoons grated lemon rind
Cake: 2 cups Homemade Biscuit Mix
           ¼ cup honey
           ½ cup raw sugar
           2 eggs
           ¼ cup water

Line a 9-inch square baking pan with waxed paper. Melt butter and combine with 1/3 cup of honey. Spread over waxed paper. Arrange fresh berries and lemon rind on top. Prepare the cake batter by mixing all remaining ingredients together until smooth. Pour over berries. Bake in a 350° oven for 40 to 45 minutes, until a toothpick inserted into the center comes out clean. Cool in pan 10 minutes, invert onto a cake plate or wire rack, peel off waxed paper, and finish cooling.

RECOMMENDATIONS

General Rule of Purchase: Select whole grain flours that have not been bromated or phosphated. Excellent choices include whole wheat flour, whole wheat pastry flour, rye flour, buckwheat flour, soy flour. Always choose unbleached white flour rather than the bleached varieties. Do not buy flour mixes dependent on white flour.

EXEMPLARY BRANDS
Whole Wheat Flour
East—*Catherine Clark's Brownberry Ovens*
Elams
Harrington's Hodgson Mill
King Arthur
Mrs. Wrights Kitchen Craft (100 percent whole wheat and graham)
Pillsbury
Robinhood

Middle—*Catherine Clark's Brownberry Ovens*
    Elams
    Gooch's (100 percent whole wheat and graham)
    Harrington's Hodgson Mill
    Hungarian Stone Ground
    Light Crust
    Mrs. Wrights Kitchen Craft (100 percent whole
       wheat and graham)
    Pillsbury
    Robinhood

West—*All-O-Wheat*
    Clinton's
    Co-op
    El Molino (100 percent whole wheat and whole
       wheat pastry)
    Elams
    Family Kitchen
    Fisher (100 percent whole wheat and graham)
    Harrington's Hodgson Mill
    Hungarian Stone Ground
    Mrs. Wrights Kitchen Craft (100 percent whole
       wheat and graham)
       Olde Mill
       Pillsbury
       Stone Buhr

Rye Flour
    Catherine Clark's Brownberry Ovens
    Cellu
    Elams
    Fisher
    Gooch's
    Harrington's Hodgson Mill
    Pillsbury
    Robinhood
    Stone Buhr

Soy Flour
    Byrd Mill
    Cellu
    El Molino

> *Elams*
> *Fisher*
> *Stone Buhr*

Buckwheat Flour
> *Catherine Clark's Brownberry Ovens*
> *Elams*
> *Harrington's Hodgson Mill*

Unbleached White Flour
> *Catherine Clark's Brownberry Ovens*
> *Cresota*
> *El Molino*
> *Elams* (with wheat germ)
> *Harrington's Hodgson Mill* (with wheat germ)
> *Hecker's*
> *King Arthur*
> *Pillsbury*
> *Stone Buhr*

Corn Starch
> All brands alike

Potato Starch
> All brands alike

Flour Products
> *Aunt Jemima* Whole Wheat Pancake Mix; Buckwheat Pancake Mix (some unbleached white flour, sugar)
> *Catherine Clark's Brownberry Ovens* Granola Bread Mix; Whole Wheat Bread Mix; Northern Rye Bread Mix (some unbleached white flour, sugar)
> *El Molino* Muffin Mix; Whole Wheat Bread Mix (some unbleached white flour); White Bread Mix (with added wheat germ)
> *Elams* Stone Ground 3 in 1 Mix; Stone Ground Whole Wheat Yeast Bread Mix
> *Fearn Soy-O* Pancake Mixes; Corn Bread and Muffin Mix
> *Krusteaz* Whole Wheat and Honey Instant Pancake Mix (some white flour, sugar)
> *Mille-Lacs* Wild Rice Pancake Mix (some white flour)
> *Stone Buhr* Pancake Mixes
> *Sunnyfield* Buckwheat Pancake Mix (some white flour,

Triti/Cay/Lee Brand Triticale Mix

N.B. *Gold Medal* flours have not been included by request of the manufacturer.

Your Daily Bread

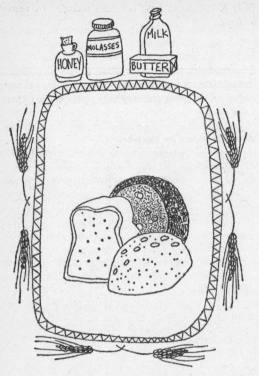

Have you ever tried to find the ingredients on the wrapper of a loaf of bread? If so, you know how often it's been in vain.

Bread is another one of those food products whose formula is standardized by the Code of Federal Regulations. Consequently, almost none of the ingredients need be listed on the label. The presumption, as we have said, is that if you care to know what has been used to produce the loaf you are free to consult the government regulations. Since very few of us are trained in nutrition or are familiar with legal terminology, the federal standards might as well be nonexistent. We hope that this section will give you a greater understanding of what's included in *your* daily bread.

According to the legal definition in those regulations, bread is "prepared by baking a kneaded yeast-leavened dough, made by moistening flour with water" *and* one or all of seventeen *categories* of optional ingredients. The product you purchase as bread will always contain flour, yeast, and usually salt. The flour may be white or whole wheat (stated on the label), bleached or unbleached (stated on the label if unbleached), treated with monocalcium phosphate or potassium bromate (two chemicals used to "improve" the baking qualities, not specified on the label), and may have gluten added (wheat protein, not on the label).

The bread may also contain more than a hundred food and chemical additives (also *not* on the label)!

The standard applies to white, enriched white, raisin and whole wheat bread and rolls, which means all these items are free from mandatory labeling. The bakery can, of course, list any or all of the ingredients it chooses, which is sometimes helpful and sometimes misleading since there is no way of knowing if this list is complete. See how the Code of Federal Regulations helps you?

Specialty breads, like rye, pumpernickel, corn, nut breads, and other unique combinations, are required to give you a full list of what's in them, but even this may be deceiving. For instance, a "rye" bread listing wheat flour and rye flour may have as little as 2 percent rye.

To further mislead you, many additives are not listed by specific names, but are grouped meaninglessly together as "emulsifiers," "dough conditioners," "coloring," etc., which reveals little useful information.

COMMON BREAD INGREDIENTS

Let's suppose for a minute the loaf of bread you pick off the shelf does have a detailed label. Following are some of the ingredients which might appear on it, with an explanation of what they mean and what to do about them.

Flour or Wheat Flour: The term "flour," unqualified, refers to bleached "white" flour which may or may not have the chemical "improvers" mentioned above. (A full description of the scientific story of the creation of flour appears in the chapter "Sifting Out the Flour.") Suffice it to say that if the bread you chose was made with "flour" (which is the same as "wheat flour" and "white flour"), it has little to offer in the way of nutrition, a lot to offer when it comes to chemical adulteration, and you should put it back immediately.

Unbleached Flour: Although this flour is certainly not untainted by chemicals, and is missing the bran and germ which is the vital center for nutrients in flour, it has escaped the final bleaching process which at least minimizes the harm done. When the choice is between white and unbleached flour, choose the latter, although it isn't much of an option.

Enriched Flour: To compensate for the rape of the wheat, white bread is often "enriched," which means of the twenty-two nutrients removed during milling the B vitamins are replaced (although riboflavin is the only one to reach and actually surpass the original level of concentration), and vitamin D, calcium, and iron salts are added. All these added vitamins are man-made.

Whole Wheat Flour: This is the flour you should be looking for on the label. In order for the bread to be named "Whole Wheat Bread" only 100 percent whole wheat flour may be used. If white flour is included it must be stated on the label. Whole wheat flour at least contains all the nutrients native to the flour—the highest quality protein, the essential B vitamins, iron, phosphorus, vitamin E—in the bran and germ which are left intact. This flour may be bleached, although it's unlikely, and it may be treated with those "improvers."

Shortening: "Shortening" means animal or vegetable fat which is hydrogenated (partially saturated) and which may (and probably does) contain emulsifiers and preservatives. Vegetable oil and butter are the preferred choices in this category.

Sugar Syrup: This may include glucose, dextrose, corn syrup, and a long list of other highly refined sugar extracts. They have no nutritional positives and a lot of negatives (which you'll find in the chapter "Sweet Things"). Honey and molasses are better for you and better for the bread too, since both increase the moisture retention and produce a loaf that stays fresher longer without any artificial help.

Dough Conditioners: A variety of chemicals are included in this listing, mostly calcium salts and enzymes, designed to increase the moisture and gas retention. This makes a more elastic dough, so that less flour stretches out over a greater volume and the baker doesn't have to use as much (and you, of course, get less).

Yeast Nutrients: These may be in the form of natural yeast foods, like malt or milk sugar, but may just as easily be chemical calcium and potassium salts. These yeast nutrients increase the yeast activity, again allowing the baker to produce a larger loaf from fewer ingredients. Yeast alone should be sufficient.

Emulsifiers: Another impressive list of chemicals (mono- and diglycerides are among these and are often listed under their specific name) added to soften the bread so the amount of natural softening agents like oil, milk, and eggs, which add to the nutritional value, can be reduced. Since oil, milk, and eggs are more costly than emulsifiers, the manufacturer's cost can be reduced too.

Fresheners: Just like it says, these additives serve to create the impression the bread is fresh long after it should be. They also prevent mold and bacterial growth. In addition to these "fresheners," sodium or calcium propionate is added to many loaves of bread to retard spoilage; both must be on the label specifically if used. Most authorities concede that bread made with clean, wholesome ingredients under proper baking conditions does not need preservatives. Avoid this deception in the loaf of bread you buy.

If no ingredients appear on the label, it's best to assume the baker would rather you didn't know. Just because a label boasts "No preservatives added" does not mean none of the other undesirable ingredients mentioned above have not been used. If no other ingredients are given, we still say they're hiding something!

WEEDING OUT THE BREAD

Now that you are aware of how to read the label, what breads are you likely to find in the supermarket that meet your new high standards? Happily, there are a few choices and the selection appears to be growing.

Thomas' breads, for one, use only unbleached and whole wheat flours and no chemical preservatives or dough conditioners in their whole wheat, as well as their raisin, and enriched breads. We avoid all enriched breads on the theory that nothing that is good to begin with needs to be enriched; however, if you haven't weaned your family away from white bread, this brand does offer a superior choice. The Gluten Bread does have nutrients added "for enrichment," but both it and the Protein Bread are made without any shortening or sweetening. Molasses is the sweetener in the Whole Wheat Bread.

Pepperidge Farm also uses only unbleached and whole wheat flours in their bread, and while in general their products are made with wholesome, natural ingredients, with the exception of the Corn and

Molasses Bread, the Sprouted Wheat Bread, and Sprouted Rye Bread all their breads contain preservatives. The *Pepperidge Farm* Sprouted Wheat and Rye breads, by the way, list all the ingredients on the front label (they are considered "specialty" breads and are thus required to do so) and it's quite an impressive list at that: no refined flour, no refined sugar, and no chemicals. They taste absolutely delicious.

The *Oroweat Baking Company* is another outfit that offers several breads that are worth recognition, like their SoyaBean, Branola, Sprouted Wheat, Honey Wheat Germ, Wheat Nugget, and Oro d'O-euvre Pumpernickel Breads. However, several of the breads in their line do contain preservatives, so check the label.

Catherine Clark's Brownberry Ovens Breads provide a choice in some eastern and middle states; but in L.A. *Good Stuff* Breads far surpass all the rest.

In response to the natural foods movement, *Arnold* is promoting a "Health Loaf Naturel" and a "Seven Grain Bread" which include unbleached and whole wheat flours, cracked wheat, soya flour (a high-protein flour), wheat germ, and no refined sugars or chemicals. The taste is not too different from ordinary whole wheat bread and the contents are far superior. The Arnold Health Loaf is a superior replacement for white bread in French toast.

We're glad to see that Safeway, one of the largest supermarket chains in the country, has marketed their own praiseworthy Soya Bread, Wheat Germ Bread, and Sprouted Grain Bread with Raisins. Many smaller chains are following their example.

Again we must stress that just because a bakery claims its bread uses "natural, unbleached flour" and "no preservatives" doesn't mean the loaf is chemical-free. If they don't tell you what else they've used, don't fall for this propaganda.

In addition to these widely distributed breads, many areas are now featuring products distributed locally that meet the requirement we're seeking. We have seen several cracked wheat breads, soy and wheat breads, banana breads and mixed grain breads in various supermarkets that will delight any bread lover. Because these are considered specialty breads they offer a complete list of ingredients so you can evaluate them for yourself. Here is one instance in which the Federal Code is working for you.

Small, square, compact loaves of thinly sliced whole grain breads with such names as roggenbrot, Old World pumpernickel, whole grain rye, etc., appear on most supermarket shelves. Again these offer a complete list of ingredients. The nutritional value of these breads, particularly when it comes to the B vitamins which are vital to your health and come primarily from whole grains, is noteworthy. Unfortunately, many of these brands include preservatives and several use caramel color which does come from a natural source but has been cited as a possible cancer contributant.

Not too many of the packaged rye breads on the market are much to speak of; however, *Munzenmaier* distributes a Danish Farm Bread made with rye flour and no chemicals that makes terrific toast.

Consumers' Report offers this hint for bread shoppers: they suggest buying the hard-crusted loaves of Italian Bread, often termed "Home Style," which are usually made with unbleached flour, no sugar, and no animal fat.

Another form of bread that uses unbleached flour and no sugar or shortening of any type—just flour, salt, and water—is the Mid-Eastern pita bread which is gaining widespread popularity all over the country. These flat, oval-shaped breads are excellent for scooping up dips and salads and, when cut in half crosswise, open to form a pocket for cheese, egg salad, or your favorite sandwich filling. You can also use them as a foundation for homemade pizza.

Sour dough bread, a San Francisco specialty, is beginning to show up in other parts of the country of late. A fermented dough starter provides the leavening gases for this bread, hence the name "sour dough." Most sour dough bread is free of noxious chemicals; however, white flour is the basis of this loaf so it cannot be depended upon for much nutritional value.

In Mexico it is tortillas rather than bread which accompany most meals. These flat, pancake-like breads of ground corn are quite popular in our own Southwest, and today most supermarkets offer canned or frozen versions that are reasonably good. Corn, water and possibly salt are the only necessary ingredients and the label provides you with this information. *Patio* frozen tortillas and *Old El Paso* canned tortillas are both acceptable examples.

Many modern supermarkets have fresh bakery sections or sell loaves of old-fashioned pumpernickel and rye in the delicatessen department. Fresh bakery bread is usually free of preservatives, but unbleached flour, dough conditioners, and emulsifiers are often an integral part of the operation. You might try asking—if there's something to boast about, most bakers will be happy to let you know.

BAKE YOUR OWN

For anyone who wants to make his own whole grain bread, all the necessary ingredients can be obtained in your supermarket. Although it sounds like a lot of work, the actual effort involved is small. What you do need is time. Yeast bread must be allowed to rise at least twice (that's two 45-minute to 1-hour periods) and bake for about the same duration. If you plan to be at home, bread-making won't take much time away from whatever else you're doing. Children enjoy joining in.

This recipe is for a basic whole wheat bread. You can vary it by adding raisins, chopped dried fruit, chopped nuts, spices, and shaping it in a hundred different ways. Many whole grain bread books are available and all general cookbooks give instructions for bread-makers which you can follow to vary this fine bread.

WHOLE WHEAT BREAD

1 envelope (1 tablespoon) yeast
1¼ cups warm water, divided
2 tablespoons honey
3 tablespoons oil
1 tablespoon salt
¼ cup wheat germ
about 3½ cups whole wheat flour

Combine yeast, ¼ cup of warm water, and honey, and mix to dissolve yeast. Let stand until mixture becomes frothy. Add remaining water, oil, and salt to yeast, then beat in wheat germ and 3¼ cups of flour. When dough leaves sides of bowl, turn out onto a well-floured board or oilcloth and knead, adding the remaining ¼ cup of flour as you knead to keep it from sticking. Knead about 5 minutes, until dough is fairly smooth. If necessary add a little more flour. Place dough in a well-greased bowl, cover with a cloth, and let rise in a warm place (an unlit oven works well) until double in size, or for 1 hour. Push down dough, knead again briefly (and again, if dough seems too moist, you can add a little flour), and shape into an oiled 4½ x 8½-inch loaf pan. Cover and let rise again for 45 minutes. Place the bread in a cold oven, set temperature at 400° and bake for 15 minutes. Reduce heat to 325° and continue baking for 30 to 35 minutes, until golden brown. When bread is done it will sound hollow when tapped. For a crisper crust, brush surface with cold water before baking. Remove hot bread from pan and cool on a wire rack. Let bread cool completely before slicing and eating. *Yield:* 1 loaf.

HANDLING BREAD

Whether you have purchased your bread in the supermarket or baked your own you'll want to preserve the freshness as long as you can. You'll be surprised to find that a loaf of bread can easily be kept for a week without the aid of preservatives, if it is prepared with whole grains and other fine ingredients in the first place.

Store bread in a reusable plastic bag to keep in the moisture. Storing bread in the refrigerator may dry it out a bit, but will prevent mold growth and is a must in warm weather. If the package suggests refrigerator storage, by all means follow this advice. Bread that is to be toasted should be stored in this manner as well.

Bread can be successfully frozen for six months or longer if closely wrapped in an airtight package. When you need a few slices, remove them from the package and let them stand at room temperature. In less than half an hour your bread will be restored to its original texture. If the bread is unsliced to begin with, wait until serving time to cut it. This prevents further drying out and the presence of surface ice crystals from the freezer. Any frozen bread can be toasted or warmed immediately.

USING STALE BREAD

If you've handled your bread properly, chances are you will be able to finish the loaf before it has molded or become dried out. If your family is small, or doesn't eat much bread, there may be several slices left that are less fresh than you'd like. If you don't want to use these for toast, French toast, bread pudding, etc., put them out on a plate at room temperature for several hours until they become good and hard and no moisture is left in them. Dry, hard bread will not mold and makes the best possible bread crumbs. Store this bread in an airtight packet for future use, or grate it immediately in the blender or with a hand grater, and store it in an airtight container in your kitchen cabinet. Each time you have an extra slice of bread you can add it to your bread-crumb jar.

RECOMMENDATIONS

General Rule of Purchase: White bread and rolls, raisin bread, and whole wheat bread and rolls may list none, or only some, rather than all of their ingredients. So-called specialty breads, including rye, pumpernickel, corn, sprouted wheat, mixed grain, etc., must give a complete list of ingredients.

Look for breads made with whole grains, honey or molasses, vegetable and nut oils, and fresh dairy products. Consult the list of ingredients to avoid white (also known as wheat) flour, hydrogenated shortening, dough conditioners, mono- and diglycerides, and preservatives or fresheners.

EXEMPLARY BRANDS
  100% Whole Grain Breads
    East—*Arnold's* Seven Grain
        B&M New England Brown Bread with Raisins (canned)
        Balduf 100% Whole Wheat with Honey; Nature's Diet Grain
        Earthgrains Earth Bread; Whole Wheat Bread
        Friends Brown Bread with Raisins (canned)
        Jewel Maid Wheat Bread
        Mandala ·.
        Monk's Whole Wheat
        Pepperidge Farm Sprouted Wheat; Sprouted Rye
        Rainbo Earth Bread
        Thomas' Whole Wheat
    Middle—*B&M* New England Brown Bread with Raisins (canned)
        Orowheat Oro d'Oeuvre Pumpernickel
    West—*B&M* New England Brown Bread (canned)
        Clinton's 100% Whole Wheat
        Co-op Whole Wheat Bread Plus
        Earthgrains Earth Bread; Whole Wheat Bread
        Good Stuff Bakeries—an exemplary line including Natural Whole Grain Bread; Honey Wheat Special; Once-A-Bread; Whole Grain Raisin Nut Bread; Natural Sour Dough Rye; Honey-

wheat Eggbread; Pumpernickel; Onion Wheat Rolls; Natural Whole Wheat Ounce-A-Bread Rolls; Whole Grain Dinner Rolls; Natural Sour Dough Rye Rolls; Pumpernickel Rolls; and Whole Wheat English Muffins

Jack Spratt's Sprouted Wheat Bread (no added fat)

Kilpatrick's Earth Bread

Nassraways Bakery Whole Wheat Pita

Natural Food Mill Bakery Sprouted Wheat Bread; Sprouted Wheat Burger Buns; 7-Grain Sprouted Wheat Bread

Orowheat Oro d'Oeuvre Pumpernickel

Pepperidge Farms Whole Wheat Bread ("New," no preservative)

Rainbo Earth Bread

Safeway Stone Ground Whole Wheat

Workingman's Bread

Your Black Muslim Bakery Natural Wheat; Whole Wheat Raisin; Whole Wheat Egg; Whole Wheat Rolls; muffins and sweet rolls

Back-up Breads—these contain some white flour but in general use other high-quality ingredients to compensate.

East—*Arnold's* Branola; Naturel; Wheat Berry

Catherine Clark's Brownberry Ovens Wheat Bread; Rye; Oatmeal; Whole Bran; Health Nut; Frozen Wheat Dough; and also, Seasoned Stuffing Mix

Holsum Old Heritage

Koeplinger's Sunny Honey Bread

Pepperidge Farm Wheat Bread

Rhodes Honey Wheat Frozen Bread Dough; Flaked Wheat Pan Rolls (frozen)

Thomas' Raisin

Middle—*Catherine Clark's Brownberry Ovens* Wheat Bread; Rye; Oatmeal; Whole Bran; Health Nut; Frozen Wheat Dough; and also, Seasoned Stuffing Mix

Orowheat Branola; Soya Bean Bread; Sprouted Wheat; Honey Wheat Germ; Wheat Nugget; Honey Wheat; Bohemian Style Pumpernickel;

also, for special diets, Low Sodium Wheat
Pepperidge Farm Wheat Bread
Rhodes Honey Wheat Frozen Bread Dough;
Flaked Wheat Pan Rolls (frozen)
West—*Albertson's* 100% Wheat; Whole Grain Natural
Clinton's Soya Bread
International Baking Company Whole Wheat Pita
Orowheat Branola; Soya Bean Bread; Sprouted
Wheat; Honey Wheat Germ; Wheat Nugget;
Honey Wheat; Bohemian Style Pumpernickel;
also, for special diets, Low Sodium Wheat
Rhodes Honey Wheat Frozen Bread Dough;
Falked Wheat Pan Rolls (frozen)
Safeway Wheat Germ; Soya Bread; Sprouted
Grain with Raisins
Standish Farms Honey Whole Grain

Tortillas
East—*Ashley's* (canned)
El Paso (canned)
El Ranchers
El Rio (canned)
Patio (frozen)
Pinata Corn
Van de Kamp Corn
Middle—*Ashley's* (canned)
El Paso (canned)
El Rio (canned)
Happy Jose's Corn
Paradise Corn
Patio (frozen)
Pinata Corn
Ramirez and Sons Corn
Ricardo's Corn
Rosarita Corn
West—*Ashley's* (canned)
Casa Sanchez Corn
Chico's Corn
El Dorado
El Encanto Bueno Brand Corn and Indian Blue
Corn

El Paso (canned)
Josie's Best (white and blue corn)
Kountry Fresh Corn
La Famosa Corn
La Fortaleya
La Tolteca Corn
Lynn Wilson's Fresh Corn
Macayo Corn
Patio (frozen)
Pepito Corn
Pinata Corn
Premium Mission Brand Corn
Ralphs Corn
Rancho Francisco Corn
Stella's Corn

Pasta: Make the Best of It

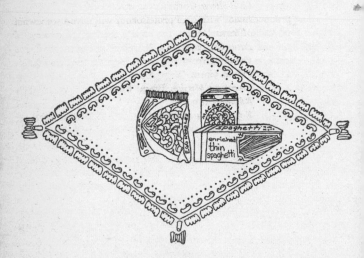

Pasta products don't have very much in the way of nutrition to recommend them to your table. They are pretty much a high-starch, low-protein food with a small amount of vitamins coming from the usually synthetic enrichment. Most adults and kids, however, love the stuff, and if it is used as a base for other nutritious foods it can be of some value.

There are two general types of pasta: macaroni and noodles. The first group includes spaghetti, macaroni, shells, lasagna, and other similar Italian type noodles; the second includes egg noodles, egg barley, and vegetable noodles (such as spinach noodles).

Pasta is classified this way because of the variation in ingredients. The ones you are likely to encounter in your supermarket are the traditional semolina–durum wheat macaroni products, and the flour and egg noodles. First let's discuss the macaroni.

MACARONI PRODUCTS

Several varieties of flour can be used to produce these starch-based foods: durum flour, regular or high protein flour; semolina; or farina. The federal regulations leave it up to the manufacturer to decide what details he provides on the label about the flour used.

Those products made with high protein flour will have a somewhat higher food value. Durum wheat, the variety used in the making of durum flour and semolina, contains a "tougher" protein, considered more desirable in the manufacture of pasta. Regular flour and farina are derived from softer wheat. This affects the physical, not nutritional, quality of the product. Any of these flours may or may not be bleached. If possible, use a product made with unbleached flours.

Many brands state right on the label "no artificial color added." This appears to be a case of petty deception since as far as we can figure from the government standard of identity, there is no provision for any added coloring in this product. No pasta product should have anything but its natural color. What it can have is added seasoning or the chemical disodium phosphate to make it quick-cooking, but these must be stated on the label.

Most major brands of macaroni are enriched with B vitamins, calcium, and iron salts. The label need only say "enriched," and it usually comes from the synthetic vitamins added to the enriched flour, although natural enrichment from wheat germ or food yeast may be used if the manufacturer chooses.

Of the brands we have investigated, these products are worth pointing out (note they list no chemical additives):

Buitoni Macaroni Products: Durum flour, high protein flour (both unbleached), wheat germ and food yeast go into the making of all Buitoni macaroni products. The wheat germ and food yeast are natural sources of B vitamin enrichment. Buitoni also offers a "20 percent protein spaghetti" made from unbleached high protein flour, wheat germ, and food yeast.

Prince's Vita Roni (Spaghetti and Macaroni): The ingredients in this package are semolina, gluten flour, soya flour, and wheat germ. Both gluten and soya flours are high in protein and the wheat germ adds a natural source of enrichment.

DeBoles (sold primarily in the natural foods section): DeBoles products are labeled "imitation" because they are made with artichoke flour along with durum semolina and soy flour. The artichoke flour

127

is derived from Jerusalem artichoke pulp and is nonstarchy, making these macaroni products lower in carbohydrates. This is one case where the imitation is a lot better than the real thing.

Hilo Spaghetti: The inclusion of wheat germ and brewers' yeast makes Hilo a more nutritional pasta.

NOODLES

The difference between noodles and macaroni products comes from the addition of eggs. Although the eggs add to the nutritional value of the product, a lower quality flour is used, so in the final analysis egg noodles are actually lower in protein than macaroni. The eggs used may be fresh or dried, whole or just yolks. Noodles made with fresh whole eggs are the best. Those with just egg yolks will have a little more vitamins, but also a lot more fat. Those which include egg whites have a slightly higher protein content.

The government standard prohibits artificial coloring and preservatives in noodles. Any other added chemicals will be given on the label. Like macaroni, most noodles are synthetically enriched.

The exceptional supermarket will stock whole wheat noodles. We have noted *Royal Whole Wheat Noodles* in supermarkets on the West Coast.

Aside from the common flat noodles, egg noodles are available in bow shapes and other whimsical forms; as egg barley; or as pastina (fine egg barley). Any vegetable puree can be added to the product, but spinach noodles are the ones most commonly available. They are the same noodle product with pureed spinach (fresh, canned or dried) added. The taste is rather pleasant, although not much like spinach, and the green color can make many dishes more attractive.

USING PASTA INTELLIGENTLY

As long as you continue to buy pasta, use it to introduce nutritious foods to your table, not as a substitute for them.

Homemade noodles and cheese can be a gourmet dish as well as a quick meal that's high in protein if you make it like this:

BAKED NOODLES AND CHEESE

8 ounces noodles, cooked
2¼ cups grated cheese
2 eggs
1 cup milk
1 teaspoon salt
½ teaspoon pepper
2 tablespoons butter

Layer noodles and 2 cups of the cheese alternately in a large, shallow baking pan or a 2–quart casserole. Beat together eggs, milk, salt, and pepper, and pour over noodles and cheese. Sprinkle with remaining ¼ cup of cheese and dot with butter. Bake in a 375° oven for 25 minutes, until set.

For interesting combinations use spinach noodles and a combination of Swiss and Parmesan cheese or use macaroni and Cheddar cheese and let freshly made bread crumbs replace the ¼ cup of cheese topping. *Yield:* 4 servings (this recipe can easily be cut in half and baked in a 1–quart casserole).

A side dish of noodles or macaroni can be enriched with a crunchy topping of chopped walnuts, sesame seeds, and wheat germ. A covering of grated cheese or a side dish of bean salad along with a pasta meal will enhance the food value.

The protein that is present can also be supplemented with lentils or other dried beans. The Egyptians have a dish called Koshery which is nothing more than a large bowl of macaroni, rice, and lentils topped with crisply fried onions and a thin, spicy tomato sauce. They consume it in great quantities. Use brown rice in your version for a dish that's really nutritious and great-tasting.

GOING ALL THE WAY

Noodles are really fun to make at home if you like to cook. Most cookbooks include recipes for homemade pasta which call for all-purpose flour and eggs. Although the taste is an improvement, the protein and vitamin content is no better than the commercial varieties (and actually is lower than some). If you really want to make some good noodles, follow the recipe, but use whole wheat flour in place of the other kind.

One recipe that we cherish produces a very wholesome, tender noodle with a noticeably fresher taste. Instead of the eggs we use yogurt.

EGGLESS NOODLES

1½ cups whole wheat flour
1 teaspoon sea salt
1 cup yogurt

Mix flour, sea salt, and enough yogurt to make a stiff dough. Squeeze and knead the dough well for 2 to 3 minutes. Roll out thinly on a floured board, let rest 5 minutes, then cut into ¼-inch slices for noodles (or to any desired size).

Spread the noodles on paper and let dry at room temperature until hard. This will take several hours. Store in a closed container. Noodles can be cooked immediately, without drying, if you do not wish to store them. Cook in boiling salted water about 10 minutes. *Yield:* Noodles!

If you don't want to go to the trouble of rolling the dough, which is not much work but does require some space, at least try some homemade egg barley. This is another kitchen project where kids excel.

EGG BARLEY

4 cups whole wheat flour
4 eggs
1 teaspoon salt
5 tablespoons water

Combine ingredients, blend with hands and knead until very stiff, about 5 minutes. Divide dough into small balls, flatten slightly, and allow to dry partially, about 1 hour. When somewhat dry, rub each lump of dough against a coarse (cheese) grater, making pea-sized pieces. Spread on paper and allow to dry thoroughly. Use as you would commercial egg barley. *Yield:* about 2 pounds; enough for 16 servings.

RECOMMENDATIONS

MACARONI

General Rule of Purchase: Most brands are similar. Label may not be complete. Whole wheat flour, unbleached flour, and enrichment with wheat germ and brewer's yeast preferred when specified.

EXEMPLARY BRANDS:
> *Buitoni*
> *De Boles* Artichoke Macaroni
> *Hale and Hardy* Whole Wheat Spaghetti; Wheat and Soya
> Spinach Macaroni
> *Hilo*
> *Prince's* Vita Roni

NOODLES

General Rule of Purchase: Most brands of plain and vegetable noodles are similar, and the label may not be specific. Again, whole wheat flour, unbleached flour, and fresh whole eggs preferred.

EXEMPLARY BRANDS:
> *Hale and Hardy* Whole Wheat, and Wheat and Soya Ribbons
> *Royal* Whole Wheat Noodles

Beans, Beans, Beans

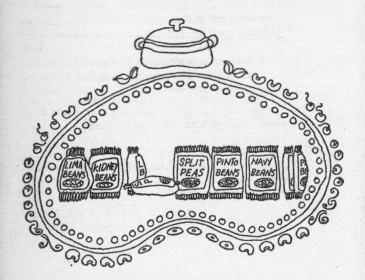

The biggest supermarket bargain in food we know of comes in a plastic bag or cardboard box with a see-through plastic window. This little gem will cost you 20¢ to 30¢ for a pound bag, enough for eight to ten servings. Each one of those servings will be rich in protein, iron, thiamine, and riboflavin. We're talking about dried legumes—beans, peas, and lentils—the prince of the food world in Europe and the Middle East where they provide a rich, tasty source of nourishment for millions of people daily.

Every supermarket devotes a section to dried legumes. The large variety is actually surprising in view of the fact that most people are unaware of their creative possibilities. A well-stocked shelf is likely to include dried split peas, lentils, kidney beans, chick peas, black beans, pigeon peas, black-eyed peas, lima beans, pinto beans, and white beans (marrow, great northern, navy, and pea). We are dismayed to find that dried soybeans, the most nutritious natural vegetable food known, are often missing from the supermarket shelf.

PROTEIN FOR PENNIES

To repeat: the price of a pound bag of dried legumes is 20¢ to 30¢. Eight to ten *highly nutritious* servings can be produced from this package. Certainly this is a food bargain you can't afford to ignore.

Beans, peas, and lentils are a primary source of protein in much of the world. By themselves they are considered an "incomplete protein," which means they lack, or are low in, certain amino acids needed by the body to synthesize protein. There are eight amino acids which cannot be made by the body and must come from food. Beans, with the exception of soybeans which are complete proteins, are defi-

PROTEIN FOR PENNIES

Food	Calories/ pound	Protein/ pound	Cost/ pound[1]
		(grams)	($)
Soybeans	1,828	154.7	.25
Split peas	1,579	109.8	.39
Lima beans	1,565	92.5	.65
Kidney beans	1,556	102.1	.53
Lentils	1,542	112.0	.39
Chick peas (garbanzos)	1,633	93.0	.59
Eggs	658	52.1	.58
Cottage cheese	481	61.7	.79
Swiss cheese	1,610	119.8	2.05
Chicken	382	57.4	.69
Halibut	454	94.8	1.59
Tuna, canned	760	111.1	1.60
Hamburger	1,216	81.2	1.09
Sirloin, bone in	1,316	71.1	2.09
Bacon	3,016	38.1	1.75
Frankfurters, all meat	1,343	59.4	1.29
Pork, loin chop	1,065	61.1	2.09
Veal, loin chop	681	72.3	2.39
Lamb, shoulder chop	1,082	58.9	2.19

1. Based on average supermarket price in June 1976.

cient in two of these amino acids. However, *whole grains, wheat, nuts, seeds, and dairy products are rich in these two amino acids and when combined with legumes offer the value of a complete protein.* This wisdom is reflected in the popular Spanish specialty of rice and beans.

BUYING FOR QUALITY

Although most peas and lentils and many beans are officially inspected before or after processing, retail packages seldom show the federal or state grade. You can, however, do your own grading.

Most dried legumes are available in see-through packages. Look in and consider these factors:

●Color—dried beans should have a bright, uniform color. Fading is an indication of long storage, which means your beans won't be fresh, will take longer to cook, and will be less tasty.

●Size—look for a package with beans of uniform size. Small beans cook faster than large ones and a variety of sizes will result in uneven cooking. By the time the larger beans are tender, the small ones will be mush.

●Defects—cracked coating, foreign materials, many discolorations, and perforations in the package itself are all signs of possible damage, decay, and a low-quality product. Buy bags of beans free of any visible defects.

BUYING FOR VARIETY

Although the exact variety varies from store to store, you will always have a broad selection to choose from. Here are some of the most popular varieties along with some suitable uses:

Black Beans (or black turtle beans): Select these beans for thick soups. Often used in Mediterranean and South American dishes.

Black-Eyed Peas (or cow peas): These are small, oval-shaped beans which are creamy white with a small black spot on one side. They are served as a main dish vegetable and are popular in southern and soul food cookery.

Garbanzo Beans (or chick peas): These beans are characterized by a nutlike flavor which lends itself to pureeing for dips and main dishes, and seasoned with salt and pepper the cooked beans are often served cold for snacking. Cranberry beans are similar to chick peas and can be used interchangeably.

Great Northern Beans: Similar to pea beans, only larger, these beans are used in soups, main dishes, and home-baked beans.

Kidney Beans: Kidney beans are red and shaped like a kidney. They lend themselves to Mexican dishes, especially chili.

Lentils: One of the oldest and most nutritious of foods is the tiny lentil. These cook in only 30 to 45 minutes and do not need soaking. Any extra cooking liquid makes excellent soup or gravy. Lentils team up well with other vegetables, grains, meat, or fruit.

Lima Beans: These are broad, flat, and come in small and large sizes. They make an excellent vegetable, casserole ingredient, and a rich soup.

Navy Beans: This general name is often applied to all small white beans, great northern, and pea beans.

Pea Beans: The favorite for homemade baked beans, these are small, oval, and white. They hold their shape particularly well, even when cooked very tender.

Pinto Beans: Relatives of the kidney beans, only beige-colored with speckles. Use as you would kidney beans.

Red and Pink Beans: Again in the kidney bean family, only more delicate in flavor.

Soybeans: Soybeans are the most virtuous of all beans. They are the only food in the vegetable kingdom that contains all the essential amino acids the body needs to synthesize protein. People often talk about masking the flavor of soybeans with gravies and lots of seasoning; we don't know why since these beans actually have quite a pleasant taste of their own. Although cookbooks dealing exclusively with soybeans have been written, soybeans can be used just as you would any other bean and require no special handling.

Dry Split Peas: Available in green and yellow (which have a less pronounced flavor), these peas have had the skin removed by mechanical processing. They are known for their use in split-pea soup, but combine well with other foods. Since they cook in a relatively short period of time and do not require soaking they can be cooked along with rice or other grains for a rich protein dish.

Dry Whole Peas: Dry peas are served in many ways and one of the nicest is just plain boiled and seasoned with butter. Unlike the split peas, these must be soaked, like other beans, before cooking.

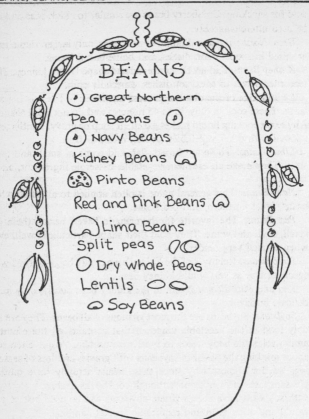

BEAN STORAGE

Store dried legumes in the package they come in, on your kitchen shelf. After the package has been opened, transfer any unused beans to a covered container. We keep a variety of beans on hand in glass jars on an open shelf. They make a very pretty kitchen display.

Once cooked, legumes can be stored in the refrigerator for at least one week, or in an airtight container in the freezer for long-term use (up to six months).

BEAN COOKING

The lengthy cooking time involved often discourages people from cooking with beans. Although time is an important consideration, the fact that there is no work involved should more than compensate. Since they store so well, you can prepare a large quantity of beans at once and avoid repeating the process often.

BASIC BEAN COOKERY

The basic preparation is as simple as this:

1. Wash the beans in cold water.
2. Dried beans and whole peas should be soaked before cooking to replace the water lost in drying and to reduce the cooking time. Lentils and split peas do not have to be soaked. Soak in three times the volume of water overnight; or bring the beans and water to a boil, cook 2 minutes, then remove from heat, cover, and let soak 2 hours (Quick-Soak Method).
3. When the soaking period is over, bring beans and water to a boil, reduce heat to a very low temperature, cover and simmer gently until tender, about 2 hours. Always cook the beans in the water they were soaked in. Add more water during cooking if beans begin to stick. Keep the heat low. Fast cooking causes the beans to break. Low heat produces whole beans and prevents sticking.
4. The exact time will vary with the variety of legume and the intended use. For dishes that call for reheating the beans, for salads, and for storage, the beans should be tender but still hold their shape. For purees and mashed bean dishes they should be quite soft. Split peas and lentils will be tender in about 45 minutes. Most other beans require 2 to 3 hours.
5. Do not add salt to the beans until they are almost tender, or, if they are to be combined with other ingredients, add the salt then. Salt hardens the legumes and makes the cooking time longer. The only thing you might want to add initially to the cooking pot is a tablespoon of oil to keep the foaming down. Old recipes suggest adding baking soda to the water. This decreases cooking time and makes the skins slip off the beans easily. It also destroys thiamine. Never add baking soda to dried beans.
6. Remember to allow room in the pot for expansion. Depending on the bean, 1 cup dry (approximately ½ pound) will yield 2 to 3 cups after cooking.

BE CREATIVE WITH BEANS

If you are going to serve the beans as an accompaniment to the main course they can be seasoned with tomatoes and Italian seasonings, chili powder, or lightly sweetened with molasses. Sautéed onion and garlic heighten the flavor.

All cooked beans can be marinated in an oil and vinegar dressing and served as a salad. Chopped scallions and parsley should be included here for a well-received dish.

Legumes in the form of soup are the most popular and, with the exception of baked beans, almost the only way they appear on most American menus. Your favorite cookbooks will supply you with plenty of recipes in this category, and the chapter "Homemade Soups" in this book will add a few more. You should take full advantage of the protein offered in these soups and make it a complete protein with the addition of grains or a garnish of chopped nuts.

If you really want to save money, though, think about serving bean dishes as a main course. In the Middle East they have a fabulous bean dish that is served in every home, sold in every restaurant, and vended on the street much as our American hot dog. The name of the dish is Falafel, and it's no more than tiny pureed bean croquettes that are deep-fried and served in the pocket of pita bread with a spicy salad and a sesame butter sauce (which adds the missing amino acids). Lately, Falafel stands have been springing up in metropolitan areas with incredible speed to great public acceptance. We will take that as a hint that many of you are looking for creative ways to introduce beans to your diet, so here are some very easy, highly nutritious, low-cost main dishes you should try out in your kitchen.

BEAN LOAF

2 cups ground cooked beans, your choice (obtained by cooking 1 cup dried beans which makes 3 cups cooked beans or 2 cups when ground)
¼ cup fresh bread crumbs, wheat germ, or a combination of the two
1 egg
2 tablespoons tomato juice
2 tablespoons catsup
¼ cup chopped onion
1½ teaspoons salt

(continued)

¼ teaspoon pepper
¼ teaspoon dried herbs
1 tablespoon oil

Combine all ingredients except the oil, pack into an oiled loaf pan or mold onto a greased baking sheet. Bake in a 350° oven 45 minutes. Baste occasionally with the oil.

Vary the loaf by adding any or all of the following: ¼ to ½ cup of grated cheese, ¼ cup of chopped olives, ¼ cup of chopped nuts, ½ cup of sautéed mushrooms. *Yield:* 4 servings.

CHILI WITHOUT CARNE

3 tablespoons oil
2 cloves garlic, finely chopped
2 large onions, chopped
2 tablespoons chile powder
¼ teaspoon cayenne pepper or pepper sauce
2 teaspoons oregano
2 teaspoons salt
2 tablespoons soy sauce
1 tablespoon brewer's yeast, optional
4 large tomatoes, diced
4 cups cooked kidney beans

Heat oil in large saucepan and sauté garlic and onion until delicately browned. Sprinkle in chili powder and cayenne and cook 1 minute. Add remaining ingredients, cover and cook gently until tomatoes melt and form a rich sauce and the chili is good and hot, 15 to 20 minutes. Mixture can be reheated as necessary. If it gets too dry, add some of the bean liquid.

Serve with brown rice and whole grain crackers. *Yield:* 4 generous servings.

MOTHER'S CHOLENT

1 cup dried lima beans
3 tablespoons chicken fat or oil
3 onions, chopped
4 potatoes, peeled and quartered
¼ cup barley
3 pounds short ribs of beef
1 tablespoon salt
1 teaspoon pepper
1 teaspoon paprika

1 teaspoon unbleached flour
Boiling water
2 carrots, cut in half

Wash beans, soak 1 hour in warm water to cover and drain. Heat fat in large heavy saucepan or Dutch oven. Add onion and sauté until golden, about 10 minutes. Add beans, potatoes, and barley, and stir. Place meat in center of pot. Combine seasoning and flour and sprinkle over meat and vegetables. Add boiling water to reach 1 inch above the ingredients. Cover and cook 5 hours over very low heat, or bake in a 300° oven for 3½ to 4 hours. Halfway through cooking add the carrots. Check the casserole every so often to see if more water is needed. The barley absorbs a good deal of liquid, so if you don't want to concern yourself with adding more water, partially cook the barley before you begin.

Serve on a cold winter day. *Yield:* 6 hearty servings.

CANNED BEANS

Beans are available in cans, cooked and ready to be seasoned in your kitchen. As a matter of fact, some are already sauced and seasoned. The price you pay for this convenience is high, almost double that of the dried beans, and with few exceptions these beans always have EDTA added. EDTA is an antioxidant which preserves color in the beans. It is linked with kidney disorders and should be avoided. The exceptions include most of the beans packed by *Busch, Progresso* Roman Beans and Fave Beans, the *El Paso* beans (most of which are preseasoned), *Pope* white Kidney Beans and Chick Peas, and *Superfine* Red Kidney Beans and Black-Eyed Peas. Some cans of *Progresso* Cannellini (white) beans have EDTA added, so be sure to check each label.

Cook your own legumes from the dried state and don't risk ingesting this chemical. You'll be rewarded with a much richer tasting bean. If you think you don't have the time, consider all the evenings you spend at home watching TV or reading a book. In the morning, before you leave the house, put the beans and water in a pot to soak. When you come home turn on the heat and you can go right on doing whatever else you like to do when you're home. Two hours later your beans will be finished and ready for use in the coming days. You can select a different bean every week and plan a creative meal around it.

BEAN SPROUTS: INDOOR FARMING

We'd like to add a word about sprouting beans here. Most of you have probably seen bean sprouts (fresh or canned) in your supermarket travels. These are the product of a germinating mung bean. (The mung bean is a variety used mostly for sprouting and is sold dried in specialty stores only.) All beans (and grains and seeds as well), unless specially treated, can be turned into fresh sprouts for salads, snacking, or cooked vegetable dishes. Once sprouted, the protein, vitamin B, and vitamin C content of the bean or seed soars.

RELATIONSHIP OF BEANS TO SPROUTS

¼ pound soybeans grows into about 1 pound of bean sprouts

	calories	protein (grams)	vitamin A (I.U.)	thiamine (mg)	riboflavin (mg)	niacin (mg)	C (mg)
¼ lb. soybeans	457	38.7	80	1.25	.36	2.5	–
1 lb. soybean sprouts	209	28.1	360	1.03	.88	3.9	58

It is very simple to make your own sprouts, in fact it's one of the earliest science projects kids do in school. There are many different methods. We use this easy one:

1. Soak beans (or any sprouting seed) in a jar with warm water to cover, overnight, or at least 8 hours.
2. Drain off water (and save it for soup) and secure a piece of cheesecloth over the mouth of the jar.
3. Rinse beans with warm water through the cheesecloth, invert and drain completely.
4. Keep the bean jar inverted at an angle to increase the surface area and allow any excess water to drain off.
5. Sprouts grow best in a dark place. A closet or kitchen cabinet is perfect. We put the jar in a bowl so any extra liquid doesn't run into the cupboard.
6. Rinse, as above, two or three times a day.

Within two to five days (depending on the variety) you will have nice shoots. Soon green will begin to appear which will add vitamin A, but the sprouts become somewhat bitter at this point. Before they turn green, when they are about ½ inch long, transfer the sprouts to a covered container and refrigerate for use over the next three or four days. Sprinkle them on salads or sandwiches, sauté them with diced

141

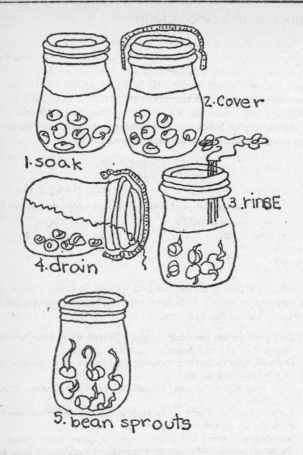

1. soak
2. Cover
3. rinse
4. drain
5. bean sprouts

vegetables for an Oriental dish, or just eat them plain. Not only are they high in food value, they're extremely low in calories.

Remember, the volume of the sprouts may be four to six times the original volume of beans, so use a jar that can accommodate the growth. Your yield will vary with the type and freshness of the dried bean, so begin with a few tablespoons the first time and you'll be able to gauge yourself by the results in the future. Try sprouting soybeans, lentils, split peas, and chick peas.

RECOMMENDATIONS

General Rule of Purchase: Buy dried beans, peas, and lentils; all brands are similar. Choose canned, precooked beans only when you can't cook your own. Check the label for non-essentials like sugar and the preservative disodium EDTA. Salt will be unavoidable, so be sure to cut down in the rest of the recipe. The label gives all ingredients; note that this product varies with the variety as well as the brand.

EXEMPLARY BRANDS:
> Kidney and Red Beans
>> *Beany Boy* Red
>> *Busch's* Red
>> *Dell'Alpe* Red Kidney
>> *Elf* Red
>> *Holleb's* Red Kidney (commercial size)
>> *Howell Mill* Kidney
>> *Janet Lee* Small Red
>> *Old El Paso* Mexe-Beans (or *Mountain Pass*) (preseasoned)
>> *Superfine* Red Kidney
>> *Trappey's* Light Red
>> *Van Camps* New Orleans Style Red Kidney (preseasoned)
>
> Pintos
>> *El Rio* Mexican Beans (preseasoned)
>> *Food King*
>> *Gebhardts* Spiced Beans (preseasoned)
>> *Howell Mill*
>> *Janet Lee*
>> *Old El Paso* (or *Mountain Pass*)
>> *Scot Lad*

Great Northern
- *American Beauty*
- *Avondale*
- *Big Top*
- *Busch's*
- *Elf*
- *Food King*
- *Foodland*
- *Gaylord*
- *Hanover*
- *Howell Mill*
- *Janet Lee*
- *Kimbell*
- *Kountry Kist*
- *Meadowdale*
- *Raggedy Ann*
- *Scot Lad*
- *Staff*
- *The Allens*

Navy
- *Busch's*
- *Elf*
- *Food King*
- *Gaylord*
- *Hanover*
- *Scot Lad*
- *The Allens*

Garbanzos
- *Ashley's of Texas*
- *Busch's*
- *Coop*
- *El Rio*
- *Garcia's*
- *Janet Lee*
- *Marconi*
- *Old El Paso* (or *Mountain Pass*)
- *Pope*
- *Raggedy Ann*

Blackeye Peas
  Garcia's
  Margaret Holmes
  Progresso
  Scot Lad
  Superfine
White Beans
  Dell'Alpe White Kidney
  Goya Cannellini; White Kidney; Small White
  Pope White Kidney
Limas or Butter Beans
  Busch's Speckled Butter Beans
  Food King Limas
  Meadowdale Butter Beans
  Raggedy Ann Butter Beans
  Seaside Cooked Dry Butterbeans
Black Beans
  Goya
  Kirby Frijoles Negros (Black Beans with Creole Seasoning)
  La Preferida
Others
  Busch's October Beans
  Cedar Creek Green Boiled Peanuts
  Dell'Alpe Fava Beans; Roman Beans; Lentils; Lupini Beans
  El Tibarito Pigeon Peas
  Gioia Fave Beans
  Hollywood Soy Beans
  Loma Linda (Green) Soy Beans·
  Peanut Patch Boiled Peanuts
  Progresso Fave Beans; Roman Beans; Lupini Beans
  Ziyad Brand Falafil Mix

Eat Your Vegetables

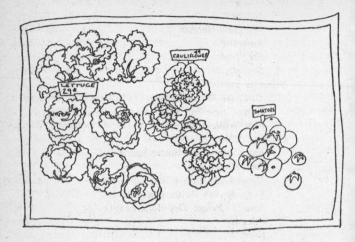

Why is it that vegetables are regarded as some sort of punishment by so many of us, when in reality they are among the most delicious foods nature has provided? Why is it that the refrain "Eat your vegetables" has become a national joke?

Perhaps because they are so rich in important vitamins and minerals, we have somehow gotten the idea that vegetables can't possibly taste good too. More likely it is because they have been so abused by the vegetable growers and manufacturers and in our own kitchens that most of their excellence has been masked or destroyed by the time they reach the plate.

Despite all objections, the reason wise mothers are so concerned about getting junior to finish his vegetables is that this class of foods makes a significant contribution to our daily vitamin and mineral intake. With the exception of vitamin D, every vegetable is well endowed with one or more of all the essential vitamins and minerals without which our body could not make use of protein, or build and sustain bones, tissues, blood, hair, nails, and all of the body organs. No one vegetable, however, is high in all these nutrients and so a wide variety of them is a necessary part of the diet.

Many factors govern the nutritive value of vegetables, among them climate, season of harvesting, soil, variety, storage, and preparation. Despite these variables there are generalizations that can be made.

•Seed vegetables, such as peas and beans, are good sources of the B vitamin thiamine and a fair source of riboflavin. They are among the best vegetable sources of protein and iron.

•All yellow, orange, and dark green vegetables are rich in vitamin A (or carotene which can be converted to vitamin A in the body). This is true whether they are root vegetables (like carrots) or leaves (like spinach).

•Green leaves are also an important source of riboflavin, vitamin C, and iron. Although vegetables generally are poor sources of calcium as compared to milk and milk products, leafy green vegetables do offer significant amounts of calcium as well.

•When they are fresh, practically all vegetables make some contribution to vitamin C intake, particularly when they are eaten raw.

•Another attractive feature of vegetables, particularly for the calorie counter, is that the average ½-cup serving of most vegetables contains only 50 calories, climbing to a high (which is still pretty low) of between 50 and 100 calories for a serving of the more starchy varieties like lima beans, peas, corn, and boiled potatoes.

•Finally, vegetables add variety to the menu. Think how drab a meal would be without the color and crispness and deep, rich flavor of a well-prepared vegetable dish or salad.

FRESH VS. FROZEN VS. CANNED

Vegetables have the most to offer nutritionally, and in most cases the richest flavor, immediately after harvesting and when eaten in the raw state. As time passes, chemical changes occur within the plant which alter the nutritional makeup and the taste. These changes are hastened by warmth, including cooking, and slowed down by cold.

Vegetables that are fresh can be transported rapidly from field to market in chilled vans to keep them at maximum quality. If they are handled properly at the store they can reach your kitchen without losing too much of their natural goodness along the way.

Frozen vegetables must go to a packaging plant from the fields, and depending on the efficiency of the manufacturer, may be frozen just at their peak, or may wait around for several days to be processed. Theoretically, those frozen almost immediately should be as rich or richer than those that are fresh in your store. The factors that keep this a theory rather than a reality are rather weighty. For one, vegetables must often wait around the packing plant several days before they are attended to. In the meantime they may be sprayed with chemicals to prevent spoiling and to keep away visiting insects. Secondly, before they are frozen, vegetables are blanched to destroy certain enzymes which cause further changes during storage. When vegetables are blanched, they are boiled for about five minutes, then rapidly cooled. Even this short heat treatment is enough to destroy some of the vitamin C and thiamine and bring about an additional loss of vitamins which seep into the water. Although very few studies have been done thus far, the enzymes the blanching is meant to destroy are thought to be very important to man and his utilization of his vegetable foods.

Cold temperatures cannot preserve vegetables indefinitely, and over time, the food value and flavor continue to diminish, although at a slow rate. There is no accurate way of knowing how long the package of frozen vegetables has been in your supermarket freezer case, and continued freezing at home only increases the chance of further loss. What's more, the buyer has little chance of discovering if the package of frozen vegetables has indeed been frozen the entire time. Often, during transfer from shipping vehicle to market to freezer showcase, vegetable packages partially or fully defrost, are refrozen, only to defrost again, possibly several times. Each time the package becomes soft, vitamins and minerals are destroyed and the vegetables run the risk of decay.

The form in which the vegetables are packed is another major consideration. Peeling, cutting, dicing, and shredding all bring about vitamin loss. Unless the vegetable is frozen whole, its nutritional contribution may be even lower than you've estimated.

Canned vegetables are widely consumed in this country and are probably the reason for the great number of "vegetable haters" we have here. To begin with, the taste of canned vegetables hardly resembles their fresh counterparts. The heat of canning has brought about color, flavor, and textural changes that render most canned vegetables drastically different and, moreover, inferior to their true state. The same loss of nutrients possible during fresh vegetable shipping and frozen vegetable storing and handling occurs with canned vegetables to say nothing of the additional loss caused by the extreme heat of the canning process itself. Most canners will naturally disagree, stating that studies have revealed only a slightly lower vitamin and mineral content in canned vegetables, as compared to fresh and frozen ones.

What they neglect to say is that most of the nutrients measured are in the *liquid* in the can, the portion that usually goes down the drain.

This is not the end of the canned vegetable story. To prevent color and texture changes, canning is more dependent on chemical additives than most other methods of vegetable handling. Bacteria don't grow well in an acid medium so a certain percent of acid is required by law in canning; therefore, if the natural acidity of the vegetable is not enough, acids must be added during processing. In foods that are too acid, baking soda must be introduced, and baking soda destroys B vitamins.

To limit the color change, chemical substances known as sequestrants are added which hold this change to a minimum. Canned beans are almost always treated this way, as the chemical EDTA on the label indicates. Vinegar and other added acids perform the same function. Vegetables packed in jars, where light can penetrate and cause further color change, are particularly prone to this mistreatment.

To keep the vegetables firm under the extreme heat and pressure of canning, chemical salts (calcium salts) are frequently added, which help maintain texture. Among the other things that are commonly added to vegetables during canning are:

salt—almost always included and mandatory on the label

MSG and spices or flavoring—on the label

artificial color—on the label

starch—particularly in creamed vegetables, on the label

flavor intensifiers—such as disodium inosinate and guanylate, on the label

butter, plus emulsifiers—with only butter on the label

water—always present, not always indicated

hydrolized vegetable protein—amino acid salts extracted from vegetables which include MSG and sodium chloride (common salt) on the label

yeast extract—on the label

149

sugar and dextrose—added for enhancing the flavor, making the vegetables a little "sweeter" than they really are. Need not be on the label.

With very few exceptions, to be discussed a little further on, canned vegetables are almost never recommended to the aware buyer.

BE FRESH WITH YOUR VEGETABLES

As a general guideline for serving vegetables to your family keep in mind that in most cases "fresh is best." And for those few times when this generalization does not hold true the alternatives will be given here.

Just because your vegetable is purchased in the natural state, that is, fresh, does not make it exactly an untainted food. Most of the vegetables grown for market are treated to heavy doses of chemical fertilizers and pesticides, whether they are slated to reach the consumer in fresh, frozen, or canned form. Residues of this chemical treatment are absorbed through the roots of the plant (where they are impossible to remove) and remain on the outside surface (where washing can decrease the amount somewhat and peeling can remove it). For many vegetables, the peel and the surface just beneath the peel are the richest source of vitamins and minerals, and when chemical treatment necessitates the removal of this outside skin it is a sad waste indeed. Vegetables with a thick, inpenetrable skin (like avocados) or a protective casing (like peas) afford their own natural protection against chemical invasion through the surface.

In order to make the vegetables attractive on the produce counter many growers and distributors wax the outside skins to give them a high color and shiny façade. This surface treatment makes it difficult to judge the quality within and is often indigestible as well. Those vegetables likely to be waxed include carrots, parsnips, cucumbers, tomatoes, potatoes, green peppers, eggplant, and rutabagas (where the problem is less serious since the outside skin is inedible to begin with). Locally grown produce is less likely to be waxed and likely to be fresher.

Along with wax, coloring matter may be added to the vegetable surface with the same deceptive purpose in mind. The shipping carton is supposed to indicate this and the produce manager in the store is legally bound to display a sign indicating the vegetables have been artificially colored. Either most produce men are ignorant of this fact or they think the consumer is and don't bother to do so. Potatoes are particularly subject to this practice and you can be sure when you see "new" potatoes with a lovely deep red blush that a little "makeup" is the cause of that rich color.

Another problem common to potatoes and onions is the growth of sprouts (or "eyes" as they are familiarly referred to in potatoes). This growth is part of the natural aging process and the knowing consumer will not buy sprouted potatoes and onions. These vegetables are frequently treated with a chemical which slows this growth and makes you think the vegetable is younger and fresher than it indeed is. Formerly, borax, a highly poisonous chemical, was used to prevent sprouting, but today maleic hydrazide has pretty much taken its place. This chemical is only a "suspected" mutagen.

Other things to watch out for when buying "natural" vegetables:

•Your celery may be bleached with ethylene gas to give it a clear color. The result of this bleaching—vitamin loss.

•Your tomatoes may be picked green and gassed in the van on the way to market so by the time they get to the store they have changed miraculously from green to bright red *overnight*. Here again, the difference in vitamins between a vine-ripened and a gassed tomato is extreme. So is the taste.

• Sorbic acid, a preservative, may be used to coat the surface of the vegetable to keep it from decaying before you have a chance to buy it. This should always be stated at the display counter. Fresh black-eyed peas seem particularly destined for this treatment.

A WORD ON ORGANIC VEGETABLES

There is such a thing as truly "natural" vegetables, ones that have been grown in chemical-free soil, without the help of chemical insect repellents; ones that have not been colored, waxed, preserved, or otherwise treated to make them seem what they are not. The label "organic" is given to these untainted vegetables and many supermarkets make a conscious effort to obtain some chemical-free produce for concerned shoppers. Unfortunately, there is no certification for organic vegetables yet (although independent concerns such as Rodale Press are presently trying to work out an effective program) and so many stores are offering as "organic," produce which is not. Many do this knowingly, while many others are themselves being cheated. If your supermarket sells organic vegetables, ask their source and try to discover what steps the store has taken to insure they are, in fact, genuine.

Remember too, organic vegetables may not be as attractive outside, but it's what's behind that pretty front that counts. This does not mean that wormy, decaying, poor-quality produce is what you should have to select from. If these signs of poor quality are what your supermarket offers as "organic" you can be certain someone is being cheated. Don't let that someone be you.

PICKING THE BEST VEGETABLES

To help you avoid some of the chemical pitfalls and select the vegetables that are the freshest, and therefore those endowed with the most nutrition and taste, the following buying guide has been assembled. The best way you have of getting vegetables that are richest in these qualities is to buy in season when the supply is ripe and plentiful. Fortunately, this is the time when the prices are lowest too. If a particular vegetable is not in season, build your menu around another. Many are in constant supply year-round due to a naturally long growing season, and there is always something seasonal that can be used to create a tasty, nutritious dish.

Artichokes (Peak season March through May)

Artichokes are grown in California and while shipped throughout the country year-round, they are at their peak from March to May. The vegetable must be cooked to be eaten and is particularly delicious either warm or cold, dipped into lemon butter, hollandaise sauce, or French dressing.

Tips: To enjoy this delicacy, pull off the leaves one at a time, dip the leaf into the sauce, then draw it between your teeth, scraping off the tender edible meat at the base. When the leaves have been removed you will reach a solid "heart" with fuzzy little leaves attached. Scrape off these leaves (called the choke) and eat the remaining heart with a knife and fork.

Look for: Compact, tightly closed heads that are heavy in relation to size, with green, fresh-looking leaves. Size is not related to quality or flavor.

Avoid: Leaves that are excessively brown or that show mold growth or worm holes. Spreading leaves indicate age, and the leaves will be tough, dry, and bitter.

Asparagus (Peak season March through June)

Asparagus are rarely available out of season.

Look for: Firm, well-rounded spears with compact tips.

Avoid: Flat stalks and tips that are open or decayed. Such asparagus will be tough and stringy.

A Tip: Although few people take advantage of this, asparagus can be eaten raw as well as cooked. When you do cook them, try pan-frying; this method conserves the flavor and bright green color as well as the nutrients.

Another Tip: To trim the ends of asparagus, break the stalk as far down as it snaps easily rather than trimming with a knife. This saves vitamins and prevents stringiness.

Avocado (Available year round with a slight peak December through June)

Actually a fruit, but treated by most people as a vegetable. Avocados are delicious diced in salads, served "on the half shell," filled with fish salads, or mashed with tomato or mayonnaise and seasonings and used as a dip or spread.

Look for: For immediate use, avocados that yield to gentle pressure on the skin. For use in a few days, buy firm fruit and let it ripen at room temperature. The skin should be of uniform color and free of cracks. Irregular brown markings, however, have no effect on the inside flesh.

Avoid: Avocados with dark, sunken spots in irregular patches and a cracked surface. These indicate decay.

Tips: Ripe avocado should be used immediately or stored in the warmest part of the refrigerator (the lower section). If bought for home ripening, leave at room temperature; it will not ripen in the refrigerator and chilling may prevent ripening in the future. To avoid darkening once the avocado has been cut, sprinkle with lemon juice, and if you plan to hold it any length of time, replace the pit and cover.

As stated before, the thick, tough skin of the avocado affords some protection against chemical sprays, making this fruit more "natural" than most.

Beans, green or wax (Peak season May through October, and particularly June and July)

Look for: Young pods that are crisp and snap easily. Color should be fresh and bright-looking.

Avoid: Pods that are limp, thick, and show brown rust spots or serious blemishes.

Tips: Trim the ends of beans by snapping rather than cutting them. Serve beans raw as a snack or salad ingredient, and when cooking, do so only until crisp-tender, not limp and soggy, for the true bean flavor.

Beets (Peak season June through August, but supplies are available year-round)

Look for: Beets should be firm with a smooth surface and lush red color. Beets that are sold in bunches are easiest to judge by the fresh appearance of the tops (beet greens). Buy beets of fairly uniform size for even cooking.

Avoid: Badly wilted tops indicate the beets are less than fresh; however, if the bulb is still firm they may be satisfactory. Soft, wet areas, scaly areas around the top, and an elongated contour indicate beets that will be tough and strong-tasting.

Tips: The fresh tops of beets should be removed and may be used immediately in salad or cooked in the water that clings during washing and seasoned in the same manner as spinach (see Greens). When beets are cooked, the color seeps into the water; to retain their redness they should be left whole, with the peel intact, until after cooking. Raw beets are excellent peeled and grated into salads.

Broccoli (Peak season October through May)

Although available in the summer months, this broccoli is not as rich or tasty as the peak season variety.

Look for: Firm stalks with dark green or purplish green compact clusters of buds. Stems should not be too thick or tough.

Avoid: Buds that are spread, yellow, or wilted, all signs of over-maturity and over-display. This broccoli will be tough and stringy. Soft, slippery spots on the buds are signs of decay.

Tips: When you trim broccoli, save the leaves and add them to your salad, or if there are enough, cook them as you would other greens.

Brussels Sprouts (Peak season September through February)

Much like miniature cabbages, this vegetable is often rendered unpalatable by overcooking. Ten minutes is sufficient to give them a nice consistency without releasing the strong flavoring acids that make them smelly and strong-tasting.

Look for: Tight, firm leaves with a bright green color, free from worm holes and blemishes.

Avoid: Those with yellow or yellow-green leaves that are soft, loose, or wilted.

Cabbage (Available year-round)

Look for: Heads that are compact and heavy with outer leaves that are deep green or red (depending on the type) and free from blemishes. The outer leaves may be loose, and are usually discarded, so too many loose leaves are wasteful. If there are no outer leaves, but the head is already trimmed, leaving it compact and lacking the characteristic color, you can be fairly certain the head comes out of storage and is not as fresh as the others. It is still satisfactory, though not as rich in vitamins, if it is not wilted or discolored.

Avoid: Outer leaves that are wilted, decayed, or yellow. Worm holes on the outside usually mean worm holes on the inside.

Tips: Cabbage is another vegetable that is often overcooked and consequently considered distasteful by many. This vegetable is extremely rich in vitamin C and you should do everything possible to make it enjoyable. This is not very difficult if you pan-fry it in oil or butter only until wilted (about 10 minutes) and sprinkle it with sesame seeds for added flavor, instead of boiling it to death as most cooks do. Also, serve cabbage raw, alone, or along with other greens in a salad. Fresh cole slaw can make a cabbage-lover out of anyone. Here is a recipe sure to do the trick.

DICKIE'S FAVORITE COLE SLAW

3 cups shredded cabbage
1 teaspoon salt
3 tablespoons raw sugar
3 tablespoons wine vinegar
¼ cup light cream or yogurt
Combine all ingredients. Serve immediately or let marinate in the refrigerator until needed. *Yield:* 1½ pints.

By the way, cole slaw is available in many supermarkets, but since it has been shredded and prepared long before you buy it—much less use it—you are paying an extravagant price for nutrients that have long since been destroyed. In addition, benzoate of soda, tartaric and citric acids may be added (shown on the label). It is cheaper, tastier, and very easy to prepare your own.

Carrots (Available year-round)

Look for: Firm, smooth, well-colored carrots that are fairly regular in shape. Crooked carrots may be just as delicious but lead to excess waste. We find thinner carrots are usually younger and sweeter. If you can find carrots with the green tops still on (and this is rare in most supermarkets), choose those with tops that are fresh-looking.

Avoid: Carrots that have large green areas at the top and those that are flabby or show soft spots.

Tips: The skin and surface just beneath the skin are particularly rich in vitamins. Unless the vegetable is old and the skin noticeably thick a good scrubbing is all that is necessary. The source of vitamin A in carrots can be made more available to the body by cooking, chopping, grating or liquefying the vegetable.

Carrots lend themselves particularly well to "candying" (see "Serving Vegetables"), if they are to be eaten cooked. Grated raw carrots are best for salads.

Cauliflower (Peak season September through November; low May through August)

Although available year-round, it is best to avoid cauliflower during the summer months when it is not really in season and is exorbitantly priced.

Look for: Compact, solid heads with white to creamy white clusters and fresh green leaves if they have not been removed.

Avoid: Heads that show many discolorations, a sign of mold and insect injury, and clusters that are spread, indicating age.

Tips: Before using cauliflower, soak the head briefly in cold, salted water. This will evacuate any lodging insects. Serve the vegetable raw as well as cooked. Particularly good raw for dunking into cheese dips.

Celery (Available year-round)

Look for: Crisp, thick stalks that snap easily. Buy those stalks with as many fresh green leaves as possible. These are delicious for flavoring soups, stews, and egg dishes.

Avoid: Limp, lifeless-looking celery which shows brown discoloration along the stalk and rust marks where they are attached at the base.

Be sure to wash celery well before using.

Chinese Cabbage (Available year-round)

This vegetable is growing in popularity. It is elongated, much like celery, with leaves emanating from a crisp, firm center stalk. It is delicious in salads.

Look for: Crisp, light green plants with no signs of decay.

Avoid: Those with wilted, yellow leaves.

Corn (Peak season May through September)

Although you will find it on the market most of the year, do not buy fresh corn out of season. Corn begins to lose its delicate sweet flavor immediately after harvesting, and unless it is really fresh or in the prime of its life, it will have tasteless starchy kernels rather than ones that are filled with sugar-sweet milk.

Look for: Ears of corn which still have the husks. Once the husk has been removed, the flavor and nutritional value of corn rapidly dissipates. The husk should be a good green color, with silk ends that are free from decay and stems that are neither discolored or dried out. When you pull back the husk, the kernels should be plump and milky. Color is not a reliable indication of quality since some varieties are whiter than others.

Avoid: Ears that have already been husked, husks that are yellow or wilted, kernels that are extremely pale, underdeveloped or shriveled, and ears with oversized kernels.

Tips: Be sure to store corn in the refrigerator and do not remove husks until just before cooking. Three minutes in boiling water is all you need to "set" the milk and have corn that is rich in flavor and nutrients. Do not salt the water as this tends to harden the kernels.

Cucumber (Available year-round with a slight peak in summer)

In most places it's hard to avoid cucumbers that have been waxed, but if you can, do. If not, be sure to peel cucumbers before using them.

Look for: Unwaxed cucumbers with a trim, even shape and a good green color. Small whitish lumps on the surface are characteristic of the vegetable. The diameter of a cucumber should not be too large; this is the sign of an overgrown vegetable.

Avoid: Overgrown cucumbers which will also have a dull color and will be turning yellow. Also those with withered ends and a mushy texture under slight pressure. If you make a poor selection you'll know immediately by the bitter flavor.

Eggplant (Available year-round with a slight peak in late summer)

Eggplant is another vegetable whose skin affords it natural protection against chemical farming. Although the skin is edible it may be necessary to remove it to rid the plant of chemical residue and an often waxed surface.

Look for: Firm eggplants that are heavy for their size with a uniform rich purple color.

Avoid: Those with dark brown spots, poor color, cracked and shriveled skin.

Tips: Although cookbooks often suggest soaking eggplant or dredging it with salt and allowing the "bitter juices" to drain off before using, this only draws out the water-soluble nutrients. A good-quality eggplant will not be bitter in the first place. Store eggplants in a cool, dry place, rather than the refrigerator.

Garlic (Available year-round)

Used mostly for seasoning, garlic is a fresh vegetable and the fresh form is best for giving your foods a garlicky taste.

Look for: Roots that have unbroken casing.

Avoid: Garlic plants with soft, brown spots—a sign of decay.

Tips: The garlic roots should be stored whole in a cool, dry place, but not in the refrigerator, and will last several weeks. To use, remove single cloves as needed and peel off the protective coating.

Greens (Available year-round)

This loose term encompasses many vegetables: spinach, kale, collard greens, turnip greens, beet greens, chard, mustard greens, broccoli leaves, chicory, endive, escarole, dandelion greens, watercress, sorrel. All can be used raw in salads or cooked.

Look for: Greens that look fresh, with a healthy green color and no apparent blemishes.

Avoid: Wilted leaves and those with coarse stems, yellow coloring, and soft, wet decay spots.

Tips: To cook greens, wash well, shake excess water from the leaves, and cook in a covered pot in only the water that clings, for 5 minutes, until wilted. Serve seasoned with salt, butter, sautéed onion, and your favorite herbs. Most greens have a slightly bitter but pleasant flavor.

Leeks (Peak season September, November, and in the spring)

Look for: Crisp, firm leeks with medium-sized necks and an even, light green color.

Avoid: Leeks with wilted, brown outer leaves and soggy roots. Leeks are particularly good served as a vegetable dish lightly steamed or sautéed in butter. If you're not on a diet, sauté wheat germ and bread crumbs in butter as well, and use to top the fresh-cooked leeks. Also recommended for flavoring soups and vegetable stews. The taste is similar to that of onion, only milder and sweeter.

Lettuce (Available year-round)

Lettuce is available year-round and in many different forms. The four main varieties are iceberg, butterhead, romaine, and leaf.

Iceberg lettuce has a nice crisp texture, but sad to say lacks much taste. This is often the most readily available form of lettuce, but do not take this as a sign it is the best. Try to use other kinds of lettuce, and other greens as well, when composing your salads.

Butterhead lettuce, including Boston and bibb, has soft leaves that are often oily (this oil *should* be natural) and quite succulent.

Romaine lettuce includes many species, all with broad, tender leaves and a loose head. This form of lettuce is usually grown and sold locally and is often the freshest.

Look for: The leaves of iceberg and romaine should be crisp, and, for other varieties, tender without being wilted. In most varieties the color will range from medium to light green, and it should always be bright.

Avoid: Iceberg lettuce that is very hard and lacks a rich color; wilted leaves which are brown at the tips, edges, and the stem end for all varieties.

Tips: Lettuce should be washed well before it is used to remove clinging sand or soil, but it should never be soaked in plain or acidulated water. This will only extract the vitamins.

Mushrooms (Available year-round with a low in August)

Look for: Young mushrooms, which will be small to medium in size. The caps (the white portion on top) should be closed around the stem or just slightly open to reveal light tan "gills" (the rows of paper-thin tissue under the cap). The cap surface should be cream-colored or white, although a light brown color is acceptable.

Avoid: Those with wide-open caps and dark gills, those seriously pitted or discolored, and those with a spongy texture.

Tips: Mushrooms absorb water easily, becoming soft and spongy. To avoid this do not soak, but clean by running briefly under water or wiping with a damp cloth. Do not peel mushrooms. Raw mushrooms are wonderful in salads, or marinated in oil-and-vinegar dressing as a salad in themselves.

Okra (Peak season June through September)

Okra is grown and marketed primarily in the South. It is the popular ingredient in "gumbo" and, when cooked, oozes a thick, gooey liquid.

Look for: Pods free from blemishes with tips that bend with very slight pressure. They should be under 4½ inches long.

Avoid: Pods that are tough, indicated by ends that are stiff and won't bend or a very hard body, and those that are pale.

Onions (Available year-round)

Onions are popular both as a seasoning and as a dish in themselves. They can be eaten raw or cooked. The most popular kinds are the ordinary globe onions used for all-purpose cooking and seasoning, the larger Spanish onions (yellow or white-skinned), and Bermuda onions (purplish red) which are somewhat sweeter and ideal for salads.

Look for: Hard, firm onions that have dry skins and small necks. The outer scales should be papery and free of soft spots.

Avoid: Onions that are wet, beginning to sprout, or show excessive green spots on the surface.

Tips: Almost everyone is familiar with onions and has a favorite way of using them. An interesting way of serving onions is one that is not known to many and requires the least amount of preparation. These are Baked Onions, similar to baked potatoes, and can be made by removing only the outer, loosest layers of skin which are already falling off, then placing the onion whole in a 400° oven and baking for

30 to 40 minutes until the outside is crisp and the inside tender. For outdoor or fireplace cookery, which is even tastier, place the onions into the ashes near the hot coals.

Parsley (Available year-round, slight peak October through December)

Parsley is the delicate herb that usually appears as a garnish, gets shoved to the side of the plate, and is ultimately discarded. A big mistake. Parsley is rich in vitamin C, A, iron, and vegetable protein, and is meant to be eaten.

Look for: Crisp, bright leaves for both the curled and flat-leaf variety. Slightly wilted leaves can be freshened by standing the stems in cold water, but this causes some vitamin C loss.

Avoid: Leaves that are yellow or brown and moist, or those that are wilted.

Tips: Extra parsley can be chopped and stored in a plastic bag in the freezer and used for seasoning other dishes. The Arabs use this herb in combination with fresh mint as the basis of a delicious salad. Here is the recipe.

TABBOULEH

½ cup cracked wheat
1½ cups water
2 cups chopped parsley
½ cup chopped mint
½ cup thinly sliced scallion, whites and green
2 cups chopped tomato
¼ cup olive oil
¼ cup lemon juice
½ teaspoon salt
¼ teaspoon pepper sauce

Soak wheat in water about 30 minutes, until tender. In a large bowl toss together parsley, mint, scallion, and tomato. Drain wheat well and add to ingredients in bowl. Pour in oil, lemon juice, sprinkle with salt and pepper sauce, and mix well. Serve on large lettuce leaf scoops. *Yield:* 6 servings.

Parsnips (Peak season October through April)

Although on the market pretty much year-round, parsnips are really a winter vegetable.

Look for: Small or medium-sized parsnips that are smooth and even-shaped, firm and free of surface blemishes.

Avoid: Large parsnips (which usually have thick woody centers), and those that are flabby (they will be tough even when cooked).

Tips: For a flavor that is sweet and nutty, parsnips should be steamed, not boiled. Remove the peel after cooking. Parsnips are a common soup vegetable, but are excellent alone served in the same way you would carrots.

Peas, green (Peak season March through June)

Peas should be bought soon after harvesting or they will lose their sweet flavor. Overripe peas have a flat, starchy taste, similar to raw peanuts.

Look for: Pods that are bright green and velvety to the touch. They should be well filled without being swollen.

Avoid: Underdeveloped pods which are swollen, flecked with gray, and have poor color.

Tips: Peas that are good are *really* good in the natural raw state, straight from the pod. Leave them in the shells until it's time to serve them and then let everyone unshell their own. This is David's favorite "appetite depressant."

Pepper, green or red (Available year-round, slight peak June through September)

Although most of the sweet peppers on the market are green, those that are fully mature (and even sweeter) have a bright red color. Peppers are an excellent source of vitamin C.

Look for: Firm, bright peppers with strong color. Remember, shininess may be misleading since peppers are frequently waxed. They should be relatively heavy for their size. A crooked shape is fine for flavor and nutrition, but may have greater waste.

Avoid: Peppers with very thin walls, apparent by the light weight and flimsy sides, those that are soft, show water spots, and those with a cracked surface.

Tips: Serve peppers raw, or blanch them in boiling water for 5 minutes, then stuff with your favorite meat, grain, cheese, or vegetable combination, and bake in a 350° oven 30 to 40 minutes, until tender. Sauté diced green pepper along with the onion when seasoning soups and sauces.

Potatoes (Available year-round)

Although the lines of demarcation are not quite clear, potatoes fall into three general categories: "new" potatoes, all-purpose potatoes, and baking potatoes.."New" usually signifies those freshly harvested and they are often not fully matured. The outer skin is usually very thin and often dyed (on those that are red). They spoil rather rapidly.

All-purpose potatoes are used for just that—boiling, mashing, frying, baking, and salads, while baking varieties are considered most desirable for producing a potato which is not mealy or dry when cooked in this manner.

Look for: Reasonably smooth, well-shaped potatoes that are firm and free of eyes or excessive sprouting. Dirty potatoes; pre-washed ones have lost some vitamins and absorbed some water. They cost more too.

Avoid: Potatoes with large cuts or bruises, large areas of green, soft spots, and lots of sprouts.

Tips: Potatoes are extremely rich in vitamin C, which is soluble (therefore lost) in water. To save the vitamin C, cook potatoes with the peel on and remove it, if you must remove it at all, after cooking. It is easier to remove then anyway, and you will not lose much more than the thin outer covering.

When you mash potatoes, add a few tablespoons of nonfat dry milk powder or yogurt to the puree for extra protein. Also, try topping baked potatoes with cottage cheese (which can be whipped in the blender to make it creamy) instead of sour cream.

Pumpkin (Available October and November)

Although used mainly for baking pies, pumpkin can be cooked and served in any way you would cook winter squash.

Look for: Firm heavy pumpkins with bright orange skin.

Tips: Cook as you would winter squash by steaming or baking. It is easier to remove the skin after cooking, although it is rather tedious any way you pick.

Radishes (Available year-round, slight peak May through July)

Look for: Medium-size radishes that are firm, round, and of good color.

Avoid: Large flabby radishes and those with yellow or decayed tops. Slight pressure will reveal undesirable spongy ones.

Spinach—See Greens

Squash, summer *(Some form available year-round)*

Although called summer squash, some form of this vegetable is available year-round. Varieties include the green zucchini and the yellow crookneck and straight-neck. All parts, including the skin, are edible.

Look for: Those with good color that are heavy for their size with a rind soft enough to puncture with a fingernail.

Avoid: Squash with a dull surface that has soft spots or a dry, tough surface. Such squash will have enlarged seeds and a dry, stringy texture. Also avoid soft, flabby squash.

Tips: Serve squash pan-fried and seasoned with herbs, or slice it thin and use it raw in salads just as you do cucumber. There is no need to peel squash.

Squash, winter *(Peak season early fall to late winter)*

There are many varieties of winter squash, including Acorn and Butternut (available year-round) and Buttercup, Hubbard, Delicious and Banana.

Look for: Squash that is heavy in relation to size with a tough, hard rind.

Sweet Potatoes and Yams *(Available year-round, low May through July)*

Yams, the more common variety of sweet potato, are moist and sweet with a bright orange color. Regular "sweets" are paler, less moist, and less frequently available.

Look for: Firm, well-shaped potatoes with a smooth, bright, and evenly colored skin. The true quality may sometimes be obscured by the waxing process and artificial coloring, which is applied to sweet potatoes as well as white potatoes.

Avoid: Potatoes with worm holes, cuts, or any surface injury. This leads to waste and rapid decay which will give your potato a bad taste. Look for decay, common in sweet potatoes, at the ends (shriveled, discolored ends are a sign of decay), at the sides in the form of sunken, discolored areas, and finally for wet, soft spots on the skin.

Tips: Sweet potatoes decay more rapidly than other potatoes and should be bought for use in the near future. Store them in a cool, dry place; not the refrigerator.

Serve sweet potatoes as you would any other potato: baked, mashed, boiled, in soups, and in stews. They are a terrific source of vitamin A and can be a real treat topped with honey, maple syrup, or even whipped cream.

Tomatoes (Peak season June through August)

Yes, tomatoes are on the market throughout the year, but the texture of most offerings closely resembles cardboard and the flavor is not even quite that good. The best-flavored tomatoes are generally the locally grown varieties. These are allowed to mature and ripen completely before being picked. They may contain as much as twice the amount of vitamin C as those tomatoes picked and shipped green or those raised in hothouses. The poorest quality tomatoes are those that are picked green and ripened in the truck by ethylene gas on the way to market. It's far better to buy them green and let them ripen in a warm place, out of direct sunlight, in your own home. One important clue to selecting vine-ripened tomatoes seems to be in the smell. As far as we have detected, vine-ripened tomatoes have a fresh tomato odor; gassed tomatoes are odorless.

Look for: Firm, plump tomatoes which have good color, no serious blemishes, and a tomato smell.

Avoid: Overripe and bruised tomatoes which are soft and watery, tomatoes which have growth cracks, and those with water-soaked spots, depressed areas, and surface mold.

Tips: When poor-quality hothouse tomatoes are all that can be found in your supermarket, it's better to do without than to spoil the image your family has of sweet, juicy, high-quality tomatoes. Save the tomato salads for the times when fine tomatoes are around. By the way, if Mexican tomatoes are available in your area, they are of excellent eating quality. Because they are smaller than domestic tomatoes, unduly restrictive import standards requiring a minimum size often make it impossible for them to be brought in.

Turnips and Rutabagas (Peak season October through March)

The most popular turnip has white flesh and purple shading at the top. Most supermarkets remove the leafy tops. Rutabagas are the yellow-fleshed large-sized cousins of the turnip. Although their season is the late fall and winter they are often coated with a paraffin layer and held in cold storage for sale in the spring. Since the skin is inedible the paraffin layer gets removed; however, if the rutabaga is covered with this wax it is best to peel it before cooking.

Look for: Turnips that are small to medium in size, firm, smooth, and fairly round. Rutabagas that are heavy for their size, firm, and round to slightly elongated.

Avoid: Large turnips with obvious fibrous roots and rutabagas with skin punctures or deep surface cuts.

GENERAL SHOPPING NOTES FOR ALL VEGETABLES

•Buy in season.

•Buy only as much as you need. Vegetables are perishable. Overbuying is wasteful.

•Don't look for bargains in vegetables. Bruised or injured vegetables decay rapidly, develop off-flavors, and will only turn your family off to eating them. Slightly overripe vegetables, tomatoes in particular, are often sold at a reduced price and can be purchased to make excellent sauces and soups.

•Handle produce carefully. Vegetables injure easily and injury leads to decay.

•Select vegetables that are fresh-looking and free from bruises and skin punctures. There are government grades and inspection procedures for vegetables; however, few states require this grading. Unless there is an official government seal, the grades offer little assurance of quality. An official shield, however, or the words "USDA inspected" or "Packed under continuous inspection of the U.S. Dept. of Agriculture" can inspire some amount of confidence.

VEGETABLE STORAGE: IN AND OUT OF THE COLD

Most vegetables keep best in the refrigerator and can be held for an average of two to five days. Root vegetables—potatoes, carrots, parsnips, onions, turnips—can be stored from one to several weeks, but keep in mind that the nutritional content of vegetables decreases with every day of storage. Those vegetables that keep best out of the refrigerator include: potatoes, sweet potatoes, onions, winter squash, eggplant, rutabagas, and turnips. These should be stored in a cool, not cold environment, such as a basement or cellar.

COOKING VEGETABLES

As we have indicated, the nutritional benefits you derive from eating most vegetables are greatest when the vegetable is eaten raw. Some, however, must be cooked to be edible, and others are often cooked for variety. If you are going to cook your vegetables you should do it properly so you can preserve the maximum food value and flavor.

Vegetables should be cooked in as little water as possible—just enough to keep them from sticking to the pot. Many vitamins are soluble in water, which means they leach out into the cooking liquid and, unless the liquid is consumed, are lost. Here are some of the cooking methods you can employ to minimize this loss.

Baking

Baking a vegetable in its skin preserves most of the food value. This method can be used with any vegetable that has both a high enough water content to keep it from drying out and little exposed surface or a protective skin. Potatoes, winter squash, and onions and other root vegetables lend themselves to baking. This method does take more time than others—45 minutes to 1 hour.

Steaming

Other than baking, this is the best and most convenient method for conserving nutrients and lends itself to all vegetables. Green vegetables cooked by steaming may not have as bright a color—a factor of little importance compared to flavor and nutritional preservation. To steam a vegetable, place it on a rack, strainer, or adjustable vegetable steamer set above gently boiling water, cover tightly, and let the steam cook the vegetable. Several vegetables can be cooked at once with this method. Vegetable steamers are available in most hardware stores and are a good investment.

Pressure Cooking

Pressure cooking preserves the nutrients in your vegetables and can considerably shorten the cooking time. Careful timing must be used with this method, however, for even one minute too long in the pressure cooker can reduce your vegetables to mush. Most vegetables cook rapidly enough to make this method inefficient. If you do choose pressure cookery, pay close attention to the manufacturer's directions.

Pan-Frying

Sautéing vegetables in melted butter or oil over high heat (similar to the Chinese wok or stir-fry cookery) produces vegetables with bright color and a crisp texture. As vitamin A is fat-soluble (it is absorbed by fat rather than water), any remaining fat should be served along with the vegetable. This type of cooking is recommended for asparagus, green beans, celery, sliced summer squash, cabbage, and root vegetables. Mushrooms and onions are traditionally cooked by this method as well.

Cooking Without Water

Leafy green vegetables should be cooked in a covered saucepan in *only* the water that clings to the leaves after washing. It takes just 3 to 5 minutes to render them soft and ready to eat. Other tender young vegetables (peas, baby carrots) can be cooked this way too by placing them in a dry saucepan and laying a few washed lettuce leaves on top. Cover the pot and let the water that seeps from the greens cook the vegetables. Keep the heat gentle to prevent scorching.

Boiling

Not really recommended, but when you use water to cook your vegetables use only enough to prevent burning—¼ cup will generally do the trick. The time the vegetable remains in the liquid will be reduced if you let the water boil first, then add the vegetables, reduce the heat, and cook covered until just tender. Start root vegetables, however, in cold water so they cook evenly. Green vegetables can be left uncovered for the first 5 minutes of cooking to let the acids which turn them an olive color escape. Never use baking soda to keep the color bright; it destroys the B vitamins.

SERVING VEGETABLES

Vegetables are delicious simply cooked until crisp-tender and served plain or with a dab of butter. For variety, many delicious seasonings can be added that take little more time than the pre-seasoned canned and frozen vegetables that are on the market. Following are some simple sauces that can be used to flavor your freshly cooked vegetables when you wish. Of course, you can experiment with your favorite herbs added to the cooking medium as well. The chapter

"Seasonings: Natural Food Enhancers" will also give you some suggestions.

HERB BUTTER FOR TOPPING OF VEGETABLES

Soften butter to room temperature. Combine with mixed dry herbs allowing ½ to 1 teaspoon of herbs per tablespoon of butter. Prepare as needed or in large amounts, wrap in foil, and store in refrigerator. At serving time remove 1 to 2 tablespoons of seasoned butter from the packet to place on top of each cup of hot vegetables. A pinch of nutmeg or dried mustard, a drop of hot pepper sauce or ¼ teaspoon of lemon juice can be added to each tablespoon of butter as well.

CANDIED VEGETABLES

To "candy" your vegetables simply melt together 1 tablespoon of honey or molasses and 1 tablespoon of butter per cup of cooked vegetables. Gently heat the cooked vegetables in the sweetened butter until coated, about 5 minutes. Spoon any remaining sauce over the vegetables in the serving dish. Longer cooking in the sauce will allow the coating to glaze the vegetables entirely. Ideal for carrots, parsnips, sweet potatoes, and winter squash.

CHEESE-TOPPED VEGETABLES

There are many ways to combine vegetables and cheese on your table. The simplest is to sprinkle a tablespoon of freshly grated cheese over each serving of the hot vegetable. For a more elaborate treatment (and more protein), top the vegetable with a homemade cheese sauce (see "Do-It-Yourself Sauces").

NUTTED VEGETABLES

Vegetables topped with chopped almonds, walnuts, or sesame seeds are delicious. Simply sprinkle the freshly chopped nuts or seeds over the cooked vegetables or pan-fry the nuts or seeds along with the vegetable in hot butter or oil. Dill seed, celery seed, caraway, poppy seed, and wheat germ add new dimensions to your vegetable dish. Try this method with green beans, cauliflower, broccoli, cabbage.

VEGETABLES WITH A FOREIGN FLAIR

To give vegetables an exotic flavor, choose seasonings associated with the country you have in mind. Italian vegetables are made by adding oregano, basil, thyme, and garlic. Mexican vegetables include chili powder, oregano, hot peppers, or pepper sauce. Ginger adds a touch of the Chinese and cumin, turmeric, coriander, and ginger or prepared curry powder and yogurt make it Indian. Chopped olives add a Greek touch.

MARINATED VEGETABLES

Vegetables can be served cold or at room temperature as well as hot. Let them stand in your favorite oil-and-vinegar dressing for 30 minutes at room temperature for a marinated salad or appetizer. Mayonnaise spiked with lemon makes an interesting topping for chilled vegetables too.

QUICK-CREAMED VEGETABLES

With the aid of a blender you can quick-cream your vegetables in seconds. Combine the cooked vegetable (spinach, carrots, cauliflower) and enough cooking liquid or milk or light cream to get the machine going (about 2 tablespoons per cup). Process until creamy. Season to taste with salt, pepper, a pinch of dry mustard, nutmeg, or other desired herbs and spices, and reheat gently.

FROZEN VEGETABLES

Guidelines for Buying Frozen Vegetables

The most important point we can make when it comes to buying frozen vegetables is never buy if you suspect the package has been totally or even partially defrosted. Packages that give when you apply pressure, or are limp, wet, or sweating, are not properly frozen. Packages covered with frost do not keep in the cold and their contents will not be sufficiently frozen either. Packages stained by the contents have at one point been defrosted and refrozen. Avoid all of these. If properly frozen most of the nutrients will be retained. Once thawing begins, food value dissipates at a much more rapid rate than refrigerated fresh vegetables. To avoid vitamin loss frozen vegetables should go directly from freezer to the pot.

The only vegetables you should purchase frozen are those that are unseasoned. Seasoned vegetables, or those in a sauce, may contain modified food starch, MSG, margarine or butter with emulsifiers, coconut oil, hydrolized vegetable protein, sugar, and artificial color. Those that are labeled "Quick Cooking" or "5-Minute Vegetables" have the chemical sodium phosphate added to make them that way. Plain frozen vegetables have nothing but the possible addition of salt. These are the ones you want for your table when good-quality fresh vegetables cannot be obtained. Often the store's own brand is the only suitable choice since many of the major brands concentrate on offering the consumer special seasonings and shortened cooking times, very expensive gimmicks designed to make you think they have something special to offer. *Seabrook, Westpac, Bel Air* and *Dulaney* all offer several vegetables with nothing added.

Vegetables that require peeling—beets, potatoes, carrots—are "specially treated" by food processors to make the job easier. Soaking in a caustic lye bath is one of these treatments, and is destructive to vitamins and minerals. Potatoes, which darken on exposure to light and air, are treated with many chemicals (kind of like embalming fluid) that you would not like to ingest, to prevent this from happening. Stay away from all of these vegetables in the frozen (as well as canned) form.

Fresh lima beans have been practically processed out of existence, so that in most places only the choice of canned or frozen beans remains. If you want to serve your limas, choose the frozen rather than the canned.

Corn that is frozen is usually obtained close to harvesting and may retain most of its original value. Purchase the corn that is frozen on the cob.

Choose vegetables that have been frozen whole over those that are sliced or diced. They may be more costly, but remember, it's vitamins and minerals you're paying for, not chemicals for once.

Grading

Most frozen vegetables are graded, even if the grade does not appear on the package. Those of top grade are usually the most expensive. If a grade is indicated, Grade A or Fancy are the freshest at packing time, Grade B or Extra Standard are slightly mature vegetables. Grade C or Standard indicate mature vegetables with a lower nutritional content which lack prime flavor. Stick with the top or second grade levels only.

VITAMIN LOSS IN VEGETABLES

vegetable	vitamin A	thiamine	riboflavin	niacin	vitamin C
(1 pound)	(I.U.)	(mg)	(mg)	(mg)	(mg)
Peas					
fresh	2900	1.58	.62	13.0	124
canned (with					
liquid)	2040	.52	.26	4.5	40
frozen	3080	1.45	.45	9.3	85
Carrots					
fresh	40920	.22	.20	2.2	29
canned (with					
liquid)	45360	.11	.11	1.6	9
Broccoli					
fresh	8840	.35	.81	3.2	400
frozen	8620	.32	.59	2.5	354
Cauliflower					
fresh	270	.50	.44	3.0	354
frozen	140	.27	.27	2.2	254
Corn kernels					
canned (with					
liquid)	1220	.12	.22	4.1	23
frozen	1590	.50	.32	7.3	38

CANNED VEGETABLES

Guidelines for Buying Canned Vegetables

The canning (and bottling) of vegetables is, as we said earlier, dependent on added chemicals and heat that is highly destructive to nutrients. Rarely should you resort to this form of vegetable. The exceptions to this rule are in the form of pimientos, which are no more than roasted red peppers and water, and canned tomatoes packed in their own liquid or in tomato puree only. Since the liquid is easily included in soups and sauces, canned tomatoes can be substituted when good fresh tomatoes are not available. If calcium salts, acid, or sweetening are added to the tomatoes, it must be stated on the label. Do not buy those brands which include these additions. *Progresso* is one of the few that doesn't.

Instant and dehydrated vegetables (mushrooms are often available in this form) should only be used for seasoning. Instant or dehydrated potatoes are totally unacceptable in a chemical-free (or nutrition-conscious) kitchen.

Note: If you purchase canned vegetables, do not buy cans that are leaking, swollen, or bulged at the end. Bulging and swelling indicate spoilage. Bad dents are harmful to the contents; avoid these cans, even if they are sold at a reduced price.

Vegetables sold in jars (like the pimientos we spoke of) depend on lids that are tightly sealed to preserve the contents. If there is any indication that the lid has been tampered with, choose another container. If you have already gotten the jar home before you discover it's been opened, return it to the store and let the manager know.

RECOMMENDATIONS

General Rule of Purchase: Fresh vegetables are always preferred over canned and frozen. For purchasing guidelines, refer to the description of the vegetable in this chapter. Avoid those fresh vegetables whose skins have been artificially colored or waxed unless you intend to peel them. Select organic vegetables where available.

If you buy canned and frozen vegetables, check the ingredients to see that only salt and water have been added. Buy these vegetables as close to the whole state as possible. Frozen vegetables are always preferred over canned, as you do not pay for added water into which many nutrients dissolve; moreover many frozen varieties have no salt added. However, when peas or limas are in the package, a trace of salt is generally added. Make sure the package is frozen solid, and, if graded, Grades A and B contain vegetables that were the freshest at packing time.

> EXEMPLARY BRANDS:
> Frozen
> East—*Acme Ideal*
> *Bel Air*
> *Country Delight*
> *Deerfield*
> *Dulaney*

Freshlike
Hanover Brands
Pictsweet
Queen of Scot
Red and White
Shop-Rite
Snowcrop
Snow-Kist
Southland
Stokely's Combination Vegetables
Top Frost
Winter Garden
and many other house brands

Middle—*Bel-Air*
Camelot
Flav-R-Pak
Hy-Vee
Janet Lee
Pictsweet
Sno-Fresh
Stillwell
Stokely's Combination Vegetables
Top Frost
V.I.P.
and many other house brands

West—*Bel Air*
Bonnie Hubbard
Camelot
Flav-R-Pak
Janet Lee
Kold Kountry Frozen
Pictsweet
Ralph's
Stokely's Combination Vegetables
V.I.P.
and many other house brands

Other Vegetable Products
Fritini Mix for Vegetable Patties
Golden's Frozen Potato Pancakes
Steakhouse Taboli Salad Mix

Nuts and Seeds

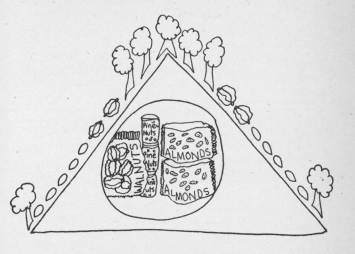

Remember the old description of a real gourmet meal, one that's complete from "soup to nuts"? Well, if you dine at our house some days that's what you might get—a complete meal of soup *and* nuts. Maybe that doesn't sound like much, but those nuts have an awful lot to offer. Most common nuts and seeds are from 10 to 25 percent protein, and a rich source of iron, thiamine, phosphorus, vitamin A, and some calcium. Begin to think of nuts and seeds as protein foods and bear in mind that while most other protein foods (meat, cheese, eggs) add saturated fats to your diet, the fat portion of nuts and seeds is highly unsaturated. Coconuts are the exception here, being high in saturated fats, but then again, they're not a good source of protein, either.

Before we get into the specifics of our nut dinner, let's look at nuts in general. A nut is defined as a dry fruit or seed with a hard, separable shell and an edible interior kernel. Included in this definition are not only the common nuts, but chestnuts and coconuts and the edible seeds like sunflower, pumpkin, and sesame (although sesame seeds are usually sold among the spices in most supermarkets). Because coconuts don't follow the general rules, they will be dealt with separately in the chapter "Picking Fruits." Peanuts are treated like nuts, although biologically speaking they belong to the same family as dry beans, split peas, and lentils.

Many of the nuts available in the supermarket are grown in this country—almonds, pecans, walnuts, filberts, macadamia nuts, and pine nuts. Pine nuts, when they are imported, are often called pignolias. Other imported varieties include pistachios, Brazil nuts, cashews, and chestnuts. Except for chestnuts, sold only in the winter, some form of these nuts can be bought year-round.

NUTS IN A NUTSHELL·

Nuts are sold shelled and unshelled, cashews being the only variety never in the shell. The shell is a natural container for the nutmeat and the best there is for maintaining freshness and preserving the nutritional value. Most nuts in the shell are not roasted. Peanuts, however, usually are roasted as indicated on the label. If unroasted peanuts are sold in your store, you should try them. They are quite different tasting, and although not to our liking, many people find them better this way.

Not only is the shell a natural guard against nutritional depletion, it is the shield of protection against chemical invasion. Although the shells of almost all nuts are treated with lye and gas to soften and loosen them, and although the shell is always bleached and possibly colored and waxed, this mistreatment doesn't penetrate the edible portion, and since you will discard the shell you needn't be too concerned about this processing. Pistachios are the exception here, and if the choice is between dyed red nuts (the natural shell is cream-colored) and no nuts at all, choose the latter.

In all cases these nuts sold in the shell should be your first choice. Although the bleaching of the shells makes it difficult to judge quality, you should look for nuts that are free from splits, cracks, holes, and surface mold.

SHELLED NUTS

Nuts removed from the shell are sold raw, as exemplified by walnuts and almonds, or roasted. Those that are raw may be whole, in pieces, or in slivers. Almonds are usually blanched; this means the outer skin, which is edible and acts as a protective coat, but is not so pretty, is removed in a hot-water bath. Raw cashews are just making their supermarket debut and are far superior in every way to the salted, greasy "cocktail" cashews.

Seeds are usually sold shelled, although sunflower seeds may be left intact. The only time we recommend shelled nuts over unshelled is when they are to be used in quantity for cooking. For instance, unless you intend to eat sunflower seeds as a snack, it would be ridiculous to consider shelling them on your own to incorporate into a recipe. For general eating, though, stick with the sunflower seeds in the shell. Not only will they remain fresher this way, but your teeth and gums will get a good workout cracking the shells.

Once the skins and shells are removed, the nut is left defenseless in the face of the inevitable chemical fumigation.

Shelled nuts are sold in plastic bags, glass jars, and cans. Those in see-through bags are subject to light degradation, but give you the opportunity to check quality. Look for plump kernels uniform in size and color. Those that appear limp, dark, shriveled, or rubbery are stale.

The vacuum-packed cans are your best buy since the nuts are well protected against light and air. With a can, of course, you have no way of judging the quality of the nut, so you'll have to experiment until you find the right brand.

There is absolutely no need to include antioxidants in the nut package, but many processors do. When any such preservative is used it will be stated on the package.

FRENCH-FRIED NUTS

The most serious step in nut adulteration comes with the roasting. It would be more accurate to call this processing "French frying" because what actually happens is the nuts are fried in a bath of grease —in oil that is continually being heated and reheated—and then heavily salted. This is what you are munching when you are served "cocktail nuts." Shelled, roasted nuts are therefore never included in our recommended list of supermarket goodies. If you only like roasted nuts, roast them at home where you can control the cooking.

HOME-ROASTED NUTS

Take nuts (or seeds for that matter) of your choice and spread on a baking sheet or shallow pan. Bake in a 350° oven for 5 to 10 minutes until lightly browned. For a richer flavor and more even browning you can add 1 teaspoon of oil per cup of nutmeats.

The same procedure can be used to roast nuts still in the shell, like unroasted peanuts. To do this, increase the baking time to 15 or 20 minutes. When they are sufficiently roasted you'll find that when you remove the shell the skin will slip right off and the meat will be delicately browned.

Jars of dry-roasted nuts, made particularly appealing for dieters and people paying attention to fat consumption, are almost as undesirable as the regular roasted ones. They boast "no oils" but many add sugar, all add salt, starch, MSG, vegetable gums, and spices, and still others add preservatives.

Macadamia nuts, although delicious, are prepared with highly saturated coconut oil which limits their desirability for many consumers.

BUYING AND STORING GUIDE

As a buying guide, 1 pound of nuts in the shell will make 1½ to 2½ cups of nutmeats once the shells are removed.

To remain fresh and crunchy, nuts must be protected from heat, air, and moisture. The best way to store them, both in the shell and out, is in a large, covered jar or container at room temperature, out of direct sunlight. Nuts in the shell can be kept out in a bowl for people to snack on for short periods of time. If your storage area gets hot, particularly in the summertime, keep the closed nut jars in the refrigerator. Opened vacuum-packed nuts should also be kept in the refrigerator. Properly stored, nuts will last for six months without losing their quality or going rancid.

A SPECIAL WORD ON CHESTNUTS

The only nut which must be cooked in some way before it can be eaten is the chestnut. These nuts are much more starchy than other nuts and not nearly as nutritionally valuable. They are, however, delicious for snacking, so we'll tell you how to roast them any way.

TO ROAST CHESTNUTS

Make a slash through the shells with a sharp knife along the flat side of the nut. Place on a baking sheet, cut side up, and roast in a 400°F oven about 20 minutes. When they are ready they will be tender when probed with a fork through the cut in the shell. To cook them over a fire use the same slitting method, only this time place the nuts on a grill and turn them occasionally during roasting.

NUTS IN YOUR MEALS

Now we're ready to discuss using those nuts in your family's meals. Because nuts are low in certain amino acids, the building blocks of protein, you can enhance the quality of your protein when you combine nuts in a meal with dried beans, milk products, grains, or even other nuts and seeds. One way to accomplish this is to add nuts, chopped or ground, to a variety of dishes. Here are some examples.

•Combine chopped nuts with other ingredients for stuffing meat, fish, or poultry.

•Add chopped nuts to all baked products—breads, cookies, cakes —as well as frostings and fillings.

•Top puddings, cooked cereal, and steamed grains with chopped walnuts, slivered almonds, or pumpkin seeds.

•Thicken soup by blending in 1 tablespoon of peanut butter (instead of flour) per quart of soup. This will give you a creamy broth with a very hearty taste.

•Use sunflower seeds as a standard salad ingredient; add a tablespoon of sesame seeds to flavor the dressing.

•When preparing fried rice and vegetables, stir in a handful of pine nuts or sunflower seeds.

•Sauté sesame seeds and slivered almonds in oil and then add vegetables for pan-frying.

•Garnish dried bean dishes with chopped nuts or add ground nuts to bean purees for making dips, bean patties, or fillings.

•Use nuts to stuff dried fruits, enhance cottage cheese and cream cheese for sandwich spreads; to enrich seafood and egg salads.

•Make pancake and dessert toppings by combining honey or maple syrup with chopped walnuts and pecans. Call it "Praline Syrup."

Aside from their use as a garnish for other dishes, nuts can be the basis of the meal itself. One of our prize dinners is in the form of this nut roast.

NUT ROAST

1¾ cups mixed nuts (walnuts, almonds, sunflower seeds, raw cashews)
1 small onion, chopped
1 tomato, chopped
2 eggs, lightly beaten
2 tablespoons wheat germ
1 tablespoon oil
1 teaspoon salt
¼ teaspoon pepper
2 teaspoons soy sauce or brewer's yeast
    or
1 teaspoon mixed herbs or thyme

Grind nuts to a powder. Combine with remaining ingredients, pack into a greased loaf pan, or shape into a loaf on a greased cookie sheet. Brush with additional oil and bake in a 350° oven for 40 minutes. *Yield:* 4 servings.

This is especially delicious with tomato sauce or onion gravy (see "Do-It-Yourself Sauces").

MORE ON NUTS

Nuts are always popular with bakers, and not only can they be added to batters for texture, they can be ground or finely chopped to replace the flour in many baked products. Next time you need a pie shell try this one:

WALNUT CRUST

Combine ¾ cup of finely ground walnuts, ½ cup of whole wheat flour, 2 tablespoons of oil and 2 tablespoons of raw sugar. Press into 9-inch pie plate. Fill and bake as usual, or for unbaked pies, bake in 375°F oven about 10 minutes, until lightly browned.

For many people who cannot tolerate milk, nuts provide a fine substitute that comes in handy for moistening cereals or making a refreshing drink.

NUT MILK

1 cup nuts (peanuts, blanched almonds, or raw cashews)
2 cups water
2 teaspoons honey

Grind nuts until powdery at high speed of blender. Add water and process until smooth. Additional water can be added to thin "milk" if desired. Stir in honey. *Yield:* about 2½ cups.

Don't forget, nuts right from the shell or package are ideal for random eating. Many people shy away from nuts because they are high in calories. In reality nuts may be a good way for dieters to cut down on their food intake. Because they are so high in fat, nuts have "staying power" or what is known as satiety value, which means a few nuts can put a curb on your appetite and keep you from overeating when you shouldn't.

NUT BUTTERS

Another form in which you can buy nuts is nut butter, peanut butter being the most available. Peanut butter, a very rich source of protein, theoretically should be no more than ground peanuts with nothing else added. When the commercial manufacturer makes peanut butter, though, he adds lots of salt and, as permitted under the federal standard of identity, additional peanut oil, making the product up to 55 percent fat. Because the oil has a tendency to separate out and collect on the top of the jar, the manufacturer also adds hardened oils (often cottonseed oil) which act as an emulsifier and keep the peanut butter smooth. Sugar and dextrose are added to impart the too-sweet taste.

The only brands of peanut butter which are free of these additives are those found in the special natural foods section or those freshly ground at the store. *Deaf Smith* brand is the very best and the soil in which the peanuts are grown is reputed to be the richest in the country. The trace minerals transferred from the soil to the nuts make this peanut butter more healthful than any other, according to some nutritionists. If the oil separates in any of these unprocessed peanut butters, all you have to do is stir it smooth again.

If unprocessed peanut butter is not available to you, you'll be astonished to find how simple it is to make excellent peanut butter at home.

HOMEMADE PEANUT BUTTER

Remove shells from peanuts to make 2 cups of nuts. Process nuts in an electric blender (or clean meat grinder) until powdery, then gradually add up to ¼ cup of peanut or safflower oil, 1 tablespoon at a time, blending completely. Stop blender from time to time to push the peanuts into the center. When the peanut butter is the consistency you like, stir in ½ teaspoon of salt and about 1 teaspoon of honey to heighten the flavor. Store this peanut butter in a covered container. When you're ready to use it, if you find the oil has separated, simply stir it smooth with a knife.

Shelling the nuts for nut butter, we'll grant you, is not the most stimulating job, but this rich nut butter will be worth it. If you have any available children, assign the task to them . . . and if they sneak a few nuts in the process they'll only profit from it.

Although not commonly marketed, raw cashews, almonds, pecans, and walnuts all make interesting nut butters. Make some in your blender, just like you did with the peanuts.

Although you can store peanut butter in a covered container on your shelf, it will keep fresher longer in the refrigerator. Remove from the refrigerator a few minutes before needed to increase the spreadability.

TAHINA

Sesame seed butter, or tahina, a Mid-Eastern specialty, is also sold in many supermarkets. This product, a puree of sesame seeds and oil, is thinner than other nut butters, very high in protein, and better used in combination with other foods than as a spread by itself. Since it is rich in both calcium and phosphorus it makes an excellent substitute for milk.

When mixed initially with other ingredients, even liquids like water, tahina thickens and becomes stiff. It is best to beat in these additions briskly with a fork to obtain a smooth consistency. As you add more liquid, the paste will thin out and become creamy and saucelike.

●Try combining equal amounts of tahina and cottage cheese for a delicious spread for crackers and raw vegetables.

●Beat 2 tablespoons of tahina and 1 tablespoon of lemon juice into 1 cup of yogurt. Season with salt, cumin, or garlic, and serve as a dip.

•Mix tahina with cooked spaghetti or noodles for a nutritious nut-flavored pasta.

•For a sweet topping combine tahina with an equal amount of honey.

Other uses for tahina, which by the way is the main ingredient in halvah, can be found in Mid-Eastern cookbooks.

RECOMMENDATIONS

Nuts and Seeds

General Rule of Purchase: Select unroasted, unsalted nuts, preferably still in the shell. When purchasing nuts and seeds in a package, both the vacuum-packed cans and see-through bags are acceptable provided they contain no preservatives or antioxidants. Read the label to see that the shells are not artificially colored; bleached shells are almost impossible to avoid. Roasted nuts are generally deep fried and highly salted; dry-roasted nuts contain sweeteners, vegetable stabilizers, and salt.

Untreated nuts and seeds are frequently located in the "health foods" section, if your supermarket has one.

EXEMPLARY BRANDS:
    Nuts
        Blue Diamond Almonds
        Cimino
        Country Fair
        Diamond Walnuts
        Jean Fisher ("No Preservative and Color" varieties)
        Nature Kist
        Planter's Southern Belle Brand
        Trophy
    Seeds
        Balance of Nature Sunflower Seeds
        Cimino
        Country Fair Sunflower Seeds

> *David's* Sunsnax Sunflower Seeds
> *Dell'Alpe* Sesame Seeds
> *El Molino* Sunflower Seeds; Sesame Seeds
> *Jean Fisher* Sunflower Seeds
> *Marbopaks* Sunflower Seeds
> *Marconi* Sesame Seeds
> *Nature Kist* Sunflower Seeds, hulled and in the shell;
> Sesame Seeds
> *Planter's* Southern Belle Brand Sunflower Seeds

Unsweetened Coconut
> *Cimino*
> *Nature Kist*

Nut Butters

General Rule of Purchase: The only acceptable nut butters contain nothing but the ground nut plus salt. Most commercial manufacturers add sugar, dextrose, and hydrogenated oil to their peanut butter, as hown on the label.

EXEMPLARY BRANDS:
Peanut Butter
> East—*Country Pure* Old Fashioned
> > *Elam's* Natural Peanut Butter with defatted
> > wheat germ (unsalted)
> > *Farm King*
> > *Hazel* Old Fashioned
> > *Hollywood* (salted and unsalted)
> > *Lucerne* Old Fashioned
> > *Mi-del* Dietetic (unsalted)
> > *Red Wing* Old Fashioned
> > *Riverside* Old Fashioned
> > *Shedd's* Old Fashioned
> > *Shopwell* Old Fashioned
> > *Smuckers* (refrigerated variety only)
>
> Middle—*Country Pure* Old Fashioned
> > *Elam's* Natural Peanut Butter with defatted
> > wheat germ (unsalted)
> > *Hazel* Old Fashioned

Hollywood (salted and unsalted)
Holsum Old Fashioned
Home Brand (refrigerated)
Lucerne Old Fashioned
Mary Sherman's Holsum

West—*Adams* Old Fashioned

All American Creamy Old Fashioned (refrigerated, salted and unsalted)
Coop Old Fashioned
Country Pure Old Fashioned
Elam's Natural Peanut Butter with defatted wheat germ (unsalted)
Hain's Raw and Toasted (unsalted)
Hollywood (salted and unsalted)
Holsum Old Fashioned
Laura Scudders' Old Fashioned
Lucerne Old Fashioned
Sunny Jim Old Fashioned
Toner

Other Nut Butters

Hain's Unsalted Sunflower Butter
Hollywood Cashew Butter (unsalted)
Joyva Sesame Tahini
Sahadi Sesame Tahini
Ziyad's Brand Tahini

Filling the Cereal Bowl: Cold Cereals

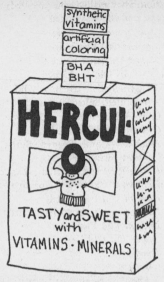

The dry breakfast cereal controversy is by no means over. In the summer of 1970, America was faced with a food scandal; the focal point of the American breakfast, served daily to men, women, and children for energy and nourishment, turned out to be a big fraud. Consumer advocate Robert Choate decried the claims of cereal manufacturers (three of whom produce 80 percent of all commercial cereals) that the product was a source of protein, vitamins, and minerals.

The result of the scandal was not a reduction in the sales of dry cereal, but a superficial effort on the part of the industry to correct its mistakes. But what can you do to enrich a product whose very nature depends on the steaming, drying, pressurization, toasting, flaking, and what-have-you of once-healthy grains like rice, corn, wheat, and oats? We say once-healthy, because after such a degree of handling all the original protein, phosphorus, and vitamins A and B can't help but be cooked out. Well, the only thing left, unless you change the entire process, is to add nutrients (synthetic ones) back. And so all that the cereal industry has done to change the picture is increase the vitamin fortification. That fortification, which costs General Mills about 0.6¢ per package, is now available to you at 15 to 20¢ more than the identical, unfortified brand.

Even if the nutritional value of these cereals was significantly improved (which it has not been), would they provide a wholesome breakfast?

To begin with, this "favorite breakfast of children" may be as much as 35 to 50 percent sugar, and that's before you add any sweetening of your own. The artificial coloring used is certainly of questionable value, particularly since one of the most popular additions, "Red 2" connection with its possible role in causing birth defects.* Then there are the preservatives BHA and BHT which extend the life of the cereal far beyond necessity. These very same preservatives are banned from baby foods in Great Britain and severely restricted in all other foods.

WHAT CHOICES CAN YOU MAKE?

Any way you look at it, dry cereal is convenient, and children love it. How can you persuade anyone to give up a combo like that? Well, you don't have to. It's merely a matter of being more selective in the choices you make.

We cannot recommend any of the American-style cereals—the flakes, "O's," crispies—that so many of us grew up on. They are all overprocessed, oversweetened, and overpriced. They do not serve the essential nutritional function of a "cereal"—that is, a breakfast food derived from whole grains with all their inherent benefits. All the time advertising has been drawing you to the cereal aisle in search of the latest "Sugar-Frosted Fortified Fake," there have been boxes of truly nutritious cereal just a few steps away which are not so well known.

Under the descriptive phrase "Swiss Breakfast Cereal," *Familia* has long been selling their brand of "muesli" (a rich blend of oat flakes, dried apple flakes, wheat and rye, millet flakes, raisins, unrefined sugar, honey, crushed almonds and wheat germ) via the supermarket. Now other brands of muesli are entering the supermarket scene as well, among them *Lutin Bircher* Muesli and the quite similar *Frutifort* from *Zwicky*. There's even a special muesli sold for babies.

---

*In January 1976 the FDA banned the future use of Red Dye No. 2 since "they cannot establish the safety of it." It will probably be replaced by another unnecessary coloring of undetermined safety, Red Dye No. 4.

Muesli is cereal as it should be. The grains are not processed; the sweetening is unrefined, much of it coming from the naturally sweet dried fruits in the package; the vitamin "enrichment" is in the form of natural wheat germ. When this cereal is mixed with milk it is transformed into a soft, rich porridge, both naturally sweet and satisfying. As a matter of fact, it's so good we sometimes sprinkle it on ice cream for a topping.

Zwicky offers other varieties of dry cereal in the form of Wheat Flakes and Millet Flakes, and *Uncle Sam* Cereal combines whole wheat flakes and flaxseed for a blend similar to the more traditional "flakes," but with no artificial color or preservatives added.

Another chemical-free breakfast food that has really caught on is "granola" (which might be labeled "Crunchy," "Super," or something akin to that preceding the granola). Granola is essentially a mixture of rolled oats, wheat germ, and sesame seeds plus nuts, coconut, and dried fruits, depending on the particular brand, lightly sweetened with honey or raw sugar and lightly toasted to preserve the nutrients. The cereal created is everything you could ask for—flavorful and crunchy—and it keeps you satisfied for hours. True, it's somewhat more expensive than the commercial cereals, but you're really getting something worthwhile for your money. As it is, granola is very simple to reproduce in your own kitchen and you can be especially creative with it, adding nuts and dried fruits to suit your fancy. The more rolled oats you use in proportion to other ingredients the less costly it will be. We always make our own granola using ingredients readily available in your supermarket. Here's one of our favorite variations:

GRANOLA

3 cups oats
½ cup wheat germ
¼ cup *each* chopped almonds, peanuts,
    pumpkin seeds, sunflower seeds
¼ cup sesame seeds
½ cup raisins
¼ cup honey
¼ cup oil
¼ teaspoon vanilla

Combine oats, wheat germ, nuts, sesame seeds, and raisins. Heat together honey, oil, and vanilla, pour over oat mixture, and mix well to coat all dry ingredients. Spread into one large or two small shallow baking pans. Bake in a 325° oven 15 to 20 minutes until lightly browned. Stir halfway through baking so ingredients at bottom have a chance to brown. Baking time varies with the oven, so check occasionally, making sure the raisins don't burn. *Yield:* about 2 pounds.

Granola and muesli are served like all dry cereals, with milk and fresh fruit. Both are especially delicious, however, when unflavored yogurt or applesauce replace the milk.

WHEAT GERM

Did you grow up thinking wheat germ was something akin to sawdust that health nuts sprinkled on everything they ate? You may have been partially right, because wheat germ actually is quite good on just about anything. As a matter of fact, although it doesn't have much in common with sawdust (except maybe its appearance), if the processed meat manufacturers added it to their frankfurters instead of some of the things they are rumored to throw in, they might be on the right track toward improving their product.

Wheat germ is the site of nourishment for the growing wheat plant. In the milling of white flour the germ, rich in B vitamins and protein, is removed.

In the Cereal Bowl . . .

Wheat germ is traditionally sold in the cereal section of your supermarket, and although its uses extend far beyond the cereal bowl, with milk and fruit it is a very tasty and healthy meal. *Kretchmer* toasted wheat germ has been the leading supermarket brand for years, and the plain, unflavored variety is a fine shopping choice. There's no need to buy wheat germ presweetened with "Sugar 'n' Honey." Add your own sweetener and you'll save on money, unwanted additives, and will be able to use your wheat germ in savory as well as sweet dishes. Other brands of wheat germ are being introduced into the supermarket these days and we've noticed *Robert's* and *Apollo* on many shelves. So far, none of the unflavored brands we've encountered have anything added, so you're free to choose as you like.

Wheat germ is more perishable than other dry cereals and once opened should be stored in the refrigerator to prevent rancidity. Up until now, the toasted kind only was available in the supermarket.

With the growth of natural foods departments in many stores, raw wheat germ is now being made available as well *(Stone Buhr, Fisher, Loma Linda)*. Although the toasted is usually preferred for taste (especially if it is to be used alone as a cereal), the raw wheat germ has more vitamins. Fewer vitamins will be lost if you purchase it raw and toast it yourself in a dry skillet over low heat.

If you don't serve wheat germ plain as a breakfast cereal, be sure to sprinkle it on top of the cereal you've selected and, if your family insists on TV-advertised brands of dry cereal, at least purchase the unsweetened kind and improve it with a tablespoon of wheat germ sprinkled on each serving.

Wheat Germ Improves Almost Everything

Try using wheat germ in some of these ways to enhance the quality of your favorite dishes:

•Add ¼ cup of wheat germ to every 1 cup of flour or bread crumbs when coating meat, fish, poultry, or vegetables, or in making crumb topping.

•Sprinkle a tablespoon of wheat germ into meat, fish, and egg salads. No one will ever know it's there.

•Add it to ground meat mixtures before shaping your meat loaf, hamburger, or meat balls.

•Sprinkle 1 heaping teaspoon of wheat germ over individual bowls of salad, both fruit and vegetable, for a crunchy garnish.

•Enhance a sandwich with a teaspoon of wheat germ layered over the bread spread.

•Add 2 tablespoons of wheat germ per cup of flour to the batter for bread, cakes, and cookies.

•Let toasted wheat germ serve as an ice cream or pudding topping.

•Rolling cheese balls, candy, or fruit in chopped nuts, dried fruit, or coconut? Why not toss in some wheat germ as well!

RECOMMENDATIONS

General Rule of Purchase: All ingredients on label. Choose those made from unprocessed oats, wheat, rye, millet, corn, fortified naturally with wheat germ, brewer's yeast, seeds, flaxseed, dried fruit and sweetened with honey, molasses, or raw sugar. Watch for artificial color and BHT and BHA preservatives. Do not be taken in by brands which claim to be "natural" and then include large quantities of refined sugar. Remember, ingredients are listed in descending order of predominance.

EXEMPLARY BRANDS:
  Wheat
  El Molino Puffed Wheat
  Hadley's Red Wheat Cereal
  Skinner's Raisin Bran
  Uncle Sam Cereal
  Zwicky Wheat Flakes
  Corn
  Hadley's Puffed Yellow Corn
  Millet
  El Molino Puffed Millet
  Hadley's Puffed Golden Millet
  Zwicky Millet Flakes
  Rice
  El Molino Puffed Rice (whole grain)
  Hadley's Puffed Brown Rice
  Granola
  Back-to-Nature Honey Granola; Honey-Almond Granola; 7-Grain Honey Granola; Honey Raisin Granola
  Natural Life Foods Honey Almond Granola
  OM Brand Honey Granola
  Pro-Vita Honey Nut Crunch; Frunola
  Muesli
  Alpen
  Familia
  Lutin Bircher Muesli
  Swissy Swiss Mixed Cereal
  Zwicky Fruitifort

Wheat Germ
  any brand, toasted or untoasted, but not presweetened
  Apollo
  Catherine Clark's Wheat Germ Nuggets
  El Molino (raw)
  Elam's (raw)
  Fisher (raw)
  Harrington's Hodgson Mills
  Hollywood
  Kretchmer
  Loma Linda (raw)
  Robert's
  Stone Buhr (raw)
Raw Bran
  El Molino
  Elam's
  Harrington's Hodgson Mills
  Jolly Joan
  Stone Buhr

The Kellogg Company has begun to disclose the sugar content of its cereals; this information will appear on cereal boxes in the near future.

Based on Kellogg's data, its products contain the following proportions of sugar, by weight:

Cereal	Percent Sugar	Cereal	Percent Sugar
All-Bran	14	Frosted Mini-Wheats	28
Apple Jacks	56	Frosted Rice	39
Bran Buds	25	Pep	14
Cocoa Krispies	46	Product 19	11
Concentrate	11	Raisin Bran	21
Corn Flakes	7	Rice Krispies	11
Country Morning	25	Special K	7
Country Morning with		Sugar Frosted Flakes	42
raisins and dates	21	Sugar Pops	39
40% Bran	18	Sugar Smacks	56
Froot Loops	53		

Courtesy Center for Science in the Public Interest

Filling the Cereal Bowl: Hot Cereals

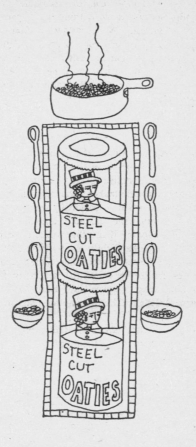

Although cold cereals are somewhat more alluring than hot cereals from the cook's standpoint, cooked cereal is a breakfast with real staying power, particularly on a cold, damp day. Unrefined grains (which is what the following cereals are made from) are your most valuable source of B vitamins and, in combination with milk, offer high-quality protein.

In the past, cookbooks advised long cooking times for hot cereal in the belief that this would improve flavor. Today, however, it has been proven that hours of cooking do nothing of the sort, and cooking beyond "doneness" only destroys the food value. Many cereals can be cooked in half the time you may have been anticipating.

Be sure you avoid the enriched cereals (this implies something was removed, which is why the enrichment is necessary) and the quick-cooking cereals (made so by enzyme treatment or the addition of disodium phosphate).

OATMEAL

Luckily, when oats are milled, the bran and germ (the richest source of vitamins and minerals in all cereals) remain in the edible portion. Oats are an inexpensive source of nutrients, and a bowl of oatmeal with butter and milk makes a warming, satisfying breakfast.

Packages of steel-cut oats are occasionally seen on the supermarket shelf. Steel-cut oats retain the maximum amount of nutrition, but often require longer cooking than other forms of oatmeal. *Quaker* Old-Fashioned Oats offers a slightly less nutritious alternate in only five minutes. Prepare the cereal according to the package directions, and if you like you can further enrich the meal by cooking the cereal in milk rather than water. *Quaker* Old-Fashioned Oats is the only common supermarket choice that puts nothing but untreated oats in the package.

Many of the "Quick Oats" do not contain additives, but are over-processed so that we cannot give them our recommendation.

WHEATENA

Wheatena is another old favorite among cereal fans that is untainted with chemicals. There's just no need to alter the natural rich flavor, decrease the cooking time (which is only five minutes), fortify the grains (already vitamin- and mineral-rich), or extend the keeping quality. Again, simply follow the package directions to prepare this cereal.

CORNMEAL

Cornmeal is a rich source of vitamin A that cooks up smooth and creamy, much like farina. Stone-ground and water-ground cornmeal, milled by the old process which is still carried on in many areas today, is far richer than the degerminated roller-ground version which requires synthetic enrichment to replace the lost elements. If you live in the southern part of the United States you should have no trouble locating the stone-ground kind with the germ intact. *Indian Head* is one brand offered in the North as well which retains the whole grain. The key word to watch for when you shop for cornmeal is "unbolted." If the word "degerminated" appears instead, this is your sign that the vitamins and minerals have been processed away. Degerminated cornmeal will have (partial) synthetic enrichment. Yellow cornmeal is a richer source of vitamin A than white.

Use cornmeal instead of farina, hominy, cream of wheat, and cream of rice, which all have the bran and germ removed.

CREAM OF RICE

For those who like cream of rice you can try your own homemade rice cereal made from brown rather than polished white rice, which is what the commercial brands use. This is how it's done:

CREAM OF BROWN RICE

Wash 2 cups of brown rice, drain well, and toast in a dry skillet until rice grains are completely dry, about 5 minutes. Grind to a powder at high speed in blender. Return rice powder to the dry skillet and toast lightly.

To cook, follow the Basic Cereal Cookery directions in this section, allotting 15 minutes cooking time. This will result in a thick porridge. Thin with milk at serving time. *Yield:* 2 cups uncooked; enough for 8 to 10 servings.

OTHER CHOICES

Other grains (see "The Grain Silo") like kasha and cracked wheat can be served for breakfast as well. Cooking in milk rather than water will provide a rich porridge for your meal. And if you have any cooked grains left from a previous meal, reheat them and serve for breakfast with hot milk and honey.

Other cereals to keep an eye out for, available in some supermarkets, not in others, include: rolled rye (the rye counterpart of oatmeal), *Roman Meal* and *Grist Mill* Cereal (a powder-packed blend of wheat germ, yeast, flaxmeal, rosehips, sunflower seed meal, rice, bran, kelp, lecithin, malt, papaya, and raw sugar) that can be served both hot and cold. Now that's the way to start a day!·

BASIC CEREAL COOKERY

Any time directions are not included with your purchase, or the given directions don't turn out the way you hoped, here is a basic guide to cereal cookery:

For fine grained cereals (cornmeal, cream of brown rice) allow ¼ cup of uncooked cereal and 1 cup of water, milk, or a combination of these for each serving. For coarser grains (oats, rye, Wheatena), increase the proportion to ½ cup of cereal. Bring liquid with a pinch of salt to a boil. Gradually sprinkle in cereal so that the liquid never ceases to boil. Reduce heat and boil gently until grain is cooked and cereal reaches desired consistency. This will vary from 5 minutes to 1 hour (for steel-cut rolled oats and whole brown rice cooked for cereal). Stir only once, unless you like your cereal gummy.

• *For the more finely ground cereals* that have a tendency to lump (like cornmeal), make a paste of cereal combined with an equal amount of cold water before you add it to the remaining liquid that has been brought to a boil.

• *For a creamy consistency* combine uncooked cereal, salt, and cold water in a saucepan and bring to boil together. Stir once, reduce the heat, and simmer until water is absorbed.

• *To create flavored cereals* and eliminate the need for sweetening, cook cereal with diced dried prunes, apricots, dates, figs, or raisins; or try slicing a fresh peeled apple into the pot and cook it along with your porridge. Sprinkle with nutmeg and cinnamon.

• *Instead of sugar* sweeten cooked cereal with honey, fruit juice, molasses, or pure maple syrup. Stir in a handful of raisins and let children search for the hidden fruit as they consume their breakfast. Or serve a savory cereal with plenty of milk, a pat of butter, and salt. Fat remains in the system longer than sugar so that adding a bit of butter to your morning meal keeps you satisfied longer. A spoonful of peanut butter will have the same effect.

• *Enhance the protein* of cereal and add variety to the texture with a topping of chopped walnuts, peanuts, sunflower seeds, and a spoonful of wheat germ.

A REMINDER

Instant cereals are hardly worth the "instant." In only five more minutes you can serve your family a breakfast that really offers them something of value.

RECOMMENDATIONS

General Rule of Purchase: Choose cereals made with whole grains enriched with wheat germ and brewer's yeast only. Check the label for treatment with enzymes or disodium phosphate to make them "quick cooking." Additional grains suitable for hot breakfast cereals are included in "The Grain Silo."

EXEMPLARY BRANDS
Oats
> never the "instant" variety
> *Buckeye* Old Fashioned Rolled Oats
> *El Molino*
> *National* Oats Company 3 Minute Brand Old Fashioned Oats; Raisin Oats with defatted wheat germ
> *Old Fashioned Mother's* Oats
> *Quaker* Old Fashioned
> *Triangle* Cream Flake Rolled Oats

Wheat
> *All-O-Wheat* Steel Cut Breakfast Wheat
> *Clinton's* 100% Whole Wheat Cereal
> *Dina-Mite* Whole Wheat Hot Cereal
> *Fisher* Zoom
> *Harrington's* Hodgson Mill Wheat-Soy Grits

    Pettijohns Rolled Whole Wheat
    Quaker Whole Wheat Hot Natural Cereal
    Wheatena

Rye
    Cream of Rye

Cornmeal—unbolted, not degerminated; stone or water ground
    Adelita
    Dixie Lily White Water Ground
    El Molino
    Elam's
    Harrington's Hodgson Mill Yellow and White
    Indian Head Yellow and White
    Olde Mill Stone Ground

Mixed Grains
    Country Harvest 100% Natural Hot Cereal
    Grist Mill
    Old Fashioned *Maltex*

Red River Cereal
    Roman Meal
    Stone Buhr Seven Grain Cereal; Quick Cooking Four Grain Cereal; Manna Golden Cereal; Hot Apple Granola

Picking Fruit

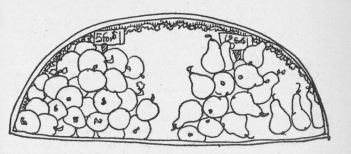

Selling your family and friends on the idea of eating fruit should not be very hard if you learn to select fruits that are ripe and ready to give their natural sweetness and juiciness. The trouble with most fruit on the market today, though, is that it is picked while still immature and thus never has a chance to develop to its fullest potential. Fruit that is harvested once it has matured can offer you a food that is as satisfying to your sweet tooth as the richest of desserts.

As with vegetables, the season for marketing fruit has been overextended to meet what is termed "consumer demands." A peach cannot be flavorful in the middle of January when nature does not favor its ripening until the beginning of June. Obviously, then, the key to buying fruit is to buy in season. To determine what the season is, consult the listings below.

The story of fruit is similar to that of vegetables in other ways as well. Fruits, too, are grown in soil that is fed chemicals to increase productivity. Fruit crops are sprayed with chemical pesticides and herbicides. The thick rind of some fruits will give the underlying flesh natural protection against these chemicals. In this group are pineapple, melons, bananas, and mangoes. For other fruits there is not much to be done but give them a thorough washing, peel them when possible, and hope for the best. Grapes and cherries are among those that are heavily sprayed with no outside skin to protect them against high levels of chemical residue.

To lengthen the growing season the plants are manipulated in ways that alter their original characteristics and bring about a change in taste and nutritional value at the same time. Modern fruit raisers' achievements include seedless lemons, grapes with elongated bodies that adhere tightly to the stems (for the purpose of making harvesting easier since grapes that fall readily from the vine are difficult to retrieve), and grapefruit the size of melons. Unfortunately, most of these "freaks" are not nearly as tasty as the original species.

To lure you to buy, even when you know a fruit is not in season, fruits are dolled-up to promise more than they can deliver. Citrus fruits have for years had coloring applied to their skins to make them more attractive. For the first time many citrus growers and packers are curtailing this process. Take advantage of this and buy oranges that may be paler, or show some green on the rind. The quality inside is just as good, you run less risk of ingesting harmful food dyes when you grate the rind into cakes, puddings, and other dishes, and moreover you're telling the fruit growers that this is the way you want your fruit.

Apples, pears, and plums are fruits that are commonly waxed to give them a glossy look on the display counter. When you purchase waxed fruits your best bet is to peel them before you eat them. For years Nikki thought she was allergic to apples—every time she ate one she was overcome by nausea and indigestion. She has since learned that a peeled apple or an unwaxed variety (a rarity indeed) has no adverse effects on her digestive system.

Bananas are one of those items picked prior to ripening and, like tomatoes, gassed in the van on the way to the store to turn them instantaneously yellow. It's better to select green bananas and let them ripen at home so you can be sure they are truly ready to eat.

Despite what your produce man tells you, many of the fruits that are not yet ripe will never reach good eating quality simply because they were immature when picked. This is frequently the case with pineapples, which may become soft but never become sweet. The guidelines in this chapter will help you determine if the fruit in your market has a good potential.

Let's now take a look at some of the fresh fruits you will come across in your supermarket and determine which are ready to be purchased.

N.B. Organic Fruits: Occasionally your produce department features fruits that are labeled "organic." Try to find out their source, and if you have reason to believe they are really organic, if they look good and are reasonably priced, these are, of course, the best choice.

Apples (Peak season October through March)

There are many varieties of apples, each with its own distinct flavor and texture which determine its use. Those commonly recommended as eating apples include Delicious, McIntosh, Stayman, Golden Delicious, Jonathan, and Winesap. Tart varieties are usually reserved for cooking (although they make fine eating too). For pies and sauce, try Gravenstein, Jonathan, Greening, and Newtown. For baking, firm-fleshed apples work best, like Rome Beauty, Northern Spy, Greening, and Winesap.

Although the peel is rich in vitamins and minerals you may want to peel the apple to eliminate the waxed coating and the pesticide residue.

Look for: Firm, crisp apples. Color is a sign of maturity in apples, high color indicating maturity, and only apples picked when mature will have good flavor and texture. Although the waxing is somewhat deceiving, be sure the apple you choose is well colored.

Avoid: Apples that yield to pressure on the skin. These will have soft, mealy flesh. Apples with bruised areas, a sign of exposure to frost.

Apricots (Peak season June and July)

Apricots have a very short season and a very short life. They must be picked at maturity or they will be tasteless and they can be kept only three or four days before they become mealy.

Look for: Plump juicy-looking apricots with a uniform golden-orange hue. When ripe they will yield to gentle pressure.

Avoid: Soft, mushy fruit and hard, pale yellow or greenish yellow apricots. They are either over- or under-mature.

Bananas (Year-round)

Bananas, unlike other fruits, develop their best eating quality after harvesting. Buy them green or partially green so you know they aren't gassed into phony ripeness.

Look for: Bananas free from surface bruises with skin intact at both tips. The stage of ripeness is indicated by the color. Ripen them at room temperature and when the yellow jacket is speckled with brown, the starch will be changed to fruit sugar and the fruit will be tender, sweet, and easy to digest.

Avoid: Bananas which are bruised, discolored, or dull and grayish which means they have been held in cold storage and will never ripen properly.

Tips: Although for years Chiquita has been telling people to keep bananas at room temperature, once they are ripe they can be stored very successfully in the refrigerator. This way you can keep bananas ready to eat for several days. Do not place them in cold storage, however, until they are as ripe as you want them. Although the skin will turn brown in the refrigerator the fruit itself will remain unchanged.

Blueberries (Peak season July through August)

Look for: Berries that are plump, firm, and dark in color. Those of light color lack flavor.

Tips: Store blueberries unwashed and uncovered in the refrigerator. Use as soon as possible; they do not last long.

Cherries (Peak season June and July)

Sweet eating cherries first begin to appear on the market in about May and remain there until late in August. Wait until June before you buy them if you want the flavor and price to be right. Tart cherries, used for pies and other desserts, are rarely sold retail; most go to the processing plant, so unless you have your own tree they'll be hard to come by.

Look for: The most important sign of maturity and sweetness in cherries is a very dark color. The surface should be bright, glossy, and plump, and the stems should have a fresh look.

Avoid: Cherries that are shriveled, with dried stems and a dull look about them. These are over-mature. Decay is common to cherries but sometimes hard to see through the deep color. Soft leaking spots and surface mold will give you the clue to decay.

Coconuts (Peak season October through December)

Coconut meat is most flavorful when it comes right from the fresh coconut. The packaged flaked coconut needs to be treated with chemicals to improve its keeping qualities, and even then it always has a flat, stale taste.

Look for: Coconuts heavy for their size that sound full of liquid when you shake them.

Avoid: Those with wet or moldy eyes (those three small circles at one end).

Tips: Before you crack it, the coconut can be held at room temperature and can be kept satisfactorily about two months. Once opened, it should be stored covered in the refrigerator and will stay fresh about one week. For longer storage, fresh-grated coconut can be submerged in coconut milk and frozen in containers.

To open a coconut: Pierce eyes with a screwdriver or ice pick. Drain liquid, then place in a 350° oven for 15 to 20 minutes. Remove from oven, tap all over with a hammer, and break open. The dark skin can be removed with a potato peeler and the white meat eaten in chunks or grated on a cheese grater or in the blender.

Cranberries (Peak season October through December)

Look for: Plump firm berries with good luster. Even the dull varieties should have good red color. Sort out any soft or leaky berries before you use them because they may give your dish an off-flavor.

Tips: Try chopping the berries with oranges and sweetening them with honey to taste for a raw cranberry relish some time.

Figs (Peak season July and August)

It is a rare but cherished time in which you can buy fresh figs. When they are available, buy them for immediate eating; they do not keep very well.

Look for: Figs that are fairly soft, but not mushy. Minor bruises can be ignored; however, any bruises which cause a break in the skin will bring on rapid deterioration.

Grapefruit (Peak season September through April)

Actually grapefruit are on the market throughout the year and although the supply may be low and the price high out of peak season, they will still be ripe and of fine quality.

Look for: Firm fruits heavy for their size. Thin-skinned fruits are juicier. A coarse skin and pointed end are signs of a thick-skinned, less juicy fruit, but it may be tasty nonetheless. Wrinkled and rough skin, though, will indicate tough, dry fruit inside. Skin defects are usually no indication of the interior, except for large, soft, wet spots.

Avoid: Grapefruit with large, water-soaked areas or soft discolored areas at the stem end. If the skin breaks easily with pressure, assume there is some decay.

Tips: Grapefruit can be stored in a cold room or the refrigerator and will keep a minimum of two weeks. Do not store in a closed bag but leave uncovered.

Grapes {Peak season July through November)

The most common varieties of grapes include Thompson seedless (early green), Tokay and Cardinal (early bright red), and Emperor (late, deep red).

Look for: Well-colored plump grapes still attached to the stem. Green grapes are sweetest when the color has a yellowish cast. Red varieties are best when good and red.

Avoid: Soft, wrinkled grapes and those that leak.

As we said before, grapes are prone to lots of chemical treatment, and unless you're into a slave trip like the Romans it's unlikely you'll resort to peeling them. The only way to avoid the adulteration here is to limit consumption.

Tips: If unexpected company drops in and you want to give them a real taste treat, wash a bunch of grapes and pop them in the freezer for half an hour. After thirty minutes serve them delicious "grape ices."

Lemons (Year-round)

Lemons are available year-round, keep well in the refrigerator for at least two weeks, and you should have some in stock at all times for making salad dressings and seasoning your foods. This way you'll never have to resort to bottled lemon juice which contains preservatives and much less of the native vitamins.

Look for: Lemons with rich yellow color and reasonably smooth skin. Choose those heavy for their size for the most juice. A paler fruit will be more acidy.

Avoid: Lemons with a dark or dull color, hard or shriveling skin and soft spots, mold, or punctures.

Tips: To get more juice, bring to room temperature or roll lemons before cutting.

Limes (Year-round, peak June and July)

Limes make a nice zippy salad dressing when used instead of lemons. They are also excellent on fish, just as a lemon is.

Look for: Glossy skin and heavy weight in relation to size.

Avoid: Dull, dry skin and irregularities on the surface.

Mangoes (Peak season May through August)

Mangoes are usually rather high-priced, but have a truly exotic taste . . . somewhat like an effervescent peach. The best way to prepare them is to remove the peel (which acts as a good protective coat) and slice the meat off the large center pit.

Look for: When ready to eat, a mango will have an orange-yellow to red surface skin and flesh that yields slightly to pressure. They can be bought green and allowed to ripen at room temperature.

Tips: To remove pulp, mark a band down one side with a sharp knife and peel back skin as necessary. The pulp can be eaten right out of the jacket with a spoon.

MELONS

Cantaloupe (Peak season June through August)

Look for: In order to be sweet the mature cantaloupe must be free of the stem with a smooth, shallow basin where the stem was. If all or part of the stem base remains or if the stem scar is jagged, the melon was not fully matured at picking time. The netting on the surface should be thick, coarse, and stand out like relief work. The skin between the netting should be a yellowish tone.

Signs of ripeness, as distinguished from maturity, include a pleasant cantaloupe odor and a slight yield to pressure at the blossom end (opposite the stem end). Even if the melon is not ripe, if it is mature it will reach excellent eating quality if held at room temperature for a few days.

Avoid: Overripe melons, indicated by a bright yellow color and softening over the entire surface. The flesh of this melon will be tasteless and watery. Small bruises will not affect eating quality; large ones will.

Tips: Once the melon is ripe, it can be stored in the refrigerator. It is best to store it in a bag to prevent the odor from penetrating other foods.

Try making some melon punch and cantaloupe butter when prices are reasonable. Recipes for these are found in the chapters "Drink Up!" and "Jams, Jellies, and Sweet Spreads."

Casaba (Peak season July to November)

This melon is shaped like a pumpkin with a somewhat pointed stem end. The surface is covered with shallow, irregular furrows running from stem to blossom end. The rind is hard and light green to yellow in color.

Look for: A golden yellow color for ripeness and a softening at the blossom end. These melons have no aroma.

Avoid: Dark, sunken water spots.

Cranshaw (Peak season August and September, although available July to October)

This melon is large, round, and pointed at the stem end. It too has shallow furrows, but the skin is much smoother than the casaba.

Look for: A deep golden yellow rind with a surface that yields to slight pressure and a pleasant aroma.

Avoid: Sunken, watersoaked areas on the rind.

Honeydew (Peak season June through September)

Honeydew has a lovely sweet flavor, much more delicate than cantaloupe. The melon itself is quite large and may be oval to round in shape. The rind is smooth and firm and ranges from creamy white to creamy yellow. The smaller round Honeyball melon has much the same characteristics, except for its size.

Look for: A soft velvety surface (the sign of maturity) and a slight softening at the blossom end, a faint, pleasant aroma, and a yellow white to creamy color (the signs of ripeness).

Avoid: Melons with a dull white or greenish white color and hard, smooth feel (signs of immaturity), large watersoaked areas (signs of injury), and punctures in the rind (which lead to decay). Small damaged areas will not lead to further deterioration if you plan to use the melon immediately.

Persian (Peak season August and September)

Persian melons look like oversized cantaloupes but are somewhat rounder with a finer netting. Choose them as you do cantaloupes.

Watermelon (Peak season May through August)

Although not totally reliable, look for these signs if the melon is uncut: a smooth surface with a slight dullness (not bright and not really dull); filled-out, rounded ends and a cream-colored underside.

Look for: In cut melons, firm, juicy flesh with a good red color and no white streaks; seeds that are dark brown or black.

Avoid: Pale-colored flesh, white streaks, and white seeds (a sign of immaturity). Overmaturity is shown by dry, mealy flesh or watery, stringy flesh.

Tips: Keep watermelon in the refrigerator. An uncut melon will keep longer than one that is cut.

Nectarines (Peak season July and August)

The nectarine combines the characteristics of a peach and a plum. The color ranges from a red blush to a completely red surface.

Look for: Good color and plumpness and a slight softening along the "seam." Some varieties have a characteristic speckling. As long as the color is rich and bright, you can expect the flavor to be sweet. If the fruit is too firm, allow it to ripen a few days at room temperature.

Avoid: Very hard dull-colored nectarines or those that are even slightly shriveled. Also look for surface decay (soft spots or mold).

Oranges (Peak season December through June)

Color is no real indication of quality when it comes to choosing oranges. Until recently the majority of oranges were artificially colored anyway. Restrictions require oranges to be fully mature before they can be shipped out of state.

Look for: Firm, heavy oranges.

Avoid: Lightweight fruits which are not juicy, and very rough surface which is a sign of a thick skin and little inside. Avoid soft spots on skin and weak areas at the ends.

Tips: It is particularly recommended that you buy uncolored oranges since the skin, grated into cookies, puddings, salad dressings, and many other dishes, imparts a delicious fresh orange flavor.

Papayas (Peak season May and June)

The papaya comes from tropical regions and is not commonly used in many households. It is easily bruised and requires careful handling; it is a bit harder to judge for quality than other fruits, but those people who like it, love it.

Look for: Fruit that is golden yellow to orange and yields to gentle pressure. This fruit is ripe for eating.

Avoid: Papayas that are quite soft (and mushy) and any dark patches which are signs of age and decay.

Tips: Keep the papaya uncovered in the refrigerator and use within three days. A nice addition to fruit salads.

Peaches (Peak season June through September)

If you've ever traveled abroad you'll know what a peach is supposed to taste like. You will rarely find one so good in your fruit department unless, perhaps, you live in Georgia.

Look for: Peaches that are fairly firm or just beginning to soften. The background color should be red with areas of yellow or at least cream color.

Avoid: Very hard peaches with green tones. These were picked immature and will never ripen properly. Don't buy very soft peaches either, unless you want them to have a watered-down taste. Large flattened bruises are surface signs of inner decay.

Pears (Peak season September through November)

The peak season for pears can be extended through the winter by keeping the pears in cold storage. Thus Anjou, Bosc, and Comice pears will be available in the store often as late as May. Bartlett pears, however, will fade from view around November.

Look for: Firm pears no matter what the variety. Bartletts should be pale to rich yellow; Anjou or Comice light to yellow green; Bosc greenish yellow to brownish yellow. Although they should be firm, they should not be hard, and if you want to be sure they will ripen, select those that are a little bit soft.

Avoid: Wilted or shriveled pears that are weak near the stem. These are immature and will never ripen. Also avoid those with spots on the sides or blossom ends which indicate a mealy pear beneath.

Pears should not be waxed, so you just need to scrub them well for eating.

Pineapples (Peak season March through June)

Pineapples are picked while still hard and must be allowed to ripen at room temperature. Unless they are mature at picking time, however, this ripening will never come about.

Look for: When pineapples are mature (but not yet ripe) they are dark green. As they ripen, the green color fades and orange and yellow take its place. When fully ripe the pineapple is gold, orange-yellow, or reddish brown, depending on the variety. It should have a fragrant odor and a slight separation of the eyes when ready to be eaten. The leaves, or spikes, should pull out without too much tugging. The fruit should be plump and heavy for its size.

Avoid: Pineapples with pointed or sunken eyes, dull yellow-green color, and a dried-out appearance—all are immature. If the eyes are dark and watery, the odor unpleasant, and the surface has many soft spots you can be fairly certain the fruit will show internal damage.

Tips: When ripe, store in the refrigerator.

Plantains (Year-round)

We're not quite sure if plantains should be listed with the fruits or vegetables; they resemble bananas in appearance but are larger and starchier and less sweet. They are best used to replace potatoes or other starchy vegetables at a meal and must be cooked to be edible.

Look for: Plantains that are yellow or speckled with brown are ready for cooking. If you're buying for the future, get them green and let them ripen at room temperature.

Tips: Plantains must be cooked before eating. Peel and slice on a diagonal and soak in salted water to prevent browning. The traditional way to prepare them (as they do in Puerto Rico) is to deep-fry them, remove them from the oil before they are browned, press them flat, and refry. The result—crunchy "plantain chips." For less frying and greater ease, we simply fry them once in a shallow layer of oil or butter until golden. Delicious for breakfast with eggs.

Plums (Peak season July through August)

Varieties of plums differ in flavor and appearance, going from green to purple red. Try several varieties.

Look for: Good color for the particular variety you are choosing, a slight glow to the skin, and fruit that yields to gentle pressure.

Avoid: Fruit with skin breaks or brown discoloration. Immature fruit, which is hard, poorly colored, and very tart, and overmature fruit which is soft, leaking, and decayed.

Raspberries, blackberries, and other small berries (Peak season June through August)

Although they differ in shape or color these small berries, which are often found growing wild in the country, are similar in general structure and buying considerations.

Look for: Good bright color for the species. The individual bumps on the berries should be plump, tender, and not mushy.

Avoid: Berries that are leaky and show mold. This is fairly easy to spot. Although the berries at the bottom of the basket are hard to see, if the container is stained or wet, you can be pretty sure there are too many spoiled berries in the batch.

Berries should not be washed until you're ready to use them. Try to use them rapidly; they do not last long. If you buy a whole lot, make some berry jam, according to the simple directions in the chapter "Jams, Jellies, and Sweet Spreads." Use them in baked goods as you would raisins, only use slightly less liquid to allow for the berry juice.

Rhubarb (Peak season March through June)

Rhubarb cannot be eaten raw, and even cooked it requires a lot of sweetening to make it tasty. Use honey and you'll be able to turn out some delicious rhubarb sauces and pies. Only the stalks are edible. Don't experiment with the leaves; they contain a substance which can be poisonous.

Look for: Select firm, crisp straight stalks with a deep-red or cherry color. This is the "field" variety. Hothouse rhubarb is lighter in color with yellow-green leaves.

Avoid: Wilted, oversized or extremely thin stalks.

Tips: Simmer rhubarb in just enough water to cover until tender. Sweeten with honey to taste and serve warm or chilled for dessert. Combine diced rhubarb with strawberries or apples for a delicious pie filling.

Strawberries (Peak season April through June)

Look for: Full red color, bright luster, and firm flesh. The stem should still be attached and the berries dry. Medium to small berries are sweeter than large ones.

Avoid: Berries with large, uncolored areas and lots of surface seeds, a dull, shrunken appearance or extreme softness.

Don't attempt to find a basket with all beautiful berries. They just don't exist. Try to look into the basket and determine if most of the lower berries are of reasonable quality, and other than that you'll pretty much have to pick out the good ones and ignore the rest. Be sure to sort out any decaying berries right away, before the mold has a chance to spread. Refrigerate them immediately.

Tangerines (Peak season November through January)

Look for: Yellow-orange tangerines. The skin is loose fitting, therefore the fruit will never feel firm.

Avoid: Very pale fruits (although small areas of green don't mean poor flavor) and skin punctures.

GENERAL BUYING NOTES

Suggestions for buying fruits are almost identical to those for purchasing vegetables.

- Buy in season when quality is high and prices lowest.
- Don't buy more than you need since fruits perish quickly.
- Don't buy damaged fruit and handle displayed fruits carefully so you don't ruin them for others.
- Buy fruits that are mature, well colored, and free of bruises, skin punctures, and decay. If a fruit "special" is on, and you plan to use the fruit for eating, make sure it is undamaged. Slightly damaged fruit is suitable for pies, purees, jams, and other cooked dishes, but only if it is used immediately. The longer you wait, the less flavor (or good flavor) and vitamins your fruit dish will have.

HANDLING HINTS

Once ripe, fruits last longest if stored in the refrigerator. Let them ripen first at room temperature though, out of direct sunlight, or they will never turn sweet and juicy. If the fruit has a strong odor (like cantaloupe), keep it in a bag so the odor doesn't penetrate other foods. Otherwise store uncovered.

The flavor is best when fruits are just slightly chilled or at room temperature, so try to take fruit from the refrigerator ahead of serving time.

Do not wash fruits until serving time if you want them to last longer. If you have children who take their own snacks from the refrigerator, teach them to wash their fruit before eating. If you can't, then keep a selection of washed fruits for them to choose from. Berries are particularly vulnerable to decay after washing, so try to save their cleaning for the last minute.

CANNED AND FROZEN FRUITS

Canning and freezing are somewhat less deleterious to fruit than to vegetables. One reason for this seems to be the natural protection of vitamins associated with the high amounts of acid in the fruits. Although peeling, cutting, and the heat of canning do decrease some of the nutrients, those that leak into the liquid are usually consumed along with the fruit rather than thrown away. Of course, if you pour the syrup out, you'll lose many of these nutrients.

The main problem with processed fruits is the high levels of sugar that are added. Fruits are rich in natural sugars and do not need additional sweetening. The reason manufacturers add sugar is to maintain the texture and to preserve the fruit. (The property of sugar is such that it creates "osmotic pressure" which keeps a balance of fluids inside and outside the fruit, thus regulating the texture; it also inhibits the growth of bacteria.) One thing we do not need in our diets is more sugar.

In a very few cases, fruits are packed in water (which is often mixed with juice or lightly sweetened without any indication on the label) which minimizes the sugar problem. You can always drain off the syrup, but then you are draining off vitamins as well. Citrus fruits are often canned in water only, and canned crushed pineapple in unsweetened pineapple juice is packaged by *Dole* and *Foodtown*.

With the exception of the actual amount of sugar added (although some indication is given by the terms "light," "heavy," and "extra heavy" syrup, which refer to the water–sugar ratio), all the ingredients added during the packing of canned and frozen fruits must be stated on the label. Likely additions include spice, natural flavorings, vinegar, and ascorbic acid (added to preserve the color). Chemical preservatives are not permitted in these products, and artificial coloring is allowed only in canned pears, cherries, and the cherries in fruit cocktail. This coloring must be indicated on the label so you can avoid it. Fruits packed in light syrup have less sugar than "medium" or "heavy pack." If you want your fruit sweeter, add honey—it's a sweetener and a syrup all in one.

Occasionally strawberries and blueberries are frozen whole with no added sugar (or anything else for that matter). These are suitable choices in the months when fresh berries are not in season.

You run the most chance of encountering additives when you purchase prepared applesauce. This product may contain water, apple juice, salt, added acids, sweetening, spices, vitamin C, acid preservatives, and coloring. All this must be on the label. Products which combine apples with berries or other fruits to make flavored applesauce are even more tainted. *Appletime* Unsweetened Applesauce and *Motts* Natural Style Applesauce are both choices containing only apples and water. If you have a blender, however, you can make an applesauce in one minute that will be much higher in vitamins and needs no additions at all (not even sweetening, although you can add honey to taste).

BLENDER APPLESAUCE

Dice apples. Peel only if waxed. Add a few pieces at a time to blender container. Puree, adding 1 tablespoon of lemon juice and enough apple juice to get the machine going. Stir in honey if desired and sprinkle on cinnamon and nutmeg. Use immediately to insure maximum vitamin retention and prevent browning.

RECOMMENDATIONS

General Rule of Purchase: Buy fruits fresh, following the guidelines in this chapter. Make organically grown fruits your top choice.

When purchasing canned fruits, choose those packed in water or their own unsweetened juice, and be sure to consume the liquid. When purchasing frozen fruits, choose those frozen plain, with nothing added. Be sure the package is solidly frozen. All ingredients should be on the label.

EXEMPLARY BRANDS:
    Canned
        Pineapple in Unsweetened Juice
            Avondale
            Del Monte
            Dole
            Featherweight
            Fine Fare

      Foodtown
      Grand Union
      Iris
      Janet Lee
      Kroger
      Maid Rite
      Mandalay
      S&W Nutradiet
      Shop Rite
      Shur Fine
      Staff
      Town House
      Waldbaums

Citrus in Unsweetened Juice

      Donald Duck Grapefruit Sections in Grapefruit Juice

      Featherweight Grapefruit and Oranges in Grapefruit and Orange Juice

      Kraft Chilled Grapefruit (in jars)

      S&W Nutradiet Grapefruit Sections in Grapefruit Juice

      Seald Sweet Grapefruit Sections in Unsweetened Juice

      Shavers Unsweetened Grapefruit

      Town House Florida Grapefruit Sections in Grapefruit Juice

Cherries in Water

      Busch's Red Sour Pitted Cherries
      Grand Union Red Tart Pitted Cherries
      Kroger Pitted Red Tart Cherries
      Lucky Leaf Red Tart Cherries
      Musselman's Cherries
      Orchard Park Red Cherries
      Shur Fine Pitted Red Sour Cherries
      Skyland Red Tart Pitted Cherries
      Staff Red Pitted Tart Cherries
      Stokely Van Camp's Red Sour Pitted Cherries
      Super Saver Red Tart Pitted Pie Cherries
      Supreme Red Tart Pie Cherries

Thank You Brand Tart Cherries

Town House Red Tart Pitted Cherries

Other Berries in Water

White Swan Blackberries

Wyman's Wild Blueberries

Apples in Water

Comstock Sliced Apples

Hood River Sliced Apples (Heavy Pack in Water, commercial size)

Other Fruits

Diet Delight Fruit packed in grape juice from concentrate, including peaches, pears, and apricots; and purple plums in water

Giant Food Juice Pack Peaches, Apricots, Pears, Grapefruit Sections, in white grape juice

Naturmade Pears, Peaches, and Apricots, in water

Old Mill Yellow Cling Peaches in Water (commercial size)

S&W Nutradiet Unsweetened Cling Peaches, Apricots, Bartlett Pears, Royal Anne Cherries, Kadota Figs, all in water

Tillie Lewis Tasti Diet Peaches, Pears and Apricots in Apple, Grape, and Pear Juice; Plums in Pear Juice; Prunes in Water

Waldbaums Peaches, Apricots, Pears in Grape Juice

Applesauce

Appletime Unsweetened

Country Pure Brand Unsweetened

Featherweight Unsweetened

Mott's Natural Style

Musselman's Natural Style

Seneca 100% Natural Unsweetened

Pumpkin

Del Monte

Libby's

Stokely Van Camp's

Frozen—all unsweetened

Bel Air Whole Strawberries; Blackberries; Boysenberries; Red Sour Pitted Cherries; Rhubarb

Big Valley Red Tart Cherries; Blueberries; Sweet Cherries

Brady's Blueberries; Blackberries

Camelot Whole Strawberries

Driscoll Whole Strawberries

Flav-R-Pak Whole Strawberries

Flavorland Blueberries; Blackberries; Pitted Tart Red Cherries; Boysenberries; Rhubarb

Gardenbowl Rhubarb

Overlake Blueberries

Red & White Whole Strawberries

Seabrook Blueberries; Dark Sweet Cherries; Honey Dew Balls; Cantaloupe Balls; Mixed Melon Balls

Shop Rite Whole Strawberries

Southland Cut Rhubarb

Stillwell Blackberries; Cherries; Sliced Peaches; Melon Balls; Whole Strawberries

Tennessee Winter Garden Whole Strawberries; Blackberries

Top Frost Blackberries; Rhubarb; Whole Strawberries

V.I.P. Foods Blueberries; Blackberries; Peaches; Whole Strawberries

Western Valley Blackberries; Rhubarb; Whole Strawberries; Dark Sweet Cherries; Blueberries; Boysenberries

Dried Fruit: Biblical Sweets

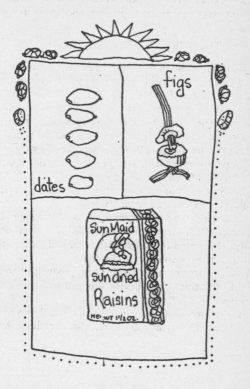

Dried fruits are a rich source of natural sugar plus all the vitamins and minerals native to the fruit when it is fresh. The drying process is one of the earliest methods of food preservation, in which about 50 percent of the water is removed from the fresh fruit while almost all the nutrients remain.

Dried fruits make excellent snacks and are the ideal substitute for candy. They are naturally sweet and offer a concentrated source of energy. Your best supply of iron, a mineral that is lacking in most diets and vital for healthy blood, can be obtained while enjoying many of these dried fruits.

Almost any fruit can be preserved by drying, although raisins, prunes, and dates are the only ones which appear in all supermarkets. Some stores carry figs, apricots, peaches, and apples as well.

ALL DRIED FRUIT IS NOT TREATED EQUALLY

The two major means of removing the moisture from the fresh fruit are sun-drying and artificial dehydration by heat evaporation. In the latter process, the fruit is usually dipped into a sulfur dioxide bath to keep it from darkening. The term "sun-dried" usually implies that no sulfur bath has been used, but this doesn't always hold true. Golden raisins always meet with sulfur dioxide, and you can be sure that any other fruits that are still quite light in color, like cream-colored apples and bright orange apricots, do too. The sulfur dioxide is declared on the label and is difficult, but possible, to avoid.

Almost all dried fruits are fumigated either during storage or importation. This seems to be unavoidable.

Dates, especially the domestic kind, are usually pasteurized to prevent molding. Corn syrup is frequently added to keep dates from drying out. Dates are already very high in natural sugar and the idea of making them even sweeter is ridiculous.

Preservatives are not necessary in these products although some dried fruit companies don't believe this and add sorbic acid as a preservative.

The use of preservatives and corn syrup must be shown on the label, and you should not buy any dried fruit that contains either.

WHAT TO BUY

Raisins

Of the popular brands, *Sun Maid* Thompson seedless raisins (except the "golden"), muscats, sultanas, and currants are sun-dried without the aid of chemicals. *S & W* raisins (the dark kinds) are also free of sulfur dioxide.

Figs

The two most popular domestic varieties of dried figs are calimyrna, the native California variety which is light in color, and mission figs, which are purplish black and less likely to be treated with sulfur. Calamata string figs, imported from Greece, are also unsulfured.

Prunes

Prunes are usually dried by artificial dehydration rather than sun-drying to control the amount of moisture left in so they remain soft. Sulfur dioxide is hard to avoid in this case.

Apricots

Most apricots are dried by dehydration, although sun-dried varieties are sometimes available in the supermarket. The sun-dried ones are tougher and call for sucking rather than chewing.

Dates

Dates needn't have any additives as is demonstrated by both the *Calavo* and *Dromedary* brands.

Organic Fruit

Many stores are including organically grown, untreated dried fruits in their stock, particularly Monukka raisins, sun-dried apricots, and dates. If you're really lucky, the supermarket in your area (like the one in ours) will also offer dried banana and dried pineapple slices—sweeter than any candy you might crave.

Grading

Dried fruits are usually graded; they may be Extra Fancy, Fancy, Extra Choice, Choice, or Standard. This grading has nothing to do with wholesomeness or food value, but is based solely on aesthetics (size, color, condition, water content).

STORAGE

Dried fruits should be stored in an airtight container at room temperature to keep them from becoming dried out. They will keep this way at least six months. If your kitchen shelf is especially warm, however, you might do better to store them in the refrigerator.

MAKING USE OF DRIED FRUITS

If your dried fruits do become hard or you want your fruit to be more like the fresh, soaking them in warm water for an hour will restore the original quality. Don't soak them any longer, though, or they'll turn watery and tasteless. Drink the liquid that the fruits have been soaked in. It is flavorful and rich in vitamins and minerals.

Dried fruits can be cooked, but unless you are cooking them to use as a puree you can achieve the same effect by pouring boiling water over the fruit, then placing it in the refrigerator to soak, water and all. In a few hours you will have "stewed" fruit.

Although the best way to eat dried fruits is out of hand, there are many other ways you can use them to enrich other dishes. We often add chopped dried fruits to:

- Cooked cereals instead of sweetener.
- Fruit salads.
- Vegetable salads, especially cucumber
- Salad.
- Cooked brown rice, along with chopped nuts, for a sweet pilaff side dish or dessert. When used as dessert, pour on some cream at serving time.
- Cookie, cake, and bread batter. If you do this, make sure the fruits are well covered with batter to protect them from the heat. Dried fruits have a very high sugar content which causes them to burn easily. It's a good idea to lower the baking temperature by 25°, especially with cookies.
- Cooked vegetables in a tomato sauce for serving over grains.
- Yogurt or cottage cheese for breakfast or lunch.

RECOMMENDATIONS

General Rule of Purchase: All ingredients on label. Choose sun-dried fruits without added sweetening or preservatives. Check the label for sulfur dioxide and sodium benzoate in particular. Dark fruits are less likely to be treated.

Additional selection in the "Health Foods" section.

EXEMPLARY BRANDS:
> Raisins
>> Most dark raisins are fine, including
>> *Albertson's*
>> *Bonner's* Muscats
>> *Cal Fruit*
>> *Camelot*
>> *Kroger*
>> *Mariani* Raisins and Zante Currants
>> *Plump & Meaty*
>> *S&W*
>> *Springfield*
>> *Sugaripe*
>> *Sun Giant*
>> *Sun Maid* Raisins, Muscats, Sultanas and Currants
>> *Sweet-n-Tasty*
>> *Town House*
>> and many other house brands
>
> Prunes
>> *Del Monte* Moist Pak (canned); Vacuum Packed
>> *Healthy Acres* Moist Pack (canned)
>> *Mariani*
>> *Sunsweet* Canned
>
> Figs
>> *Calamata* String
>
> Dates
>> *Bardo* Pitted
>> *Calavo*
>> *Dromedary* Pitted (Whole only)
>> *Gold Cup*
>> *Mariani*
>> *Sun Giant* Whole (in container only)
>
> Other
>> *Kanana* Banana Flakes (canned)

Drink Up!

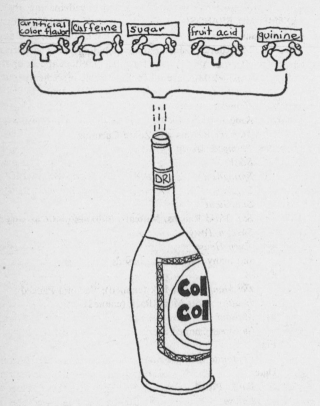

CARBONATED BEVERAGES

To someone born and raised in the "Pepsi Generation" it's hard to imagine a time when no one drank soda. Of course, it isn't news to anyone that soft drinks are bad for your health. In every eight ounces of soda you get five teaspoons of sugar. As if this isn't enough, the problem is compounded by the addition of acidifying agents, from natural fruit acids to phosphoric acid. This combination of fruit acid and sugar is a major contributant to enamel erosion of teeth. This holds true for all sweetened fruit beverages, including juices.

Caffeine in cola is no surprise to most people either. The government standard for cola allows for 20 to 36 mg. of caffeine in every six ounces—almost one third the caffeine content of coffee! How many times six ounces of cola do you or your children consume in a day?

The cola label need not mention caffeine, but its use in soft drinks extends to many other sodas, where fortunately it does appear on the list of ingredients. Many of the other undesirable ingredients found in soda are revealed on the label as well, including artificial flavor; artificial color; quinine; and a choice of twenty-three preservatives.

What you don't find out about, however, is the chemical process used to introduce the gassiness into the water; the acids added to create the acidity; the buffering agents added to counteract the acidity; the stabilizers and emulsifiers; the foaming agents and the defoaming agents. Brominated vegetable oil, one of the most popular emulsifiers, long suspected of playing a role in cardiac lesions, has recently been removed from the GRAS list.

This alarming cast of chemicals helps create club soda as well as flavored sodas.

THE ALTERNATIVES

Apple Juice

Apple juice is the new food-consciousness answer to soda, that is, the pure kind, with no sugar or preservatives added. There are many brands on the market, some richer and more flavorful than others. Local brands often cost less and are of good quality. If you can buy the unpasteurized or unfiltered kind in your supermarket, do. It won't look as nice since there is fruit sediment lingering around the bottom, but with a quick shake the taste is great. Of course there's more to apple juice than the refreshing taste (unlike soda) and you'll be rewarded with the minerals iron, potassium, magnesium, and silicon.

Orange Juice

Fresh: The main attraction in orange juice, as well as all citrus juices, is vitamin C. Unfortunately, this vitamin is sensitive to light and air and dissipates rapidly once the fruit is cut. Naturally, orange and grapefruit juices are best freshly squeezed. It's really quite easy to do and if you keep a juicer out on the counter (a hand one is inexpensive and does a fine job), you can squeeze a glass whenever you like in seconds.

Frozen vs. Prepared: Ready-squeezed juice in a bottle or container and the frozen orange juice concentrate both have their selling and unselling points. Frozen concentrate probably stacks up better on the nutrition score; it contains no added chemicals, and most brands are unsweetened. If sugar is added, the label will say so. The vitamin C content of this juice comes close to the fresh if the concentrate is kept frozen until preparation. If you let the concentrate thaw before preparation, however, flavor and vitamins begin to diminish. The pulp is usually strained out of frozen orange juice, which does remove some other nutritionally desirable substances known as bioflavonoids. And the natural water in the oranges is superior to the tap water you add when you reconstitute the juice.

Simple chilled orange juice in a container is nothing more than freshly squeezed juice with nothing added or changed, except that time has and is diminishing the vitamin C content. Unless you live in a citrus-producing state, orange juice in this form is rarely offered. What you can purchase is pasteurized orange juice. Pasteurizing inactivates enzymes to reduce spoilage and changes the flavor somewhat. If anything other than pure orange juice is present (sugar or preservatives), the label will say so. *Tropicana* does a funny number, we've noticed. Some containers say ".1 percent sodium benzoate added as preservative," while others state "no sugar or preservative added," so be sure to read the label in your area. While you're at it, always be sure you read the fine print when it comes to buying ready-squeezed orange juice. Our supermarket carries several varieties which read "100 PERCENT PURE ORANGE JUICE from concentrate." If that's the case, you might as well save money (and the vitamin C) and reconstitute it yourself.

Canned Juice: With these choices available don't waste your time on the canned citrus juices. The heat of canning destroys most of the vitamin C (so many processors kindly add some lab-manufactured vitamins back), and the taste is hardly recognizable as juice.

In all cases, make sure what you are buying is 100 percent pure juice. Watered-down orange juice goes under such titles as "orange juice drink blend," "orange juice drink," "orange drink," and "orange-flavored drink."

WHAT YOU DRINK WITH YOUR DRINK

Beverage (100 grams or 3½ ounces)	Calories	Carbohydrate (grams)	Calcium (mg)	Potassium (mg)	Iron (mg)	Vit. A (I.U.)	Vit. C (mg)
Apple juice	47	11.9	6	101	.1	—	—
Beer	42	3.8	5	25	—	—	—
Cola	39	10	—	—	—	—	—
Grape juice bottled	66	16.6	11	116	.3	—	—
Lemonade	44	11.4	1	16	—	—	7
Limeade	41	11.0	1	13	—	—	2
Orange juice fresh	45	10.4	11	200	.2	200	50
canned	48	11.2	10	199	.4	200	40
from concentrate	45	10.7	9	186	.1	200	45
Pineapple juice canned	55	13.5	15	149	.3	50	9
Prune juice	77	19.0	14	235	4.1	—	2
Tomato juice	19	4.3	7	227	.9	800	16
Wine	85	4.2	9	92	.4	—	—

Grape Juice

When we were kids (before soda discovered TV) we were all dedicated Howdy Doody fans and, by transference, avid consumers of Howdy's sponsor *Welch's* Grape Juice. Perhaps Buffalo Bob exaggerated a bit when he extolled the benefits of drinking grape juice, but at least in the drinking of grape juice there's no harm done. Pure, unsweetened grape juice is nothing more than the juice extracted from heating grapes and applying hydraulic pressure. The European version, imported in many places and available in supermarkets, although quite costly, is actually more nutritious than our own; abroad the juice is extracted from the fruit by cold pressing which conserves more of the vitamins. If you're buying *Welch's*, stick to the original deep purple juice; some of the newer white and rose-colored grape juices are not quite so untainted. Avoid the frozen concentrate; it's synthetically enriched and contains sugar.

Pineapple Juice

Pineapple juice is another healthy refresher. Most varieties are unsweetened and if not, the label will say so. Unsweetened pineapple juice is almost always enriched with vitamin C. Although we're not big on synthetic vitamin enrichment, this is still a better beverage than most.

Prune Juice

Prune juice has some unfortunate associations, but if you try some you'll find it's really quite tasty. This juice is thicker than others, really more like a nectar (although by government definition a nectar has a lot more than just juice in it). If the consistency bothers you, thin it down with some ice. *Sunsweet,* almost a synonym for prune juice, is an excellent choice; other brands may have added acid from a natural fruit source, honey, or vitamin C enrichment. These are all unnecessary, but not terrible. Why vitamin C is included is a mystery to us, since prunes are not a source of this vitamin in the first place. They are, however, an excellent source of natural iron, which is lacking in most of our diets.

As with prune juice, a water extract can be made from any dried fruit and is very easily done at home. Here's how:

DRIED FRUIT NECTAR

Cover dried fruit of your choice (apricots, prunes, figs, peaches, etc.) with water, allowing 2 pints of water for each pound of fruit. Cook over very low heat in a covered saucepan for 45 minutes. Transfer to a jar and refrigerate until needed. At serving time strain out fruit and serve juice in small glasses garnished with a slice of lemon. For a thicker nectar, puree the liquid with a few pieces of the softened fruit. Use remaining fruit in cereal and in baking. *Yield:* about 1⅓ cups of juice per pound of fruit.

Tomato Juice

Except for the addition of salt (present in almost all brands), tomato juice is nothing more than the liquid from drained, cooked tomatoes, which is usually homogenized to make it smooth. A few salt-free varieties are available too, for those interested in reducing salt intake.

Brands labeled "seasoned" or "cocktail" have such extras as Worcestershire sauce, sugar, citric acid, spices, and flavorings, making them much less natural and much less desirable. If you want your tomato juice seasoned, squeeze in some juice from a fresh lemon or make this cocktail in your blender.

TOMATO JUICE COCKTAIL

3 cups tomato juice
2 thin slices onion
1-inch-wide strip green pepper
2 thin slices lemon, with peel
4 sprigs parsley
½ teaspoon oregano
¼ teaspoon pepper

Combine all ingredients in blender container and process at high speed until smooth. Chill. Serve over ice. *Yield:* 6 ½-cup servings.

Carrot Juice

Canned carrot juice is less prevalent than other vegetable juices, but *Eveready* Carrot Juice made by *Dole* offers a delightful meal accompaniment or midday pickup that contains nothing but the juice from carrots. *Hollywood* carrot and other vegetable juices too are found primarily in the natural foods department and are also pure juice and nothing more. Carrot juice is very rich in vitamin A.

BEWARE OF FRUIT DRINKS, ADES, NECTARS, AND PUNCH

If the label says fruit drink, ade, nectar, punch, don't read any further, just continue along the aisle. A "juice-drink" is 50 percent juice, an "ade" 25 percent juice, and a "drink" only 10 percent juice. No mandatory amount of juice is set for the others, but all contain added sugar, water, and almost always artificial color, flavor, and preservatives, all of which appear on the label. There are usually buffers, stabilizers, emulsifiers, and weighting oils which do not have to be listed. This holds true for canned, bottled, and frozen concentrate varieties.

If you like fruit drinks, it's cheaper and safer to buy the real juice and water it down yourself at home. Fresh lemonade is so easy to prepare; children can make their own.

LEMONADE BY THE GLASS

Squeeze the juice of one lemon into a large glass. Add 1 to 2 tablespoons of honey and stir to dissolve. Add ice cubes and enough water to fill the glass and stir to blend.

As for other homemade juice-drinks, buy some fresh fruit or fruit juices and try your hand at some of these:

ORANGEADE

2 cups orange juice
½ cup lemon juice
½ cup honey
1 cup water
Combine all ingredients and stir or shake to dissolve honey. Serve over cracked ice and garnish with orange slices if desired. *Yield:* 4 servings.

MELON PUNCH

1 medium cantaloupe (2 cups diced pulp) ·
1 banana
Juice of 1 orange
Combine all ingredients in blender container and puree until smooth. Serve in small glasses with lots of ice. *Yield:* 4 servings.

SPICED CIDER

4 slices lemon, cut in halves
12 cloves
2 quarts apple juice or cider
¾ cup molasses
2 2-inch sticks cinnamon
⅓ cup lemon juice

Stud lemon slices with cloves. Combine apple juice or cider, molasses, cinnamon, and lemon slices in a large saucepan. Bring to boil, reduce heat, and simmer 15 minutes. Remove cinnamon sticks. Add lemon juice. Serve hot in mugs. *Yield:* 8 servings.

WATER

In the end, there's always water.

The stuff that comes out of your tap is an almost free drink, depending on the waterworks rate in your area, although with all the things added to purify and enrich the water supply we're not quite sure how natural to consider water anymore. Most supermarkets offer bottled alternatives to tap water, which may be more suitable tastewise for straight drinking, and if you choose wisely will have no additives.

Our opinion wavers when it comes to bottled water, for although it most often comes from a lesser contaminated source, there are almost no controls over what goes into the bottle, and container handling and sealing may be less than hygienic. This problem may become even more critical in the future as water pollution continues to increase. If you want to minimize the pollutants in your water and avoid paying the high price of bottled brands you can boil tap water and store it in the refrigerator for cooking and drinking.

Spring Water

Claims that spring water is therapeutic are thus far unfounded, but at least bottled spring water doesn't contain the chemicals added to the city water supply. There are presently hundreds of brands of bottled spring water on the market, and not all are reputable. *Consumer's Union* tested two of the major East Coast brands (*Deer Park* Mountain Spring Water and *Great Bear* Water) and two major West Coast brands (*Arrowheat Puritas* Spring Water and *Sparkletts* Crystal Fresh Drinking Water) and found them all suitably low in bacteria, so you can feel pretty safe with these.

Mineral Water

Softened city water is low in natural minerals and high in sodium (not too good for low-salt dieters). Water rich in natural minerals is beneficial for teeth, bones, and heart. If you don't live in a hard-water area (and the hardest natural waters come from Arizona, New Mexico, Wyoming, Utah, South Dakota, Nebraska, Iowa, Wisconsin, and Indiana), you might want to buy bottled mineral water in your supermarket. Check the label to make certain these salts are natural to the water and not in the form of added fortification. The imported mineral waters, like *Perrier* and *Vichy*, are excellent.

ALCOHOLIC BEVERAGES

While different states have different laws regarding the sale of alcoholic beverages, beer is a supermarket staple and wine is common in many places. The wide variety of chemical processes that can be used in creating these beverages and the number of brands on the market make it virtually impossible for us to offer any general guidelines or specific recommendations.*

Wine-making costs can be considerably reduced through chemical shortcuts. Although the actual ingredients may be natural (pulverized fruit and yeast), various practices employed to correct cloudiness, precipitation, off color, odor and flavor, frequently create a highly chemicalized beverage. If the wine is not sweet enough, additional sugar is added; if it is not acid enough, tartaric acid is introduced. Chalk can reduce acidity. Glycerine gives it body, and sulfur prevents any disagreeable changes. More than seventy chemical additives are permitted by law in its creation. According to the *Larousse*, French dictionary of gastronomy, these chemical processes "present many disadvantages, especially when several are done simultaneously, and they may be dangerous to the consumer." Buying imported wine is no guarantee of purity, for even in France wines produced for export are allowed certain adulteration not permitted in the beverage prepared for domestic enjoyment.

The same situation exists within the beer industry. The brew can be as simple as brewing water, corn, hops, barley-malt and yeast (as *Rheingold* beer claims), but not all brands are. Many include anti-gushing agents like EDTA to prevent the liquid from "gushing out"

*As of January 1, 1977 the FDA will require all alcoholic beverages to be labeled as to ingredient content.

when the bottle is opened, preservatives, foam stabilizers, coloring and filtering agents.

Because both wine and beer are so localized, we are recommending that you write a letter to the bottler or packer of your favorite brand asking what raw materials are used in production and what chemical processes are employed in its manufacture. If you are not satisfied with the answer, switch brands.

COFFEE

Everybody who drinks coffee knows about the caffeine and drinks it anyway. For anyone interested, caffeine has no taste and can be removed, as in *Sanka*. Of course, you'll lose the "coffee kick," which is why many people drink it in the first place.*

The coffee counter in your supermarket offers many choices both in style and brand. The essential flavoring in coffee comes from caffeol, a volatile substance which is lost by exposure to air. In order for caffeol to be released, the beans must be ground. So, to maintain maximum flavor, freshly ground beans are best. Whole coffee beans are available at the supermarket. You have a choice of purchasing a hand grinder and grinding the beans each time you make coffee for a really fresh brew, or using your supermarket's grinding machines. If you have your coffee ground in advance, be sure to store it in a tightly covered jar in the refrigerator to preserve the freshness.

Ground coffee oxidizes (loses its flavor and becomes flat and rancid) quickly. If you buy pre-ground coffee, choose the brands which come in vacuum cans. This will afford partial protection, at least until you open it. Although it's less economical, if you're a coffee aficionado, you'll have longer-lasting flavor if you buy small cans. Be sure to store opened cans tightly covered in the refrigerator.

Tips for Making Good Coffee

Tannin is the other ingredient of concern to coffee drinkers. Tannin is a bitter-tasting acid which increases as coffee brews, becoming

*"The National Cancer Institute said Sunday a chemical used last year in making decaffeinated coffee causes cancer of the liver in mice.

"The findings about the chemical, called trichloroethylene or TCE, 'serve as a warning of possible cancer danger to humans,' the institute said.

"The institute also warned against using three possible substitutes for TCE, one of which the makers of decaffeinated coffee switched to, until all safety testing has been completed."—*The New York Times,* June 13, 1976.

unpalatable once coffee boils. To avoid excess tannin in your coffee:
- Make sure never to boil coffee.
- Maintain the least contact between the coffee and boiling water. This will also keep caffeine down to a minimum. The drip method accomplishes this more effectively than percolator-brewed coffee. The *Melita* works on this principle, and for anyone who prefers fresh-brewed coffee to instant, using a Melita gives you brewed coffee in almost as short a time. Drip coffee (and the Melita brew) makes a thinner beverage, which takes some getting used to.
- Don't let perked coffee stand with the coffee grounds. Remove them as soon as coffee is perked.

Instant Coffee

Instant coffee is made from finely pulverized, concentrated coffee and supposedly contains less caffeine. Nothing is added (except to those brands which boast reduced acidity) to the regular instant or the freeze-dried instant. The one problem with these forms of coffee, according to *Consumer Reports,* is that they are generally made from low-grade beans. Their test panel ranks the following brands highest in taste and economy: *Safeway, Chase and Sanborn* Freeze-Dried, *Better Nut* Freeze-Dried Coffee Nuggets, *Stewart's* Freeze Dried, *A&P, Chock Full O'Nuts,* and *Finast.*

COFFEE SUBSTITUTES

Several coffee substitutes, which taste and smell surprisingly like coffee without the caffeine (or the coffee stimulation), are sold in the supermarket. *Instant Postum* has been on the market for years and is a beverage made from bran, wheat, and molasses. *Pero,* another long-known coffee substitute, has recently been introduced to the supermarket shelf. Like Postum, it is a drink which tastes like coffee and is made entirely from ground and roasted cereal grains. Chicory, a dried, ground, roasted root, is added to coffee, especially in the South, for flavor. It's kind of strong, but if you go for that taste you can try it by itself if you're looking for a coffee replacement.

TEA

Tea runs a close second to coffee in popularity when it comes to hot drinks, and although the problem is less serious, it also contains some

caffeine and a good deal of tannin. Black tea and green tea characterize the leaves used to create all varieties of tea. Black tea is fermented
to remove some of the tannin. Like coffee, the tannin and caffeine are
kept to a minimum when tea is brewed quickly with freshly boiled
water. While this may overcome the problem of the tea leaves themselves, there is still some degree of concern about the tea bag. The
metals used to secure the bag are viewed as harmful by many, and that
innocent-looking encasement is actually a carrier of harmful dyes.
Why not use loose tea leaves? A variety of loose teas is available in
your supermarket. For less than a dollar you can purchase an individual tea strainer (or you can use a small mesh juice strainer), and brew
fresh tea in individual glasses or by the pot. Buy a few kinds and you
can change your tea to suit your mood. *Constant Comment* offers a
delicately spiced mixture for mild tea lovers and *Twinings,* the English company, has tins of Darjeeling, English Breakfast, Earl Grey,
Orange Pekoe, and Lapsang Souchong among its diverse choices.
Other brands distributed in your area will offer a similar selection.

Tea has another advantage over coffee—it's much easier to drink
it black. For those who insist on sweetening their beverage, honey
makes a much tastier tea than sugar.

Herb Teas

Aside from the traditional tea-leaf teas, delicious teas can be prepared from herbs. Herb teas have no caffeine and many are believed
to have healing qualities. While the taste for herb tea must sometimes
be acquired, as an incurable tea drinker, Nikki can testify that the
acquisition is a simple one. Herb tea is made just like other teas, by
pouring boiling water over fresh or dry leaves (or flowers) and allowing the brew to steep for three to five minutes. Some of the herbs which
come highly recommended include basil, sage, aniseed, fennel, marjoram, and mint.

Tea can be made from many different things. We have a Hungarian
friend who has a unique suggestion for making tea from walnuts.
Inside the shell of a walnut is a woody dividing membrane. Save these
pieces and add a heaping teaspoon to each cup of water, allow them
to boil together for five minutes and then let the shell fragments settle
to the bottom. When the tea has cooled somewhat it is ready to drink.
Subsequent boiling makes the tea even stronger. We've heard this

method works with pieces of pecan shells, and the skin of almonds as well; we'll let you try these for yourself.

Pompadour, imported from West Germany and distributed in many supermarkets, offers acceptable herb tea bags with some strange-sounding names. *Fixmille* is actually camomile tea, *Fixbutter* is rose hips and *Fixminz,* mint tea. They make a most enjoyable cup of tea.

Instant Tea

Instant tea (particularly the iced, flavored kind) is an adulterated waste of money. In addition to the finely ground tea leaves, which are the basis of the beverage, all the flavored brands contain either malto dextrin to protect the flavor, or they derive their appeal from citric acid, artificial color and flavor, caramel color, vegetable oil, and BHA (a preservative). Don't be sucked in by the proud claim of "Natural Flavor" that instant tea manufacturers brandish on the label. The flavor may be natural, but not much else is. When this tea comes already prepared in the bottle you not only purchase these same chemicals, but you pay a lot of money for someone else to add the water.

If you want iced tea, brew double-strength tea (and here you can add any leftover tea that has been brewed previously), add honey and lemon to taste, and serve over ice. Add the sweetening while the tea is hot to make for easier dissolving.

HOT CHOCOLATE AND COCOA

Caffeine is bad enough when you're an adult; certainly no one wants to offer it to children. Chocolate and cocoa contain caffeine from the cocoa bean, so let's keep this in mind and cut down on the amount of cocoa we serve our kids. When you do buy cocoa select plain cocoa rather than "Dutch" cocoa. Dutched or Dutch process cocoa isn't made from special chocolate imported from Holland (which is what we always thought). As it turns out, the "Dutch" is a euphemism for "treated with alkali."

The best brand on the market to date is *Hershey's* Cocoa. In addition to being untreated, it is unsweetened so you can add your own honey or raw sugar. Prepared cocoa mixes, on the other hand, are the unfortunate victims of a long list of unwarranted and unwanted additives.

Cara-Coa is a beverage powder similar to cocoa, but made from carob rather than cocoa beans. Carob, the fruit of a Mediterranean evergreen tree, tastes remarkably like chocolate but contains no caffeine.

As another healthy alternative to cocoa try serving Hot Wheat Drink for breakfast or as a snack on a chilly winter day.

HOT WHEAT DRINK

For each serving combine 6 ounces of milk with 1 heaping teaspoon of wheat germ and 1 teaspoon of honey in a saucepan. Add a stick of cinnamon to the pot and place over low heat. When the milk is just about to boil, remove from heat and serve. Wheat germ may be strained out if you wish, but it will settle to the bottom of the cup anyway and can always be promoted as a special treat to be eaten with a spoon.

RECOMMENDATIONS

JUICE

General Rule of Purchase: All ingredients on label. Buy those that are unsweetened. Watch for citric acid, synthetic enrichment, and sodium benzoate preservatives.

EXEMPLARY BRANDS
Apple Juice
unsweetened and unfiltered best
Apple & Eve
Appletime
Bonnie Hubbard Unsweetened, Unfiltered
Coop Partially Filtered
Country Pure
Health-Aide
Heinke's Unfiltered

    Martinelli's Pure, Old Fashioned Unfiltered; Sparkling

    Mott's Country Style

    Red Cheek

    Springfield Pure, Unfiltered

    Tree Top Pure

Citrus Juice

    Buy fresh citrus fruits for squeezing

    Fresh, chilled juice

    Fresh, pasteurized juice (check that these are not "from concentrate")

    Unsweetened frozen concentrate—all similar

    Unsweetened canned—all similar

Grape Juice

    all unsweetened brands

    Seneca

    Welch's Purple and Red

    many house brands

Pineapple Juice

    canned; all brands enriched and similar

Prune Juice—unsweetened

    Del Monte

    Shedd's

    Sunsweet

    many house brands

Mixed Fruit Juices

    Bessey's Unsweetened Prune, Date, and Fig Juice

    Health-Aide Apricot-Apple, Boysenberry-Apple

    Heinke's Black Cherry, Peach, Apricot, Pomegranate

    Sunsweet Prune-Apple, Apricot, Apple, Prune

    Tree Top Pear-Grape, Pear-Apple

Tomato Juice—All brands are similar and contain salt, except those mentioned below:

    Campbell's Low Sodium V-8

    Diet Delight

    Featherweight

    S&W Nutradiet Tomato and Vegetable Juice Cocktail

Other Vegetable Juices

    Busch's Kraut Juice

    Eveready Carrot Juice

> *Hollywood* Carrot Juice
> *Meeter's* Kraut Juice

WATER

General Rule of Purchase: Check that no mineral salts are added.

> EXEMPLARY BRANDS:
> Spring Water
> > *Arrowhead Puritas*
> > *Deer Park*
> > *Great Bear*
> > *Hinckley & Schmidt*
> > *Ramona*
> > *Sparkletts*
> > *Tulpehocken*
> Mineral Water
> > *Perrier*
> > *Vichy*

COFFEE

> EXEMPLARY BRANDS:
> Beans—all brands similar
> Regular Ground—all brands similar
> Instant—all brands similar except those with reduced acidity
> Coffee Substitutes—Instant *Postum*
> > *Pero*

TEA

General Rule of Purchase: Herb teas, which are caffeine-free, are preferred. Loose tea is preferred over tea bags.

> EXEMPLARY BRANDS:
> Herb Tea
> > *Balance of Nature*
> > *Celestial Seasoning*

    Healthway
    Healthy Acres Papaya Mint; Alfalfa
    Hunza Pure Natural Herb Teas, including Papaya, Alfalfa, Cammomile, Peppermint, Rosehips, Sassafras
    Pompadour Fixmille; Fixbutter; Fixmint
    S&W Ozark Hillbilly Mountain Brew Sassafras
    Squaw Tea
    Tisa Instant Fruit Beverage Cubes (these contain turbinado sugar)
    V.I.P. Papaya-Mint; Peppermint
  Loose Leaf Tea
    all brands similar
    Bigelow and *Twinings* offer many varieties, some of which combine leaf and herb teas in one

HOT CHOCOLATE AND COCOA

General Rule of Purchase: Buy unsweetened brands. Check the label and select those that are not treated with alkali ("Dutched").

    EXEMPLARY BRANDS:
      Cara-Coa (carob)
        Hershey's Unsweetened Cocoa

Sweet Things

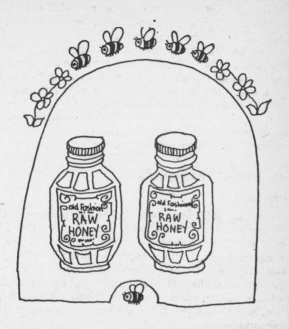

Many of us, ourselves included, meet our downfall when it comes to sweets. Sugar is one of the most harmful nonfoods on the market. We classify it as a nonfood since it contributes absolutely nothing to the body (except calories, and few of us regard calories as a positive addition), and it may do some serious harm. Sugar has been linked in some way to almost every major disease—diabetes, heart ailments, cancer. On a less drastic scale it is the cause of lots of excess poundage, and no matter what you may think about the harmful effects of chemical food additives, you can be sure of one thing in regard to sugar: SUGAR ROTS TEETH!

The human body has no nutritional need for refined table sugar yet it is added to the least likely foods. You will discover sugar is an ingredient in canned soups, sauces, canned vegetables, baked beans, pickles, processed meats, fried rice mixtures, peanut butter, catsup, crackers and almost all "convenience" foods.

If you disregard all the other advice proffered in this book, you should at least eliminate the deadly threesome—white flour, white bread, and white sugar—from your diet.

We have no cure for a sweet tooth, and know that to simply say "Stop eating sugar" without offering a replacement is unlikely to change anyone's eating habits. So, if you're going to keep eating sweets, at least choose a sweetener that can add a little something to your food intake, like honey or molasses.

Take a pitcher of water to dinner. You can minimize the effect of sugar on your teeth by brushing your teeth or rinsing out your mouth with water shortly after you're finished eating.

THE "OTHER" SWEETENERS

Molasses

The original sugarcane is well supplied with B vitamins, calcium, phosphorus, and iron. In the Mid-East, the cane is pressed through a roller and the juice is savored as a rich energy drink. In our country the sugarcane goes through a highly chemicalized refining process which strips away all the nutrients and produces sparkling white crystals of sugar. The residue that remains after refining is known as blackstrap molasses and contains all the original nutrients. It is quite strong, almost bitter. *Brer Rabbit* Blackstrap Molasses is available in many supermarkets.

Unsulfured Molasses

Unsulfured molasses (also known as West Indies and Barbados) differs from the blackstrap in that it is not a by-product of sugar refining but is manufactured for the molasses itself. This form of molasses is mellow and quite pleasing, imparting a taffylike taste when combined with other foods. The same healthy elements remain in the unsulfured molasses as in the blackstrap. *Crosby's* Barbados and *Grandma's* Old-Fashioned Molasses offer two more supermarket alternatives to white sugar.

Honey

The most universal substitute for sugar is honey. Honey is the natural nectar of a flower converted to a rich, golden syrup by hordes of hard-working bees. The latest selling trick is to tack an organic label onto honey jars. Don't be misled by a brand claiming to be "organic" and upping its prices. All honey is pretty free of pesticide residue, mainly because bees are highly sensitive to pesticides and either steer clear of sprayed plants or don't live long enough to tell about it. What you do want to check for when you buy honey is that the brand you select is 100 percent pure "unfiltered," "raw," or "uncooked." This honey has not be subjected to heating and possesses all the native nutrients and heat-sensitive enzymes.

In crystallized or granulated form, honey makes a smooth, creamy spread. This form of honey is labeled "granulated," "creamed," "spun," or "spread." Sometimes part of the comb is left intact. Many people consider the comb a rare delicacy.

All honey does not taste the same, which is why the label may read "Buckwheat," "Clover," "Blended," etc. The name and distinguishing flavor come from the flower the bees fed on. Blended honey is usually the least expensive and least distinctive. If you're not really into honey it is a fine all-purpose sweetener. If you'd like to explore the more exotic flavors that are becoming more and more apparent in the supermarket you can expect to find:

Clover Honey: Light and delicate, excellent for sweetening beverages and delicate cakes and cookies.

Alfalfa Honey: Still rather mellow in taste, well suited to most dishes.

Greek Honey: Most honey imported from Greece comes from bees fed on thyme. The resulting honey is very rich with a sweet, soothing but somewhat medicinal flavor. Delicious spread on thick slabs of bread.

Irish Honey: The characteristic flower in Irish honey is heather and it produces another thick, rich, but rather mild nectar.

Buckwheat Honey: Favored by Russian cooks, this honey is dark and more robust than the others. Excellent for bread-making.

Beware of very inexpensive brands that seem unusually thin when poured. A dishonest manufacturer often adulterates "pure honey" with sugar and corn syrup, or derives his honey from bees fed on sugar-water rather than the sweet, nourishing nectar the bees extract from living flowers.

Unfiltered honey may be cloudy and on storage may develop crystals. This is just a sign that you have really purchased unfiltered honey, and it can easily be reversed by standing the honey jar in a bowl of warm water (no hotter than the hand can bear) until all the crystals are melted.

Honey lasts a very long time (unless you use it up quickly as we do) and should be stored at room temperature, not in the refrigerator.

"Raw" Sugar

The so-called unrefined sugar is a highly controversial product, shunned by the more orthodox advocates of natural foods. Genuine unrefined sugar is a soft, dark, "impure" product that still has 30 to 40 percent of the original nutritional value of the sugarcane. The question is, is the unrefined sugar in this country really unrefined? According to Rodale Press, raw sugar was made illegal in this country in 1948 as a result of unsanitary conditions and contamination. According to Fred Rohe, a leading natural foods merchant, "raw" sugar as sold to the public is actually refined sugar which has molasses added. (Highly refined sugar with molasses added, by the way, is commercial brown sugar.)

We've seen raw sugar abroad and indeed it is quite different from the version offered in this country. Unrefined, we guarantee you, ours is not; partially refined it *may* be. Avoid all sugar whenever you can, and use it only when a substitute will not do . . . then, select the "raw" or "unrefined." Even if it is not the natural thing, chemical analysis does indicate the presence of some of the original nutrients; it has not been exposed to the "whitening" process that ordinary sugar crystals go through, and it is free of any anticaking chemical to make it "free-flowing."

Sugar-in-the-Raw is the latest commercial attempt at raw sugar on the mass-market level. The price, however, is outrageous, and the packaging is ecologically unsound—a pound box of sugar made up of individually wrapped envelopes containing 1 teaspoon of sugar each. "Raw" sugar (also referred to as turbinado and demerara) is packaged in bulk just like other sugars. Buy it this way.

Maple Syrup

Included on our list of sugar substitutes is maple syrup, the 100 percent pure kind that contains no added sugar, corn syrup, coloring, or flavoring. Among the "Maple-Flavored Syrup," the "Maple-Blended Syrup," "Pancake Syrup" and the "Imitation Maple Syrup" on the supermarket shelf, all blends of cane or corn syrup with very little maple and a sodium benzoate preservative, you'll usually find one brand of the real thing. One hundred percent pure maple syrup is not refined and retains its native nutrients which include iron and calcium. Canadian brands, like *Camp*, come highly recommended since formaldehyde pellets, often inserted into domestic trees to increase the maple syrup flow, are prohibited in Canada.

Corn Syrup

Corn syrup, like refined sugar, appears frequently on the label of many commercial food items. Corn syrup is a mixture of refined sugar, partially digested starches, and water. The light corn syrup is usually flavored with sugar, salt, and vanilla, while the dark syrup has another sugar syrup, salt, and a preservative added. Corn syrup is often artificially flavored and colored to create "Pancake Syrup." Like sugar, corn syrup is pure carbohydrate, offering the body calories and nothing more. Corn syrup is often used instead of sugar, especially in candy and ice cream making, because it controls crystal formation in frozen foods, adds body, and retains moisture in baked goods. Honey can do exactly the same things, and you should use it to replace corn syrup when included in a recipe. So should the food industry.

COOKING WITHOUT SUGAR

Honey can be used successfully in almost every recipe to replace sugar. If a sauce recipe calls for a spoonful of sugar, substitute an equal amount of honey. Let a spoonful of honey be the sweetening in your tea. Even in baked goods honey is an ideal sugar replacement.

•For each cup of sugar called for in the recipe substitute ¾ cup of honey and decrease the liquid by ¼ cup. If there is no liquid ingredient, add ¼ cup of flour for each ¾ cup of honey you use. Honey is a more concentrated sweetener than sugar, hence the decrease in amount. Baked goods made with honey (and molasses too) will keep much longer than other baked goods, remaining moist long after other cakes have gone stale.

•When baking with molasses, retain ¼ to ½ the sugar ("raw" sugar, that is) and let the rest of the measure be molasses. For each cup of molasses you include add ½ teaspoon of baking soda (to neutralize the acidity) and omit the baking powder. For each cup of molasses reduce the liquid in the recipe by ¼ cup.

•"Raw" sugar can be used just like the refined cane sugar, and maple syrup is best used according to specific recipe directions.

To make measuring easier when using these sticky syrups measure shortening first, then measure the sweetener in the same measuring unit . . . it will slide right out.

HOMEMADE BLENDED SYRUPS

If you find that straight molasses or honey is too strong by itself and pure maple syrup is unavailable, you can create your own unadulterated table syrups. These are some of the concoctions you can mix up in your kitchen:

BLENDED BREAKFAST SYRUP

Blend together: ½ cup molasses
½ cup honey
½ teaspoon vanilla
Pinch of salt

Chopped pecans or walnuts make a nice addition to this syrup.

ORANGE BUTTER TOPPING

½ cup butter, softened at room temperature
1 cup honey
6 tablespoons (½ 6-ounce can) frozen orange juice concentrate, thawed, undiluted

Beat honey, 2 tablespoons at a time, into butter until thoroughly blended. Gradually beat in undiluted orange concentrate. Use on pancakes, French toast, or waffles, and if you have any left over, store in refrigerator. To reuse, soften at room temperature and beat to reblend into a uniform mixture.

MOLASSES BUTTER SAUCE

Combine ¾ cup of molasses and ⅓ cup of butter in a small saucepan. Heat, stirring occasionally, until smooth and well blended. Serve warm.

RECOMMENDATIONS

General Rule of Purchase: Do not buy white sugar, but choose honey, molasses, maple syrup, sorghum, and "raw" (turbinado or demerara) sugar instead. In selecting honey, make sure the brand you buy is unfiltered and raw, or uncooked. For highest flavor and quality, select one of the flower honeys rather than "blended" honey. Purchase granulated (creamed, spun, or honey spread) for spreading on bread. Select 100 percent pure maple syrup (Canadian brands preferred) for topping pancakes, etc.

EXEMPLARY BRANDS:
Honey—all uncooked varieties similar
Molasses
> Blackstrap is higher in nutrients.
> *BrerRabbit* Blackstrap
> *Crosby's* Barbados (unsulfured)
> *Datetree* Blackstrap
> *Grandma's* Old Fashioned (unsulfured)
> *Holiday* Blackstrap
> *Plantation* Blackstrap

Maple Syrup
> *Camp*
> *Fancifood*
> *Jones*
> *MacDonald's*
> *Mille Lacs*
> *Vermont Farms*
> *Vermont Maple Orchard*

Sorghum
> *Benton County* Gold
> *Waconia*

Seasonings: Natural Food Enhancers

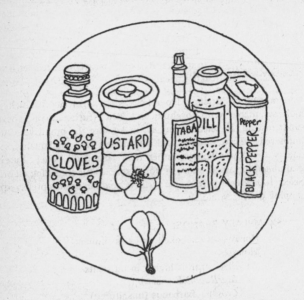

Flavor enhancers in the form of fresh and dried herbs, spices, and extracts are the key to rich-tasting, aromatic dishes that lure people into the kitchen to see what's cooking. These seasonings are mostly derived from living or once living plants and lend their characteristic flavor to whatever foods they are introduced to. The term "natural flavoring" includes these herbs, spices, and extracts.

SALT

Oversalting is a serious problem in this country where almost every commercially prepared product has "salt added." Sodium chloride is the harmful element in salt, and common table salt is virtually 99.99 percent sodium chloride. One way you can cut down on salt additives is simply by using less. Salt is a natural ingredient in all foods and the need for more is an acquired taste. Since vegetables contain less salt, a nonmeat eater might feel a need for more salt than a meat eater. To compensate for less salt, increase the use of other herbs and spices. Keep in mind that garlic, onion, and celery salt all add additional salt to your daily intake, so select pure herbs and spices—minus the salt.

The most common form of salt on the supermarket shelf is a product referred to as "table salt." In the purifying process all the native minerals are stripped away, but it is usually enriched with iodine plus dextrose to stabilize it, sodium bicarbonate to keep it white and chemical anticaking agents to keep it "free-flowing." *Morton's Special Salt* is the only brand of table salt we know of with no additives, but it has nothing to offer either.

Salt is a mineral and, when extracted from the sea and not highly refined or treated, is rich in native minerals which replace about 20 percent of the sodium chloride of table salt. However sea salt is still "salt" and should not be used as a salt substitute. Occasionally sea salt is available in the supermarket, and when it is, you should buy it. It is used in cooking and at the table just as regular salt.

Despite what other sources say, "kosher salt" is as highly refined as ordinary table salt and is treated with the same chemicals during manufacturing to remove mineral "impurities."

FRESH SEASONINGS

Fresh seasonings not only enhance the taste but add nutrients to your food. Because they are derived from plant sources, many of them are rich in vitamins and minerals. Look over this guide to using fresh seasonings and incorporate them into your recipes.

Garlic and Onion

The two most widely used flavoring agents are garlic and onion. Both are sold fresh, and in the form of ground dried powder and salt. Stick with the fresh. Nothing approaches the taste of these vegetables in their original form. Chop, mince, grate, or press as needed for enhancing your food: 1 clove of garlic and 1 tablespoon of chopped or grated onion can substitute for ¼ teaspoon of the powder in a recipe.

Ginger

Fresh ginger root is being offered in many supermarkets these days and is wonderful for making pungent dishes, especially for Chinese and Indian specialties. For every ¼ teaspoon of ground ginger called for in a recipe use a 1-inch piece of the fresh ginger root chopped finely or grated. Ginger can get quite fiery, so start with a little and add more to taste. Fresh ginger grated into the dressing really perks up a fruit or vegetable salad.

Hot Peppers

In certain parts of the country hot (chili) peppers are a common supermarket commodity. Be careful when you use them. Not only are they hot to taste, but fresh chili pulp will burn the skin too. To prepare chilis for cooking:

Wash and dry the pods, skewer on a long-handled fork and toast on top of the stove, turning so they blister on all sides. When the skin is evenly blistered and puffed away from the pulp you can lay the pods on a cloth, sprinkle them lightly with water, and cover them with another cloth so they steam. The skins can then be pulled away easily and the seeds and veins removed. Use all of the pulp, but only a few of the seeds.

The seeds and veins are the hottest part, so take it easy. Don't be a show-off when it comes to chili. If you put one of the seeds on your lips or tongue we assure you you'll never be tempted to try it again.

Lemon

Lemon juice is added to many sauces, soups, salad dressings, meat, fruit and vegetable dishes to enliven their flavor. Half a fresh lemon will serve you far better than bottled lemon juice which is rather flat tasting and preserved with chemicals.

FRESH HERBS

Herbs are nothing more complicated than aromatic leaves and sometimes flowers that are both edible and flavorful. To preserve the flavor and aroma they are frequently dried, but many of them are just as popular in the fresh form and far richer this way.

Celery Leaves

The fresh leafy tops of celery are excellent for perking up soups; an essential ingredient in homemade chicken broth. If you have more leaves than you can use, you'll find home-drying a great money-saving trick.

Wash the leaves under cold water to clean and pat dry with absorbent paper. Spread on paper (wax, parchment) and let dry slowly, exposed to the air at room temperature until crumbly. Do not dry in direct sunlight. Store these and all your home-dried herbs in a tightly covered jar for future use.

Chives

Chives are sold as a growing plant. The plant is usually jammed into a tiny container and dies because the roots are too plentiful for the pot. You can have a long-lasting source of this herb in your kitchen if you replant it in a larger pot and continually cut the tops so your chive shoots remain upright. Chives are a member of the onion family, although much milder, and can be used uncooked to flavor cheese dips, sauces, and spreads. Try adding chives to cottage cheese, sour cream, and mayonnaise to accentuate the taste.

Dill

Fresh dill makes everything taste like spring. You probably know dill in the taste of dill pickles. Its use extends to soup (particularly potato and white bean) and salads as well. We like to add fresh dill and lemon to fish salads, or combine the chopped herb with sour cream for a fish sauce.

Mint

Mint may be sold fresh or dried in your market. Add the leaves to yogurt for a refreshing salad. Also good in fruit mixtures and steeped in boiling water for a Mid-Eastern tea. For an instant breath refresher, chew a few mint leaves.

Parsley

Fresh parsley, often used as a garnish only to be pushed to the side of the plate, is actually a fine source of vitamins A and C and vegetable protein. It is also rich in chlorophyll to make your breath nice and sweet—both cheaper and healthier than mouthwash. Use fresh parsley to season soups, salads, stuffings, bread crumb coatings and thousands of other meat and vegetable dishes. To store this herb, wash, chop and keep in a plastic bag in the freezer. When you need a spoonful, dip into the freezer stock; it thaws almost instantaneously. The dried form doesn't compare for flavor or nutrition.

DRIED HERBS

Those herbs not readily available fresh are dried and bottled for your convenience. While not as fresh-tasting in this form, if properly prepared, the flavor and aroma can be satisfactorily retained. The potency is much greater in the dried form. As a general guide for interchanging fresh and dried herbs allow ⅓ to ½ teaspoon of dried herbs to replace 1 tablespoon of fresh.

Basil

This dried leaf is a natural companion for tomatoes. Use it in tomato sauces, vegetable casseroles, and fresh tomato salads.

Bay Leaves

While the leaf itself is not eaten it imparts flavor and aroma to soups and tomato dishes and pickling liquors. Also recommended in fish chowders. Add one leaf to the pot when you begin cooking. Remove before serving.

Chervil

The French are particularly fond of chervil, and it is one of the traditional components of "fines herbes." It is much less common in American kitchens but we find it one of the best flavoring ingredients for salad dressing. Use it just as you would parsley.

Chives

When fresh chives are unavailable, freeze-dried chives are the best substitute. In this form the herb retains a maximum of flavor and when added to a liquid medium rehydrates readily. Use them in any way that you would the fresh.

Marjoram

The traditional way of using marjoram is in lamb dishes. It is also good on string beans and limas, and for a unique taste you might try adding some to poultry stuffing.

Oregano

The essential ingredient in all Italian dishes, so any time you want to impart Italian flavor be sure to include this herb. Also used in Greek and Mexican food.

Rosemary

Rosemary is a sweetish herb that is sold dried and resembles small spikes. We add it along with basil, oregano, and marjoram to Italian dishes. It can be used in soups and stews, lamb, and chicken dishes, and we've heard it's great in gin drinks too.

Sage

Again, a valuable stuffing enhancer, particularly favored with pork products. Steeped in hot water it is supposedly an excellent medicinal beverage for alleviating colds.

Thyme

Of "parsley, sage, rosemary and" fame, this herb is associated most often with poultry.

CARING FOR HERBS

All dried herbs should be stored in airtight containers away from heat. Most cooks keep their herb (and spice) shelf within easy reach of the stove, a handy place except that heat dissipates the flavor and quality of your seasonings. Try to have a permanent storage place in a cooler part of your kitchen.

Always buy the form of dried herb closest to the whole-leaf state, avoiding finely crushed leaves whenever possible. The crumbling of the leaves releases the essential flavoring oils; therefore it is best to crush the leaves between your fingers just before introducing them to the pot.

SPICES AND SEEDS

Spices are the dried flavoring elements produced from the buds, flower, fruit, bark, and root of the plant. Many are sold already blended as curry powder, chili powder, pumpkin pie spice, etc. Although sometimes sold in the whole form, most of them are preground before they reach the market. Unless you use a particular spice in huge quantities buy the smallest jars available; the flavor diminishes with age and exposure to air. Store tightly covered in a cool, dry place as you do herbs. When the characteristic odor of your spices and herbs is no longer pungent it is time to replace them. Most spices are unadulterated (although they may be sprayed with fumigants to prevent bug habitation at the processing plant). Any tampering should be on the label.

Some of the more common spices are discussed below. We have included seeds here as well. Seeds come from the dried fruit or seed of a plant and differ from spices in that the seeds usually refer to the aromatic product of plants of temperate zones, while spices come from plants of tropical origin. (Use that tidbit at your next cocktail party.)

Allspice

Allspice is the product of one plant only, although its name might imply that it is a mixture of more than one spice. The flavor resembles a blend of cinnamon, nutmeg, and cloves. The whole form is used in pickling; when ground it adds flavor to baked goods and puddings. Try placing the powdered form in stored clothing as a moth preventive.

Caraway Seed

This is the flavor so many of us associate with rye bread. These seeds are delicious in sauerkraut, cooked cabbage dishes, and on potatoes. We add them to cottage cheese for flavoring dips, and David loves them in scrambled eggs.

Cardamom

Cardamom is sold both whole and ground and is often quite costly. It is a common ingredient in Indian dishes and the Danish add the ground seeds to pastry. Chewing cardamom seeds is a good cover-up for liquor on the breath.

Cayenne

This fiery red powder from small red peppers can be used to spark anything. A pinch even helps sweet dishes. Use sparingly though, it's very hot.

Celery Seed

Use just as you would celery leaves. When stuffing vegetables with cream cheese, mix in some celery seeds and you'll have a more flavorful spread. A teaspoon can be added to salad dressing for a fresh flavor, particularly fruit dressings.

Chili Powder

This spice is made from chili peppers blended with other spices and can be either mild or hot. Use it in Mexican dishes and bean stews.

Cinnamon

The best way to buy cinnamon is in stick form. A 1-inch stick of cinnamon equals 1 teaspoon of ground. Use the whole sticks as stirrers or straws in hot spiced punch, tea, coffee, and milk. Ground cinnamon, of course, goes into cakes, pies, and puddings. You needn't save it for sweet dishes though. Add some to rice to give it an arousing aroma.

Cloves

Cloves are highly fragrant nail-shaped buds which again are used in pickling (mostly fruits). Meat is often studded with cloves to add flavor in roasting. Ground, it is frequently used in baking. We find cloves go especially well in dishes that include lentils. They also make a good project for children and a wonderful inexpensive gift item when used to fashion pomander balls. For directions and more details, see "Ecology at Home."

Curry Powder

Curry powder is another spice blend and can be added to white sauce to flavor leftover meat, vegetables, and eggs. Curry, however, is more than just curry powder and for most effective use of curry spices consult an Indian cookbook. Improper use of curry powder is one sure way to turn people off to Indian food, which is delicious.

Fennel

Although this spice is not among the most popular, we mention it as it can add variety to some of your favorite dishes by imparting a licorice-like flavor. It's quite interesting in apple pie. Also in boiled fish dishes. Highly recommended for those who like licorice, to be brewed like tea and served as a hot drink.

Ginger

In addition to the fresh root, ginger is available dried and ground. This is a spice with a real bite, so taste your dish as you proceed. Use ground ginger in baking (for gingerbread), particularly in combination with fruit fillings.

Mustard

Dried mustard powder is the base for prepared mustards. Gradually beat water into the powder to creamy consistency and you've made your own hot mustard. It is our favorite flavoring ingredient in salad dressing. Add ¼ teaspoon along with the other seasonings for a sharp (but favorably so) taste. Add to cheese dishes as well.

Nutmeg

When Columbus set sail for the East Indies nutmeg was one of the spices he was searching for. Nutmeg should always be used in the ground form, alone on vegetables like cauliflower, spinach, and broccoli, combined with cinnamon on berries, bananas, eggnog, and custard.

Paprika

Sweet red peppers are the source of this popular spice, famed more for its use in coloring rather than flavoring food. Its mild flavor recommends it for use on egg salad, cream cheese, and sweet corn for color contrast. Also makes tomato sauces redder. If fresh, paprika is an excellent source of vitamin C.

Pepper

Pepper goes with everything—in small amounts. Too much (and this is true of all "hot" spices) can damage the stomach lining. Invest in a pepper mill and season meat, fish, poultry, egg, and vegetable dishes with the freshly ground peppercorns before serving. Pepper that is purchased ready-ground is flat and lifeless. By the way, a lavish sprinkling of ground pepper is another moth repellent used throughout the world.

MSG

Monosodium glutamate is a natural flavor enhancer which has no taste of its own but brings out natural food flavors and helps them to blend into one another. All foods have a natural amount of MSG in them. The huge amounts of MSG that are added unnaturally to foods have been linked to physical reactions including headaches, sweating, chills, hot flashes, and temporary paralysis. Evidence against the product is not conclusive, but it is pretty weighty. We suggest you ignore MSG when it is called for in the list of ingredients in a recipe; don't buy seasoned salts (which contain lots of MSG) or prepared foods which depend on the inclusion of MSG for flavor either.

VERY BRIEF ADVICE ON SEASONING

The best way to judge the right amount of seasoning is by taste. By all means, taste as you go along. A pot that has not been sampled during cooking usually reflects this neglect.

FLAVOR EXTRACTS

Flavoring extracts are sold in two forms: pure extract and imitation flavoring. The pure offers real flavor (from vanilla beans, almonds, lemon, etc.) diluted with ethyl alcohol. Imitation flavoring is based on a chemical compound which simulates a real flavor and should always be avoided. Even "pure" vanilla extract may not be quite as pure as its name implies. It may be doctored with glycerin, propylene glycol, sugar, dextrose, and corn syrup, without mentioning any of this on the label.

Because most of the imported vanilla beans used by manufacturers are treated with glycerin in their homeland, traces are almost universal in the common supermarket extracts.

All varieties of other pure flavor extracts must provide full ingredient disclosure on the label.

Alternatives to Extracts

●A real vanilla bean imparts a much richer flavor than the extract. To flavor hot liquids and puddings, split the bean and cook it in the liquid. Remove it when you've finished cooking. To flavor other items, like cookies and cakes, split the bean, scrape out the seeds, and use the scrapings in the batter. Use about 1 inch of the bean instead of 1 teaspoon of extract. By the way, the aroma alone of fresh vanilla beans is worth the purchase price.

●Grind almonds to a powder and use 1 teaspoon of this to give baked dishes a hint of almond flavor and aroma. Replaces ¼ teaspoon of almond extract.

●Instead of lemon or orange extract, fresh fruit flavors can be introduced to your dishes from the juice and rind of lemons and oranges. Use the juice in sauces, syrups, and salad dressing. Grate the rind into puddings and cakes and sweet-flavored vegetables (like carrots, yams, and squash): ¼ teaspoon of grated rind is the equivalent of about 1 teaspoon of extract, and the flavor will be carried a long way.

Never settle for cheap imitations when it comes to flavoring your foods. It's deep, rich flavor you want to bring to your table, not chemicals; if the real thing is not to be found, the flavor of the food itself will always be better than the manufacturer's attempt at chemical duplication.

PREPARED SEASONINGS

These prepared flavoring products are worthy of mention.

Horseradish

Horseradish can be found fresh for grating into fish, meat, and sauces for flavoring; the most common form of this root, however, is in a jar, grated, salted, and mixed with vinegar (and occasionally beet juice for red color). Nothing else need be added to retain the fresh root flavor; *Gold's, Bauer's,* and *Schorr's* all abide by this.

This seasoning is not used in cooking so much as it is alongside fish (especially gefilte fish) to give it a pungent flavor. It can be added to white sauce or sour cream for serving with cold lamb, roast beef, fish, or vegetables. Use about ¼ cup of drained horseradish for each cup of sauce for a distinct flavor.

Liquid Pepper

Liquid pepper, also known as pepper sauce or hot sauce, is the mash of tiny red-hot peppers blended with vinegar. Some manufacturers add vegetable gums or other thickeners to the hot sauce; this is totally unnecessary. Stick to the brands that have no additives like *Tabasco* and *Frank's* Hot Sauce.

Soy Sauce

Valuable for enhancing Oriental dishes, and imparting a rich "meaty" taste to vegetable patties and soups. In the purest form this flavoring aid is nothing more than soybeans, water, wheat, and salt. This product is often known as "tamari" soy sauce in natural foods circles and may be available in the natural foods section of your supermarket. Imported Japanese soy sauce, probably located in the gourmet section, is equally as good. The American simulation of soy sauce is unfortunately doctored with sugar, caramel coloring, and preservatives.

Worcestershire Sauce

Lea & Perrins, "the original Worcestershire Sauce," is original in every sense of the word. While other brands add corn syrup, artificial coloring, artificial flavoring, and stabilizers in the form of gums like gum tragacanth to their flavoring sauce, *Lea & Perrins* sauce is made with fresh spices, including shallots and tamarinds (a tropical fruit whose pulp is used for preparing chutneys and curries and whose juice is used in pickling), plus molasses and vinegar and no synthetics at all.

Lea & Perrins Worcestershire Sauce and pure soy sauce should be used to replace all browning aids and steak sauces called for in your cooking.

RECOMMENDATIONS

HERBS AND SPICES

General Rule of Purchase: Make fresh flavor enhancers your first choice, then dried herbs and spices; all brands are similar. Buy closest to the whole form and make sure you select the pure herb or spice, not the "salt." All ingredients on label.

If you want an all-around seasoned salt, find one without added starch, dextrose, or MSG.

EXEMPLARY BRANDS:
Hollywood Vegetable Seasoned Salt
Jane's Krazy Mixed-Up Salt
Spike Seasoning
Vege-Sal

FLAVORING EXTRACTS

General Rule of Purchase: Buy pure, not imitation extracts. Vanilla extract will not list all ingredients and usually contains additives, including some form of sweetening. Other pure extracts reveal all ingredients on label.

PREPARED SEASONING PRODUCTS

General Rule of Purchase: Check labels closely in selecting prepared seasoning products. No chemicals need be added, although many often are. All ingredients on label.

EXEMPLARY BRANDS:
  Liquid Pepper (Hot Sauce)
    A.B. Hot Sauce
    Crystal Red Hot Sauce
    Frank's Hot Sauce
    La Preferida Louisiana Hot Sauce
    Tabasco
    Tennessee Sunshine Hot Pepper Sauce
    Texas Pete Hot Sauce
    White Swan Red Hot Sauce
  Soy Sauce—Check for sodium benzoate preservative and caramel coloring
    Kikkoman Salt Reduced Soy Sauce
    Reeses Vintage Aged Soy Sauce
    "Tamari"
    many imported Japanese varieties
  Horseradish
    Bauer's
    Gold's
    Schorr's
    Silver Spring
    Sitler's
  Worcestershire Sauce
    Crosse & Blackwell
    Lea & Perrins

N.B. For additional information, see specific seasonings in this chapter.

Leavening Agents:
Baking Soda, Baking Powder, Yeast, Etc.

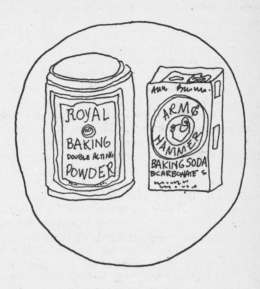

When you do any home baking you will invariably follow the directions given in the recipe for leavening the batter without giving much thought to the leavening ingredient itself. There are actually four different convenient methods of leavening baked goods though, and a little knowledge about them can help improve the physical and nutritional quality of your baked goods. We'll try not to get too technical.

BAKING SODA

Baking soda works by the simple release of carbon dioxide (a leavening gas) caused by the reaction between the baking soda and an acid ingredient in the recipe like buttermilk, vinegar, molasses, or fruit juices. Baking soda itself is nothing more than a basic salt, bicarbonate of soda, which is a chemical long used and accepted as a food item. Arm & Hammer seems to have a monopoly on this product.

In addition to its use as a leavening agent, baking soda is a fantastic nonpolluting cleaner. To learn more about this, turn to the chapter "Ecology at Home."

BAKING POWDER

Baking powder is another chemical leavening agent that works on the principle of carbon dioxide gas. The ingredients here become a bit more complex because the leavening comes from the interaction of the basic salt (baking soda), which is one of the ingredients in the leavener, and an acid salt furnished not by a food ingredient, but by another chemical ingredient in the baking powder. The use of a chemical acid and base produces a more controlled reaction than the food acid plus baking soda does. Some form of starch, usually cornstarch, keeps the powder from caking or absorbing moisture and reacting in the can. Baking powder must have liquid added in order for the release of carbon dioxide to take place.

You will notice that there are three types of baking powder available in your supermarket. Each is named for the acid salt it uses.

Tartrate depends on cream of tartar and tartaric acid. Tartaric acid is, interestingly, a by-product of wine-making. This type of baking powder releases most of its leavening gas at room temperature on contact with liquid, and when it is used the batter must be baked immediately or the gas will escape before it can be trapped in the dough and the product will not be well leavened.

Phosphate contains calcium acid phosphate, which may also be combined with sodium acid pyrophosphate, both metal salts of partially neutralized acids. Two thirds of the gas is released at room temperature on contact with liquid and the rest will not be released until heat is applied, making it a little slower-acting than the tartrate. It is used widely in prepared flour products and mixes and less commonly by homemakers.

SAS-Phosphate or double-acting baking powder only releases a small portion of its carbon dioxide at room temperature and most of it is not activated until heat is applied. Because of this, the batter can be delayed or even refrigerated for baking later in the day. The acid salts here (again metal salts) are calcium acid phosphate and sodium aluminum sulfate.

WHAT TO USE AND WHY

All chemical leavening agents (baking powder and soda) affect the acidity of the batter, and thiamine retention, a vitamin extremely sensitive to heat in an alkaline medium, becomes a problem. When the amount of acid cannot perfectly balance the basic ingredients, some of the B vitamin is destroyed. You run this risk any time baking powder or soda is used, so do not depend on these leavened products as a good source of this vitamin.

One additional, more serious problem exists with the use of baking powder, however, and that is the residue, or salts which are formed during the reaction between the acid and the base. Baking powder is used to increase the palatability of baked goods by creating a light, airy product. Many people feel the residues left are too harmful to warrant this luxury. This problem is most crucial in relation to the SAS or double-acting baking powder. For many years the question of toxicity in relation to aluminum has been posed and never really settled. Recently, Israeli researchers have been investigating the subject and have shown considerable damage in rats when aluminum salts were administered. As the scientists said, "Although what is true of rats is not necessarily true of man, it would seem advisable to suspend the widespread use of aluminum salts in man pending further studies of this problem." Who are we to argue.

Play it safe and stick with the so-called fast-acting baking powders, the tartrate and phosphate types. Solve the problem of the fast action by adding the liquid at the end and getting your batter into the oven right away. *Royal* and *Swansdown* are both tartrate baking powders; *Rumford, Dr. Price, Happy Family,* and *Jewel* are all phosphate brands.

YEAST

In addition to these "chemical leavening agents" there are "biological leavening agents" which ferment and give off carbon dioxide. The most common in this category is yeast, which you can purchase in your local supermarket. Two forms of yeast are available: compressed yeast cakes and active dry yeast. The compressed yeast cake is less popular, must be refrigerated, and must be used within a week or two, although it can be preserved for several months by freezing. If it crumbles easily it is still good.

Active dry yeast is more commonly found in the supermarket, and while it need not be refrigerated, it should be kept in a cool place. Make a note of the expiration date on the package and use it before then or chances are your bread will be as flat as matzoh. Recently, some manufacturers have taken to adding the antioxidant BHA to the yeast, probably to lengthen the expiration period; try to buy an untreated brand.

There is no secret involved in yeast baking, merely time, during which you can busy yourself with household chores and activities. Yeast needs warmth in which to grow, the ideal being 90 to 105°F. When the temperature is much higher the yeast grows too quickly and expires before the leavening gas has a chance to become entrapped in the dough. At colder temperatures it lies dormant.

Many recipes call for dissolving the yeast in ¼ cup of lukewarm water, scalding the milk in the recipe, letting it cool, and then adding it to the yeast. This method gives excellent results, indeed we often use it; however, it is more efficient and just as good to dissolve the yeast in water equal to the entire amount of liquid called for, and add the proper amount of dry milk powder along with the flour. This way there's no need to scald the milk.

Yeast feeds on simple sugars, and generally a little sweetening is added to the dissolving yeast to let it eat and grow. Honey and molasses are best.

When your yeast mixture bubbles a bit or becomes frothy on top, this is your sign that it is alive and ready to grow and leaven your bread. Follow all recipe directions for mixing and resting the dough to give the yeast time to do its work. Once the dough reaches about 130° F in the oven the yeast will die and the bread will rise no further.

Occasionally you may come across a recipe that tells you to add the yeast to the flour straight away, then pour in the scalding-hot liquid, a method which may elicit fear in experienced bread-makers who realize such extreme temperatures would destroy the yeast. Recent research has shown this method to be superior to the former, for the flour acts as a buffer and you don't risk killing the yeast if the liquid is too hot. The only problem is, if for some other reason the yeast is dead (due to improper storage or age), which is uncommon but not impossible, you won't realize it until you've used all your ingredients and spent time waiting for the dough to expand (which it never will). We're old-fashioned and stick to the traditional method, but if you trust your yeast, go ahead and follow the modern yeast-mixing directions.

A NATURAL LEAVENING AGENT

By the way, eggs are the most natural of all leavening agents, and cookies and muffins can be made quite successfully using no other source of leavening. Where the recipe calls for eggs, add only the yolk. After all other ingredients in the recipe have been included, beat the remaining egg white(s) until stiff peaks form. Then fold gently into the batter and bake as directed in the recipe. The final product will be a bit heavier than usual, but heavy cookies and muffins are much more filling anyway and you'll eat less.

RECOMMENDATIONS

BAKING SODA

General Rule of Purchase: Buy freely; all brands are the same.

BAKING POWDER

General Rule of Purchase: Choose those which have no aluminum compounds, generally the single-acting tartrate or phosphate brands. Remember, baking powder, as well as baking soda, has a high sodium content unless otherwise noted.

> EXEMPLARY BRANDS:
> Tartrate—*Royal*
> *Swansdown*
> Phosphate—*Dr. Price*
> *Happy Family*
> *Jewel*
> *Rumford*
> Salt-Reduced—*Cellu*

YEAST

General Rule of Purchase: Choose yeast cakes or active dry yeast with no preservatives (BHT/BHA). Do not confuse baking yeast with food, or nutritional, yeast.

EXEMPLARY BRANDS:
El Molino Active Dry Yeast
Fleischman's Active Dry Yeast for Bakers (2-pound tin only)
National Yeast Cakes
Red Star Active Dry Yeast

Salad Dressing, Oil and Vinegar

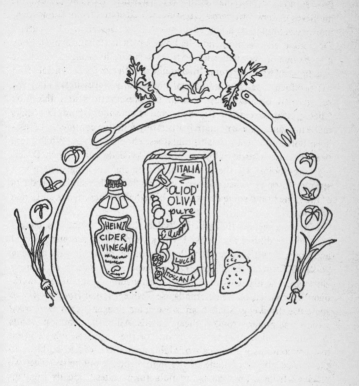

Few people these days make their own salad dressing. They prefer the prepared, bottled dressings on the supermarket shelf. We don't know just what it is that makes them so attractive. It certainly isn't the ingredients, since most oil and vinegar type dressings contain an acid ingredient (like vinegar or lemon juice), vegetable oil (a blend of oils including cottonseed oil), salt, sugar, other "suitable seasoning or flavoring" (and just what that secret blend of spices is may remain a mystery, but MSG is likely to be one of them), stabilizers in the form of pectin or vegetable gum, and a preservative known familiarly as

EDTA which is linked to kidney damage. Sounds more like it belongs in a test tube than a salad bowl. The only oil and vinegar dressing we have seen in the supermarket that is consistently free of all undesirable additives is *Porky Manero's* Dressing, which comes from Connecticut and is distributed to a few select stores only. *Bernstein's* Vinaigrette Dressing is also recommendable; however, their Italian, Danish Blue, and Roquefort contain such extras as sugar, hydrolized vegetable protein, and xanthan gum. Intermingled with the fresh vegetables in the produce case is an additional find, *Marie's* dressings. They are refrigerated because they contain no preservatives and the Blue Cheese, Italian Garlic, Rancher, and Thousand Island Dressings make imaginative use of ingredients rarely found in commercial dressings: buttermilk, sour cream, tomatoes, chopped olives. While these dressings use natural coloring, *Marie's* Avocado and French Dressings are spoiled by the inclusion of artificial coloring. There is a strange lesson to be learned here: you can find within similar products of the same brand some items with objectionable ingredients and some without.

Mayonnaise and the generic "salad dressing," which is merely mayonnaise diluted and cooked with a starch paste, are primarily oil and vinegar and seasonings with the addition of whole eggs and egg yolks to form an emulsion. The government standard of identity eliminates the necessity of showing the consumer just what the ingredient list consists of. Some brands use fresh eggs (like *Hollywood*) and some use dried egg. Some brands use cider vinegar (again *Hollywood*) and some prefer stronger, cheaper acids. All of the common brands use sugar and cottonseed oil as one of the vegetable oils. The oil usually contains a chemical to inhibit crystallization. In addition to the undesirability of some of the ingredients, a publicity leaflet we received from a mayonnaise manufacturer states: "ideally [mayonnaise] should be consumed within sixty days of purchase." This statement seems rather nonsensical for a "semiperishable" product like mayonnaise since you have no way of knowing how long the jar has been on the store shelf.

AVOIDING "TEST TUBE" DRESSINGS

Do not despair! It is amazingly simple to prepare your own salad dressing. The chapter "House Dressings" is devoted to helping you overcome any resistance. The average homemade preparation takes two minutes.

Before you prepare your dressing, though, there are two essential ingredients you should purchase with discretion: the oil and the vinegar.

BUYING OIL

The same oil that you purchase for cooking can be used in preparing salad dressing; here are some guidelines for making that purchase.

Something referred to as "Pure Vegetable Oil" is a common product in the supermarket. All the varieties of oil used to create this blend should be stated (in decreasing order) on the label. You'll find cottonseed oil is near the top of the list in most of these. We do not feel cottonseed oil is suitable for human consumption! Cotton is not generally regarded as an edible crop, thus it is treated with heavy doses of chemical sprays. The residue of this spray may be transmitted to the oil. Stay away from any product which contains cottonseed oil (including margarine, prepared salad dressings, marinated vegetables, and canned fish).

Corn and safflower oil have been well publicized as excellent sources of polyunsaturates. This is true. They also appear to be excellent sources of added chemicals. With the exception of the oils sold in the natural foods section of the supermarket we have not yet come across a brand of corn or safflower oil which does not contain an antioxidant (isopropyl citrate, BHA, BHT, citric acid, polysorbate 80) and an antifoaming agent (methyl silicone), both indicated on the label. If your store offers one, by all means buy it.

Peanut oil, on the other hand, is an excellent all-purpose oil, and both *Planters* and *Skippy* offer a chemically free choice. The labels suggest you store the oil in the refrigerator and warn you that it may become cloudy. This warning will give you the satisfaction of knowing your oil has not been "winterized"—a process which filters out the cloud-causing crystals, taking with them native nutrients. Do as the label says. If you use the oil fairly quickly, though, there is no need to store it in the refrigerator unless your kitchen cabinet is particularly warm. We have kept peanut oil unrefrigerated several weeks without having it go rancid.

One reason oils turn rancid is the refining process. Unrefined oils contain vitamin E, a natural antioxidant. When the oil is refined, this vitamin is destroyed. Olive oil, although more highly saturated than other vegetable oils, is the only unrefined oil available on the market. Olive oil is cold-pressed, which means instead of removing the oil from the plant by means of heat or a solvent, the olive is pressed to extract the natural oils. The refining of other oils removes most of the characteristic color and taste. Not so with olive oil, which retains the pungent, slightly bitter flavor of the olive and makes it desirable for flavoring salad dressings and certain Mediterranean dishes. Not everyone likes the flavor of olive oil and the quality of the oil may determine your attitude toward it. The highest quality oils have a more delicate flavor. Experiment with the imported Italian, French, Greek, and Spanish olive oils to find one that suits your taste.

Soybean oil is another suitable for cooking and salad-making. It is available without preservatives.

If there is a natural foods section in your supermarket, additional oils are likely to be offered there. Sunflower seed oil, soybean oil, walnut oil, wheat germ oil (all without preservatives) are good sources of unsaturated fat.

OIL VS. FAT

Oils can successfully be substituted for all other fats in cooking. We use oil for all sautéing, frying, basting, and greasing pans for baking. We often substitute oil for butter when we bake. This replacement is quite simple: for each cup of butter called for, use ⅞ cup (a scant cup) of oil. Many recipes call for melting the shortening anyway, and by using oil you avoid this step.

Semi-plastic vegetable shortening (the kind that comes in a can) is another fat, once unsaturated, which now has hydrogen bonds added back to make it solid at room temperature and thereby saturated (also referred to as hydrogenated). Not only that, but it's a can full of emulsifiers, stabilizers, bleaching agents, coloring agents, and preservatives. Use oil or softened butter instead, or for a homemade replica of "vegetable shortening" mix equal parts of oil and butter and whip in the blender.

On the shelf with the oils you're likely to find another fat substitute in the form of an aerosol spray designed to keep food from sticking to the skillet. This product is 97 percent Freon, a compressed propellant (used in cooling systems) which, if inhaled can cause, and has caused, anguished death. You should also keep in mind that anything purchased in an aerosol can (toothpaste, cheese, window spray) is not only unduly expensive but ecologically unsound.

Your pan will have a similar, permanent, nonstick effect if you "season" your skillet by wiping it with an oiled paper towel before cooking and after washing. Clean with a soapy sponge rather than harsh soap pads or abrasives.

VINEGAR

Vinegar is the most common source of acid, or tanginess, in salad dressing. All varieties are made by diluting acid from fermented grains or fruit with water. Plain white vinegar is derived from malt, rye, and barley, and is too strong for most tastes. We prefer to use it as a cleaner.

Cider vinegar is less tart and adds a slightly sweet taste to salad dressing. Wine vinegar is the most popular choice (although we rather like cider vinegar) and is available red, white, and flavored with herbs and spices. We choose red because of the nice color it imparts to the salad dressing; the flavors of the red and white are identical.

Unless the whole herb is still present in the vinegar bottle, as it is in imported, flavored vinegars, stick to the unflavored kind. It is easy enough to add your own garlic, thyme, or basil, if suitable to your recipe, and the result will be a much fresher flavor.

NOW THAT YOU HAVE THE RAW MATERIALS

Turn to the chapter "House Dressings" and begin to create your own.

RECOMMENDATIONS

PREPARED DRESSING

General Rule of Purchase: Mayonnaise, "salad dressing," and "oil and vinegar" concoctions may all have unlabeled ingredients in the form of sweeteners and food seasoning or flavoring.

Watch the label for citric acid and EDTA; in the "oil and vinegar" and "salad dressing" styles, look for a variety of emulsifiers including vegetable gums, pectin, propylene glycol ester or alginic acid, sodium carboxymethylcellulose. These all appear on the label.

Where specified, fresh eggs are preferred over dried and frozen, and specific nut or vegetable oils over just plain vegetable oil.

Since almost all varieties contain unnecessary sweeteners, over-salting, and oil of indeterminate purity, our best advice is make your own.

EXEMPLARY BRANDS: (Purity of oil is unknown unless stated.)

East—*BAMA* Mayonnaise (sugar)

Bernstein's French Vinaigrette Dressing

Blue Plate Mayonnaise (sugar)

Cain's Mayonnaise (sugar)

Hollywood Safflower Mayonnaise (honey, high-quality oil)

Kroger Italian Dressing (sugar, corn sweetener)

La Preferida Jalapeno Mayonnaise (sugar)

Marie's Blue Cheese, Italian Garlic, Rancher (sugar), and Thousand Island Dressings (sugar)

Marzetti Sunny Italian Dressing (sugar)

Mi-Del Mayonnaise (no sugar or salt)

Mullen's French Dressing (sugar)

Old Dutch Sweet and Sour Dressing (sugar, no oil)

Porky Manero's Salad Dressing

Tropic Bee Honey and Apple Cider Vinegar Dressing (honey, no oil or salt)

Middle—*Albert's* Finest Italian Dressing; French Dressing (sugar)

Albertson's Mayonnaise (sugar)

Bernstein's French Vinaigrette Dressing

Camelot Mayonnaise (sugar)

Cardini Original Caesar Dressing Mix (you add oil and vinegar)

Dorothy Lynch Home Style Dressing (sugar)

Food Club Mayonnaise (sugar, frozen egg yolks)

Hollywood Safflower Mayonnaise (honey, high-quality oil)

Kitchen Klatter Country Style Dressing (sugar)

Marie's Blue Cheese, Italian Garlic, Rancher (sugar), and Thousand Island Dressings (sugar)

Mrs. Clark's Italian Dressing (sugar)

Mrs. Clark's Mayonnaise; Salad Dressing (sugar)

Mullen's French Dressing (sugar)

Sona Safflower Mayonnaise (honey, high-quality oil)

Tropic Bee Honey & Apple Cider Vinegar Dressing (honey, no oil or salt)

West—*Albertson's* Mayonnaise (sugar)

Bernstein's French Vinaigrette Dressing

Bonnie Hubbard Mayonnaise and Salad Dressing (sugar)

Camelot Mayonnaise (sugar)

Coop Mayonnaise and Salad Dressing (sugar)

Hale n' Hardy French Dressing (high-quality oil); Herb Dressing (turbinado sugar, high-quality oil)

Hollywood 7 Herb Dressing (high-quality oil)

Hollywood Safflower Mayonnaise and Eggless Imitation Mayonnaise (honey, high-quality oil)

Hunza Mayonnaise (honey, high-quality oil)

Las Hierbas Exotic Herbs French Dressing

Laura Scudder Mayonnaise (sugar)

Marie's Blue Cheese, Italian Garlic, Rancher (sugar), and Thousand Island Dressings (sugar)

Nickabod's Fisherman's Wharf Avocado Dressing; Blue Cheese Dressing; Roquefort Dressing; 3 in 1 Tartar Sauce

Von's Mayonnaise (sugar)

OIL

General Rule of Purchase: Choose specific nut and vegetable oils. Label lists all constituent oils and additives. Watch for cottonseed oil, isopropyl citrate, BHT, BHA, citric acid, polysorbate 80, and methyl silicone. Avoid oil in *clear, semi-rigid* plastic containers; they are made from PVC.*

Check the "health food" aisle for additional selections.

*The FDA is presently considering proposals to prohibit certain "food contact materials," particularly packaging made from vinyl chloride like the clear, semirigid bottles and containers.

EXEMPLARY BRANDS:

Peanut
> *Planters*
> *Rokeach*
> *Skippy*

Corn
> *A&P*
> *Albertson's*
> *Caruso*
> *Fleischman's* (sometimes has preservatives)
> *Grand Union*
> *Hains*
> *Heritage House*
> *Hollywood*
> *Jewel Maid*
> *Kroger*
> *Nu Made*
> *Springfield*
> *Weis*

Soybean
> *Balance of Nature*
> *Bonnie Hubbard* Vegetable Salad Oil
> *C.H.B.* Salad Oil
> *Contadina* Vegetable Oil
> *Coop*
> *Gingham* Salad Oil
> *Good Day* Salad Oil
> *Hains*
> *Hillcrest*
> *Hollywood*
> *Hunza*
> *Lake Farm Ridge*

Safflower
> *Balance of Nature*
> *Hains*
> *Hollywood*
> *Hunza*

Mixed Oil
   Caruso Blended (Soya, Corn, and Olive)
   Balance of Nature Blended (Safflower, Soy, Sesame, and Sunflower)
Olive Oil—buy freely

VINEGAR

General Rule of Purchase: All brands similar. Choose unseasoned cider or wine vinegar for best flavor.

The Sad State of Soups and Sauces

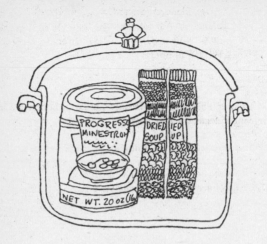

Most manufactured soups and sauces have a multitude of additives to keep them fresh-tasting and fresh-looking, to make them just the right consistency, and to keep the manufacturer's costs down. Real ingredients like fresh dairy products and high-quality meat and vegetables all cost money. On the other hand, flavor enhancers and intensifiers like MSG and disodium inosinate and guanylate are particularly popular with commercial soup-makers, as are heavy doses of salt, because they mask the lack of rich, natural taste. How can you "beef-up" soup with meat so inferior it can't be sold on the general market? No wonder they use all those additives. You are always better off preparing your own soups and, with a few exceptions, your own sauces.

CANNED SOUP

Soup brands vary greatly from market to market, so read the label. If it reads like a cookbook recipe you might consider buying it; if it reads like a chemistry textbook, leave it alone. *Progresso* offers several soup choices you might want to consider, like their Minestrone, Lentil, Macaroni and Bean, and Tomato Soup Italiano. They do, however, add MSG to some of their other soups. MSG is an ingredient you may very well find in your cookbook, but in the light of current evidence you should leave it out. To give you an idea of what an acceptable soup label features, this is a rundown of the ingredients in a can of *Progresso* Lentil Soup:

water, lentils, spinach, celery, onions, tomato paste, shortening, olive oil, Romano cheese, salt, spices.

Another acceptable choice, this one in a jar rather than a can, is *Mother's* Egg-Enriched Schav. Schav is a cold soup made from sour leaves, akin to grass.

Remember, even if there's nothing in the can you wouldn't use in your own kitchen, the quality of the ingredients may not be the same. Those vegetables, meats, and other soup-makings which don't quite make the grade for other products all go into the commercial soup pot.

DRIED SOUP

The dry soup mixes are not much more encouraging. Those that are free of additives are nothing more than an assortment of dried beans and dehydrated vegetables. Some brands contain a small packet of spices as well. The packet is where most of the undesirable ingredients are found. You can always remove the spice packet and substitute fresh vegetable or meat stock or seasoning of your own.

In the dried soup category *Goodman's* Vegetable Soup Mix with Mushrooms is a fine example of a real soup. So is their Split-Pea Soup if you throw out the spice packet, but it would be much cheaper to just buy a box of split peas and turn to the chapter "Homemade Soups." *De Looks* Minestrone offers a nice variety of beans and barley in just the right proportion for preparing a fresh minestrone following the recipe on the package.

The chapter "Homemade Soups" will help you supplement this list with many other homemade soups, some that take only minutes more than the readymade brands to fix. You'll find them much less expensive to prepare and far more welcome on your table.

PACKAGED SAUCES AND GRAVIES

Sauces are a highly cherished convenience food in many homes. A covering of sauce can enhance or disguise almost anything, so naturally you want it to be as flavorful as can be. Because sauces are used so widely you also want them to be as wholesome as possible.

Packaged and canned sauce mixes and gravies are the two pre-made alternatives, and we're sad to say there is not a single packaged sauce mix worthy of your kitchen. All rely on chemicals for flavor, color, texture, and freshness, and most of them require the costly addition of milk or tomato paste. A one-cup package, selling for 25¢ to 30¢, which calls for these added ingredients gets to be quite expensive. When you come right down to it you can prepare a fine sauce base with the added ingredients alone and eliminate the mix altogether (which is just what we'll show you how to do shortly). But first, the canned sauces.

CANNED SAUCE

Canned spaghetti sauce is the most popular item in this category. Although fresh homemade tomato sauce is much more tasty and only takes twenty minutes to prepare, many people still depend on the prepared version for a quick and simple meal. There are fortunately

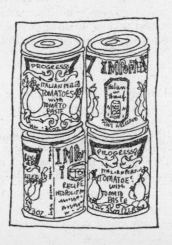

some brands that are free of artificial color and flavor, preservatives, starchy thickeners, and other extenders (like corn syrup).

Aunt Millie's Sauces are at the top of the recommended list, with no undesirable ingredients at all, including sugar, which is found in every other brand. If Aunt Millie can do it, why can't others?

Ronzoni Tomato Sauces run a close second, with sugar the only questionable ingredient. Their white clam sauce is also praiseworthy. worthy.

Consider too, the simple canned tomato sauces consisting of tomatoes plus seasoning only, like *Contadina* or *La Preferida,* as well as many house labels. These can easily be enriched with oil, fresh mushrooms, peppers, and cheese or meat to taste.

Sauces which contain meat or meat flavoring or cheese are more likely to have chemicals added to prevent these foods from becoming rancid and the quality of these added foods is often questionable. The meat is usually quite fatty and the amount is often far lower than the corresponding cost. By government regulations Spaghetti Sauce with Meat must contain only 6 percent meat. If you want meat or cheese in your sauce, add it at home.

HOT SAUCES

Several companies manufacture prepared spicy sauces that can enhance a meal, especially Mexican dishes. All ingredients are on the label and some appealing sauces include *Ortega* Taco and Green Chile Sauces, *Las Palmas* Chile and Enchilada Sauces, *Old El Paso* Taco Sauce, *Pace* Picante Sauce, *Rio Grande* Enchilada Sauce, and *Pedro Pride's* Salsita Mexicana.

TOMATO PASTE AND PUREE

Tomato paste and puree are common ingredients in canned and homemade soups and sauces. Tomato puree is a highly concentrated liquid extract of fresh tomatoes. Only salt is added.

Tomato paste is a concentrated tomato puree which may contain spices and flavoring (and these should be natural, not artificial flavoring ingredients). Baking soda may be added to tomato paste to neutralize the acidity. This will appear on the label and you should avoid these brands. No preservatives or artificial coloring are permitted. There are many brands in your supermarket that meet these specifications, but if you're in doubt, try *Progresso, Pope,* or *Contadina.* All are excellent.

Now see the chapter, "Do-It-Yourself Sauces," for some basic instruction in sauce making.

RECOMMENDATIONS

SOUPS

General Rule of Purchase: All ingredients are given on the label. Most brands display a long list of chemicals plus highly refined starch thickeners which give the soup "body" so that fewer high-quality raw ingredients need be added. Look for one that doesn't. Salt is ubiquitous, sugar and MSG are unfortunate, and where meat is included, consider the fact that bacon, pork, and other cured meats all contain nitrite preservatives.

EXEMPLARY BRANDS:
Canned
American Beauty Tall Boy Tomato (sugar, cracker meal)

Campbell's Pea (sugar, white flour); Tomato (sugar, white flour)

Gold's Shav

Hadden House Minestrone; Black Bean; Gazpacho (cornstarch)

Louis Henry Real Turtle Soup

Progresso Lentil; Tomato with Pasta Shells; Tomato Soup Italiano; Macaroni and Bean; Minestrone

Reese Mushroom (cornstarch); Minestrone

Rex Mardi Gras Crayfish Bisque (cornstarch, white bread); Shrimp Okra Gumbo (cornstarch)

Rokeach Shav

Dry
De Looks Minestrone; Bean Chowder Mix; Pasta Fazool Soup Mix: Mushroom Barley

Goodman's Vegetable Soup Mix with Mushrooms

Frozen
>> *Magic Garden* Frozen Condensed Minestrone; Lentil;
>> Whole Wheat Noodle; Matzoh Ball

SAUCES

General Rule of Purchase: All ingredients are given on label. Avoid those with added starch, sugar, MSG, flavor enhancers, and any other chemicals. All contain salt.

EXEMPLARY BRANDS:
>> Plain Tomato Sauce
>>> *Contadina* Tomato
>>> *F & P Tomato* (commercial size)
>>> *Iris* Tomato
>>> *Janet Lee* Tomato
>>> *Just Rite* Creole
>>> *Kearn's* Tomato
>>> *La Preferida* Tomato
>>> *National* Tomato
>>> *Old El Paso* Tomato
>>> *Progresso* Pizza
>>> *Shop Rite* Spanish Style Tomato
>>> *Staff* Tomato
>>> and many other house brands
>> Mexican Style Tomato Sauce (spicy)
>>> *Las Palmas* Green Chile Salsa; Enchilada Sauce; Red
>>> Chile Sauce
>>> *Old El Paso* Taco Sauce
>>> *Ortega* Taco Sauce; Green Chile Salsa
>>> *Pace* Picante Sauce
>>> *Pedro's Pride* Salsita Mexicana
>>> *Rio Grande* Hot Enchilada Sauce
>> Prepared Tomato Sauce
>>> *Aunt Millie's* Spaghetti Sauces
>>> *Cipriani's* Spaghetti Sauce (Meatless and with Mushrooms)
>>> *Contadina* All Purpose Italian Sauce (sugar)

Guidos Meatless Spaghetti Sauce; Pizza Sauce; Meat Flavor Sauce; Italian Cooking Sauce

Homestead Mushroom Gravy Spaghetti Sauce (frozen)

P & R Spaghetti Sauce; Meatless Sauce with Mushrooms

Ronzoni Marinara (sugar); Meatless Spaghetti (sugar)

Stanghellini's Lucca Mushroom Sauce with Beef (sugar)

Other Sauces

Aunt Penny's White Sauce (modified food starch)

Ronzoni White Clam Sauce

Tomato Puree—buy freely

Tomato Paste—any brand without baking soda

Condiments and Other Sundry Items

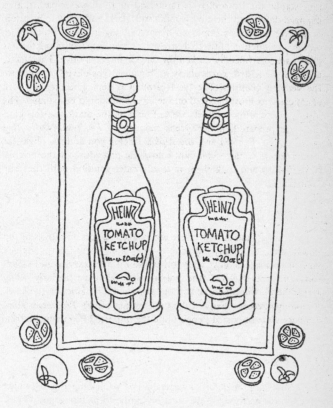

Sometimes it's not the main dish but the garnish that you add to the plate that makes a meal appetizing. Jars of these condiments—and here we're referring to such items as peppers, relishes, pickled salads, olives, pickles—adorn the supermarket shelves. Some are filled with chemicals; others are packed with fine fresh vegetables and spices. We'll try to take a look here at some of the most popular selections and advise you on what to look for on the label of your favorites.

OLIVES

In the Mediterranean countries, where olives are practically a dietary staple, the fresh olive is immersed in a salt-water bath that is changed daily until the olive is mild, soft, dark, and ready to be eaten. A quicker method is employed in the canning industry which relies on the introduction of lye to destroy the bitter taste factor and ferrous gluconate to artificially darken the once light green olive. Then lactic acid may be added, particularly in "Spanish type olives" to improve the keeping qualities. The lye treatment is kept a secret, but both chemical salts must be listed on the label and should be avoided. The most praiseworthy products we've found on the market in this category are prepared in the Greek manner by *Progresso, Dell 'Alpe, Argolis, Sica, Victoria* and *Big Alpha*. In case you find the olives too strong for your taste you can follow the procedure of the original olive-makers and soak them in a salt-water solution until they suit your palate.

PEPPERS

Both sweet and hot peppers are packed in jars for dressing up salads, dips, or simply enjoying as they are. Many brands include vinegar and spices only, while others find it necessary to add stabilizers and preservatives (the polysorbates being particularly widespread here). Choose those without any chemical names on the label. Recommended are many of the varieties put out by *Progresso, Towie* Peppers, *Star* Imported Peppers and the Imported Pepperoncini from *S & W*.

PICKLED SALADS

Relishes and small diced vegetables in a pickling liquid (which includes salt and spices) are great on antipasto platters, sandwiches, or as a side dish with meats. Here again, beware of preservatives (polysorbates and EDTA), calcium chloride, alum, gum tragacanth, and artificial color. *Progresso* and *Star* head the recommended list with several marinated vegetable combinations, and *S & W* offers a Mixed Vegetables Gardinera which can spice up your kitchen shelf. Several smaller companies, which distribute their products within their locale, present additional choices, so be sure to investigate the label of any other pickled salads you encounter.

You can supplement this list with some marinated vegetables of your own. These can be made easily by soaking raw or partially cooked vegetables in a brine of equal quantities of oil and vinegar along with your favorite herbs and spices—basil, oregano, pickling spice, cloves, garlic—for several hours or overnight. A slightly more elaborate method for making these marinated salads (which, by the way, make excellent appetizers) is given in this Mushrooms Marinade.

MUSHROOMS MARINADE

½ pound small mushrooms
⅓ cup olive oil
3 tablespoons wine vinegar
2 tablespoons lemon juice
¾ teaspoon salt
½ teaspoon pepper sauce
Pinch thyme
2 cups water
3 tablespoons finely chopped parsley

Wipe mushrooms with a damp cloth; trim off bottom of stem and cut in half lengthwise. In small saucepan, combine olive oil, wine vinegar, lemon juice, salt, pepper sauce, thyme, and water. Bring to a boil; simmer 5 minutes to blend flavors. Add mushrooms to boiling liquid; cook slowly for 5 minutes or until barely tender. Let cool in liquid. Chill with chopped parsley; drain before serving. *Yield:* 3 cups.

As for the relishes, they are really nothing more than finely diced vegetables in a spicy salad dressing. Some of the salad dressings in the chapter "House Dressings" will do quite well here. Until you get to that chapter, concentrate on the Garden Tomato Relish which will complement a barbecue beautifully.

GARDEN TOMATO RELISH

2 pounds firm ripe tomatoes
1 green pepper
1 cucumber
¼ cup oil

(continued)

⅓ cup wine vinegar
½ teaspoon hot pepper sauce
2 tablespoons finely chopped onion
1 teaspoon salt
½ teaspoon crushed mint
½ teaspoon basil
½ teaspoon honey
¼ teaspoon dry mustard

·Core tomatoes and dice. Remove seeds from pepper and chop. Peel cucumber, if waxed, and slice thinly. Combine remaining ingredients and pour over vegetables in salad bowl. Toss lightly, cover, and chill at least 1 hour before serving. *Yield:* 6 to 8 servings.

PICKLES

Perhaps the biggest American delicatessen specialty, the pickle is found more often today in a jar than in the old-fashioned pickle barrel. A traditional pickle is the result of the natural fermentation of a cucumber in a salt solution over several months. To make it a "dill" the appropriate herbs are added. Sour pickles are transferred to a vinegar-spice solution after the initial fermentation, while "sweets" go into a sweet, spicy liquor. The natural acids should be sufficient to inhibit mold.

One major problem in pickling is the softening of the pickle, and to compensate, alum, a firming agent, is almost universally added to the pickling brine. If you select your pickles from the pickle barrel this relatively mild chemical will be the only unfortunate processing your pickle has been through. Jarred pickles, however, are a different story, and it is a real find to encounter a brand that does not include a chemical additive to retard foam formation (which does not have to appear on the label) and a polysorbate emulsifier (which is listed on the label) used to keep the flavoring oils evenly distributed throughout.

Pickle Yourself

If your craving for pickles can't be satisfied without the inclusion of these chemicals from the offerings in your supermarket, follow this recipe and make some pickles of your own. When freshly made, these pickles will be nice and crisp, and those that are not consumed immediately can be stored in the refrigerator where they will stay crisp for one to two weeks.

HOMEMADE PICKLE SLICES

2 large cucumbers, unwaxed
1 small onion, chopped
1 tablespoon salt
¼ cup wine vinegar
2 tablespoons honey
½ teaspoon dry mustard

Slice cucumbers thinly and layer with onion in a large bowl. Sprinkle with salt. Combine remaining ingredients and pour over cucumbers. Let stand at room temperature 1 hour, then transfer to a jar and refrigerate until needed. *Yield:* about 3 cups including pickling liquid.

MISCELLANY

We're certain there are many other items you'd like to see included in this section. Keep on checking the labels and you're bound to come up with some others that are entirely free of chemicals. In the meantime you can add to your safe shopping list:

Progresso Eggplant Caponata, a canned eggplant and tomato mélange that is delicious in Salade Niçoise, antipastos, and on hero sandwiches.

Sunbrand Major Grey's Mango Chutney which can be added to sweet and sour sauces and served along with barbecued meats, nut cutlets, or any Indian dish. *Sunbrand* also puts out a bottled curry sauce that's worth trying. The *Sunbrand* products are costly, but they last a very long time.

Store all opened condiments in the refrigerator and they will keep beautifully without the chemical preservatives the food industry is so fond of adding.

CATSUP

We now move away from these prepared salads and on to those condiments which are used to enhance or mask food flavors; such old friends as catsup and mustard. We have already spoken of such flavor enhancers as horseradish and soy sauce. The chapter "Seasonings:

Natural Food Enhancers" will help you select these items for the garnishing of fish, lamb stews, boiled beef, eggs, rice, Chinese foods, bean stews, poultry, and hamburgers.

Catsup is so popular in America that the USDA has included a "recipe" for it in the Federal Food Code. The product, which need not list any ingredients, is composed of the concentrated liquid from ripe red tomatoes seasoned with salt, vinegar, onion, garlic, "secret" spices and flavoring, all theoretically from natural sources, and sugar, dextrose, and/or glucose. In lesser quality products the liquid comes from the residue of tomato canning or juice making and this will be stated on the label. The sweetening agents are unfortunate, but unavoidable. At least the catsup manufacturers forgo the chemicals in this product.

Catsup, used as part of a recipe, can spark the flavor of many foods. Use it this way, as a seasoning, not to mask the flavor of ill-prepared foods.

MUSTARD

Mustard is another item that can both enhance or cover up natural food flavors. All the bottle of prepared mustard you buy need have in it is mustard seeds, vinegar, salt, and spices. Most labels don't tell you what these "spices" are since they consider it a "secret formula." One name that often appears on the label is turmeric—this is not a chemical, but a perfectly acceptable spice often added to foods to highlight the yellow hue. Those ingredients which are not necessary include wheat flour, vegetable oil, and propylene glycol alginate. Those products labeled "Mustard Sauce" are more likely to contain these unwanted additions.

Among those recommended are *Gulden's, French's* (which says nothing on the label), and most of the imported Dijon Mustards (which are very hot).

BARBECUE SAUCE

The final item we'd like to deal with here is barbecue sauce. For various reasons (artificial coloring, flavoring, sugar, preservatives) we have yet to discover a brand on our supermarket shelf that we can suggest you buy. It's so simple to prepare your own, though, you'd probably be throwing out your money if you could find one anyway.

Instead, make up a batch of your own barbecue sauce from one of these:

BASIC BARBECUE SAUCE WITH VARIATIONS

1 cup molasses
1 cup mustard
1 cup vinegar (wine or cider)
Combine molasses and mustard; mix thoroughly. Stir in vinegar. Cover and refrigerate. *Yield:* 3 cups sauce.
Variations:
> *Tomato Barbecue Sauce:* Add 1 cup catsup to Basic Barbecue Sauce. Makes 1 quart.
> *Herb Barbecue Sauce:* Add ¼ teaspoon each, marjoram, oregano, basil, and thyme to 2 cups of Basic Barbecue Sauce.
> *Zesty Barbecue Sauce:* Add ¼ cup of catsup, ¼ cup of oil, 2 tablespoons of soy sauce, and ½ teaspoon of hot pepper sauce to 1 cup of Basic Barbecue Sauce.

For glazing a ham or turkey, try this mixture:
MOLASSES MUSTARD GLAZE

Combine ⅓ cup of molasses and ⅓ cup of mustard. Brush on roast occasionally during last 45 minutes of cooking time.

For Duck (or chicken) with Orange Sauce, baste the bird with this combination:
ORANGE BASTING SAUCE

Combine 1 cup of orange juice, ¼ cup of oil, and ¼ cup of honey.

RECOMMENDATIONS

General Rule of Purchase: This is a catch-all grouping. To make your purchase, read the label; all ingredients are given. Watch for EDTA, sodium benzoate or benzoic acid, and polysorbate preservatives; calcium chloride; gum tragacanth; artificial color. Most of these items are highly salted. Sugar can be avoided in all but the "sweet and sour" or "chow chow" type relishes. Although we choose to eliminate them personally, lactic acid (in green olives) and ferrous gluconate (in black olives) are probably harmless additives.

EXEMPLARY BRANDS

Olives

Argolis Calamata Olives; Green Cracked Olives

Big Alpha Greek Olives; Oil Cured Olives

Dell'Alpe Oil Cured Olives; Vine Cured Olives; Boneless Crushed Olives

Progresso Olive Condite; Oil Cured Olives

Sica Calamata Olives; Green Cracked Olives

Victoria Oil Cured Olives; Olive Condite; Olive Appetizer; Sicilian Olives

Peppers

Albert's Hot Salad Peppers

Big Alpha Hot Peppers

Bruce's Gringo Hot Pepper Points

Clem's Festive Foods Jalapeno Peppers

Clemente Jacques Jalapeno Peppers

Dell'Alpe Imported Pepperoncini

Drehers Hot Cherry Peppers

Evangeline Hot Cherry Peppers

Fancifood Cherry Peppers; Pepperoncini; Chili Peppers; Wax Peppers

Faro Pickled Jalapeno Peppers

La Preferida Green Pickled Jalapeno and Serrano Peppers

Marconi Pepperoncini; Sport Peppers

Mario's Greek Pepperoncini

Old El Paso Jalapeno Relish

Pedros Pride Green Pickled Jalapeno Peppers.

Progresso Tuscan Peppers

Reese Hot Finger Peppers

Roddenbery's Banana Peppers (hot and semi-hot)

S&W Pepperoncini

Snakpak Cherry Peppers; Hot Mix; Pepperoncini

Star Imported Peppers

    Towie Peppers
    Town House Cherry Peppers
    Victoria Pepperoncini; Pepper Salad
Pickled Vegetables
    Argolis Imported Volvi Wild Onions; Giardiniera
    Big Alpha Eggplants in Oil and Vinegar
    Delli'Alpe Stuffed Eggplant; Hot and Mild Giardiniera
    Fancifood Hot Medley
    Hadden House Baby Hot Okra; Pick-a-Dilly Mix;
       Pickled Baby Corn
    Hengstenberg Cornichons; Sliced Gherkins
    Krakus Polish Pickles
    Marconi Garden Mix; Whole Eggplant
    Monterey Gold Cauliflower
    Nalley's Pepper Valley Pickled Cauliflower
    Open Kettle Italian Vegetable Medley
    Paisley Farm Dilled Broccoli Clusters
    Progresso Eggplants in Vinegar; Marinated Mush-
       rooms; Pepper Piccalilli; Petite Marinated Aspara-
       gus; Giardiniera
    S&W Mixed Vegetables Giardiniera
    Schorr's Home Style Half Sour Pickles; Sour Garlic
       Pickles
    Schorr's Home Style Special Mixed Pickled Vegetables
    Sico Giardiniera; Stuffed Eggplants
    Snakpak Italian Mix; Pickled Cauliflower
    Talko Texas Crisp Okra Pickles
    Town House Mixed Vegetables Giardiniera; Pickled
       Cauliflower
    Victoria Giardiniera; Cauliflower
    Waldbaum's Pickles
Relish (all contain sugar)
    Balliet's Pepper Hash
    Braswell Artichoke Pickles; Pepper Relish; Artichoke
       Relish
    Country Made Artichoke Pickles
    Mountain Farm Old Fashioned Mild and Hot Chow
       Chow; Open Tomato Relish
    Mrs. Campbell's Sweet Chow Chow; Extra Hot Chow
       Chow

Open Kettle Mexican Corn Relish

Mustard

Ba-Tampte

Boetje's

Cox's Jalapeno Mustard

Dam Mill

Dijon

Food Club with Horseradish

Foodland Spicy Brown

French's

Fugelhoffer German Style

Gulden's

Heinz Horseradish Mustard

Koops Extra Strong

Kosciusko Real

Kraft Horseradish Mustard

La Hacienda Jalapeno Mustard

La Preferida Jalapeno Mustard

Medford

Retland

Catsup and Chili Sauce—all brands similar (and all have sugar)

Barbeque Sauce

Dillard's

Jim Coursey's Old Fashioned (mild and medium)

Miscellany

Albert's Seafood Sauce; Garlic Spread; Tartar Sauce

Argolis Grape Vine Leaves in Brine

Big Alpha Grape Leaves in Brine

Fancifood Grape Leaves in Brine

Mancini Fried Peppers with Onions

Old El Paso Tomatoes and Jalapeno Peppers

Ortega Tomatoes and Green Chilis

Progresso Pepper Salad; Eggplant Caponata; Antipasto; Fried Sweet Pepper with Onions

Sahadi Grape Leaves in Brine

Sharwood's Bengal Hot Chutney; Mango Chutney (sugar)

Sico Grape Vine Leaves in Brine
Smithers English Chutney Sauce (sugar)
Sunbrand Major Grey's Mango Chutney (sugar)
Pimientos—buy freely

Jams, Jellies, and Sweet Spreads

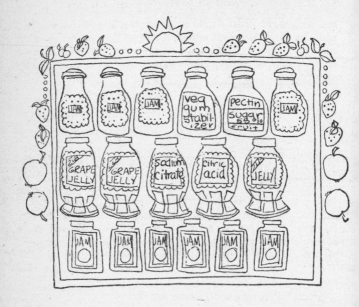

Even the jam companies these days are trying to get into the natural foods movement. Several have taken to promoting their product as pure jam, free from preservatives, artificial color, and artificial flavor. To give you the impression that they are different, they distribute their product not in the jam department, but in the produce department, usually in a refrigerator showcase. In reality, these jams are no different from many others which do not use such misleading advertising, for any jam that does use artificial color, flavor, or preservatives is required to say so on the label.

According to the federal food standard established by the U.S. Department of Agriculture no product considered a pure jam or jelly can contain artificial flavor except apple and crabapple jellies (which can have added flavor) or artificial coloring (again red or green color can be added to apple, crabapple, or pineapple jellies). In those cases where they are permitted they must inform you on the label. Preservatives are permitted, although not used in many brands, and these too will be indicated on the jar for you to reject. Check around and you'll find many brands, located right on the jam shelf, that do not use these additives and feel no need to boast about it. The reason they don't stress the point is that these jams, including the "no preservative, no artificial color, no artificial flavor" variety, are chock full of the very unnatural refined sugar.

JAM AND JELLY: MORE THAN HALF SUGAR

The big problem with these sweet spreads is the sugar. The case against sugar has been stated elsewhere in this book, and although small amounts have been tolerated in other products it is no minor ingredient here. If you purchase the commercial jams and jellies you'll be getting a product that's *55 percent sweetener* and only 45 percent fruit or fruit juice. The most common sweetening ingredient used in jelly-making is sugar, often in combination with corn syrup. Honey, or honey plus sugar can be used according to the Federal Code; however, no major brand has used this option it seems, for honey is the only one of these sweeteners which must be indicated on the label. The reason they don't use honey . . . it's more expensive! And most people haven't shown that they care.

Because of the high level of sugar and the overprocessing, a jar of jam doesn't have much in the way of nutritional offerings. A well-prepared jam from fresh fruit and honey or even a honey-raw sugar combination could contribute some vitamins to your diet. Most jams, however, are made from frozen or canned, not fresh fruit; most jellies are made from a strained extraction of frozen or canned fruit (which means the liquid portion) usually with added water.

Is this the formula for your favorite jam?

Sugar + Frozen or Canned Fruit + Pectin + Acid + Antifoaming Agent + Benzoic Acid = JAM

It could be!

The Optional Ingredients

Large-scale jelly-making isn't quite that simple anyway. Pectin is a natural fruit ingredient which causes a jelly to gel. To produce clear fruit juices for jellies the pectin is filtered out. To make up for the resulting pectin deficiencies most jams and jellies must have pectin added; in fact, in amounts more than sufficient to compensate for the loss.

In order for the pectin to work well it must be in an acid medium, so chemical acid salts as well as citric acid (not the kind that comes naturally from lemons, but more often the kind that is manufactured from fungi that are grown on sugar solutions) are added to the mixture. If you want to know more about pectin, read the label on a jar of prepared pectin in your supermarket. Chances are it will say: "water, lactic acid (assists gel), pectin, citric acid (assists gel), potassium citrate (controls acidity), and sodium metabisulphite (preservative)."

The formation of foam during manufacture is another problem common to highly acid foods. Chemical antifoaming agents are consequently the next thing to be included in the formula.

Finally, to give the fruit spreads the appearance of freshness, benzoic acid or sodium benzoate may be added. This is not true in all jars and you will always be advised of this on the label.

In a few cases jellies are spiced, and again the label will let you know. And whenever you encounter mint flavor and green color you can be pretty sure phony coloring and flavoring agents went into the jar. The label will tell you for sure.

Since only the preservative and the occasional inclusion of spice or other flavoring or coloring matter need be stated clearly on the label, there is no way of knowing what the manufacturer has included in his product from the remaining optional choices. You can be pretty certain, though, that the sweetener/fruit ratio is close to 55:45, the legal minimum. The label may tell you some of the ingredients, but remember they are under no obligation to give a list that's complete. Also, there's no telling if the fruit or fruit juice is fresh or not, so you might as well assume it isn't.

A Few Choices

The picture is not very promising for the jam and jelly lovers. No major brands make use of the honey option. Certain companies which distribute primarily in natural foods stores do, and these are beginning to appear in the supermarket. *Balanced* and *Sherman's Arcadia* are two popular brands and both are tasty. We actually found a pit in the black cherry jam one morning.

As for the others, *Hero,* imported from Switzerland, is composed of sugar and fruit only, which is nothing to rave about but does have some merits considering what some other manufacturers add.

As an additional, but we're sure unnecessary, warning, don't turn to the artificially sweetened brands out of desperation. If anything, they are far worse, for aside from the synthetic sweetening that is permitted, the list of chemicals and thickening agents in the optional ingredient section of the federal standard for these spreads is pretty long.

Some Alternatives

Why not resort to simple homemade sweet spreads instead? We're not advocating a big homemade jelly-making project, although if you're into it, it's fun to do and by far the best jam or jelly around. There are lots of simple replacements, like:

•Making a "peanut butter and" sandwich with fresh banana or pear slices.

•Sweetening sliced berries with a little honey, mashing them with a fork, and using this wherever you might use jam.

•Sweetening a sandwich with diced dried fruits.

•Substituting a paste of ground raisins, apples, bananas, dried fruits, and nuts.

•Making a simple jam by cooking diced fruits with honey until thickened, and storing the rich pulp in the refrigerator to use just like jam. This recipe for homemade Blueberry Jam will give you the idea. Try it with other fruits if you like.

BLUEBERRY JAM

1½ cups blueberries
1 tablespoon lemon juice
¼ cup honey

Combine all ingredients in a saucepan. Bring to boil and let boil for 20 minutes. Stir occasionally to prevent scorching. Pour into a clean (sterilized) jar and chill. It will thicken on cooling. *Yield:* about 1 cup.

FRUIT BUTTER AND FRUIT BUTTER-MAKING

Fruit butters are another popular sweet spread, apple butter being the most available example. The product, again defined by a government standard, is a smooth, semisolid blend of fruit and sweetening, this time in a ratio of 5 parts fruit to 2 parts sweetener. The fruit ingredient comes from cooking fresh, frozen, canned, or dried fruit, and may be diluted with fruit juice (as noted on the label). The sweetening can include sugar, sugar syrup, dextrose, and all the other common sweetening agents, including honey. Again, only honey need be mentioned on the label, so at least you'll know if the good product is to be found. In actuality though, as you know if you've ever prepared any homemade apple butter, nine times out of ten you don't need any more sweetening than the apples have to offer. If you've never made any apple butter, now is a good time to try. All you have to do is dice up the apples (you don't even have to bother removing the peel), add just enough water to the pot to keep them from sticking (about ¼ cup), and simmer gently over low heat until the pulp is thick and dark, for about an hour to an hour and a half.

If you'd like to get into more elaborate "butter"-making do try this Cantaloupe Butter. It makes a lovely gift you can be sure you won't find in any store.

CANTALOUPE BUTTER

2 cups diced cantaloupe pulp (1 medium cantaloupe)
½ cup honey
1 orange, peeled and diced with all the juice
Juice of 1 lime
1 stick cinnamon

Combine all ingredients in a saucepan, bring to boil, reduce heat, and cook gently 1 to 1½ hours, until thick. Keep in mind when cold the mixture will thicken slightly. Pour into a clean (sterilized) jar. Seal or store in refrigerator. *Yield:* About 2/3 cup; 1 small jar.

RECOMMENDATIONS

General Rule of Purchase: The best place to look for suitable jams, jellies, and fruit butters is in the natural foods section of the supermarket. Choose those sweetened with honey, and unsweetened fruit butters. Many ingredients do not appear on the label, but any artificial coloring, flavoring, or preservatives will be listed. Most jams and jellies do not have these three additives, so don't think those which boast about their absence and charge higher prices are any better—they're still 55 percent sugar.

To avoid the concentrated sugar, try some of the substitutes suggested in the text.

EXEMPLARY BRANDS
> *Balance of Nature* Preserves
> *Balanced* Jams and Jellies
> *Datetree* Rose Hips Preserves
> *Downey's* Honey Butter; Cinnamon Honey Butter
> *Fruitcrest* Grape Jelly (30 percent, rather than 55 percent, sugar)
> *Jenny Brown* Applebutter
> *Max Ams* Honey Jelly; Honey Prune Spread
> *Schimmel,* Brand Lekvar (Prune Apple Butter)
> *Sherman's Arcadia*

Sorting Out the Crackers

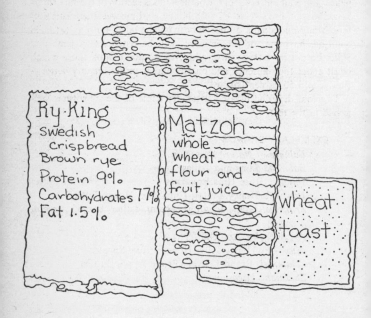

The Scandinavians have a name for crackers which really tells you what they are—"flat breads." Use them for everyday eating and you'll find the choice of breads acceptable to your inner ecology greatly expanded.

There are dozens of varieties of crackers on the market and quite a few of them are completely free of refined products (that is, white flour and white sugar), hydrogenated shortening, and any chemical bleaching, flavoring, coloring, and preservatives. To make them even more appealing, crackers keep indefinitely.

You may have to do a little searching, for there are several places in the supermarket where these healthy crackers may be located. There is generally a portion of one shelf set aside specifically for crackers, the size of which varies in each supermarket. Sometimes they are intermingled with the cookies, other times stores display them on the small shelves above the meat counter. In addition to this cracker display, you will often find other selections in the diet foods section and the natural foods section. On one of these shelves you should find just what you're looking for.

BUYING CRACKERS

Everything that is used to prepare crackers must be stated on the label, so be sure to read the list of ingredients before making your purchase. Here are some of the things you'll want to keep an eye out for and, if you find them, eliminate the box from your list of possibilities:

 white flour
 wheat flour (which is simply white flour)
 "enrichment"
 sugar, dextrose, or corn syrup
 hydrogenated shortening/margarine/butter (with BHA added)
 artificial color
 artificial flavor
 citric acid
 yeast nutrients
 sodium propionate or disodium acetate added as preservative
 BHT or BHA added as preservative

You are looking for brands that use the finest natural ingredients, which means whole grain flours, vegetable oils, honey, and seeds. Some crackers may be as simple as whole wheat flour and water. Others are leavened and lightly sweetened. Most contain salt, but there are a few salt-free choices too.

Melba Toast

Melba toast is a traditional dieter's choice, but in reality there are many crackers which are equally low in calories. Although the *Devonsheer* people bill their melba toast as "natural" all their melba toast contains some enriched white flour and hydrogenated vegetable shortening. This line of melba toast, which includes wheat, rye, and pumpernickel, is, however, free of coloring, preservatives, and other synthetics used by competitors. *Devonsheer* also puts out Brown Rice

Wafers and Allgrane Wheat Wafers. The Wheat Wafers are made from 100 percent whole wheat, use no sugar or shortening, and are available with and without salt.

Matzoh

Matzoh no longer appears just on Jewish holidays. It is offered year-round in many areas and for those who are unfamiliar with the product, matzoh is an unleavened cracker made from flour, liquid, and salt. When eaten alone it has a bland, rather undistinguished taste; add butter and salt and you have a real treat. More flavorful varieties do include the addition of egg and often onion.

Streit's offers a whole wheat matzoh and a matzoh made with unbleached flour and water as the liquid. *Horowitz Bros. & Margareten* produce a whole wheat matzoh made with whole grain flour and unsweetened apple juice (the label says fruit juice). These are your best choices.

A Jewish cookbook will suggest many ways to use the cracker in cooking, like making stuffing, matzoh brie, and potato pudding.

Flatbread

Flatbreads are similar to matzoh, but are usually paper-thin and one box lasts for ages. The crackers may be too fragile to take a spread (unless it's very soft and spreadable), but they are good carriers for firm cheeses. There are numerous brands of flatbreads, many imported from the Scandinavian countries. They appear under such titles as *Master* Old Country Hardtack, *Finn Crisp,* and *Ideal* Crackers. *Wasa Ry-King* makes a flatbread which is a bit more sturdy and heavier than the average flatbread. The *Ry-King* flatbread comes in "lite," "golden," and "brown rye" and "whole wheat."

Holgrain products are often found amidst the diet foods in the supermarket and offer a chance to sample rice crackers made from brown rice flour. These, like the flatbreads, are paper-thin and tend to get pliable with age. You can recrisp them, as you can any cracker, in the oven set at 300° for five to ten minutes.

Other Fine Crackers

This is, of course, only a guideline as to what fine crackers your supermarket has available to replace the traditional white flour, heavily salted, highly chemicalized cocktail and soup crackers. Some other choices you can add to your list include:

Venus Wheat Wafers, with and without salt. These, by the way, are sold in almost every supermarket and natural foods store; for about 5¢ more in the latter.

Feather River Rice Cakes, made from brown rice, when available, are generally located in the "health food" aisle.

Finn Crisp Rye Wafers, available plain and with caraway seeds.

Ralston Purina Original Rye Krisp. Make sure it says "Original."

Ak-Mak Armenian Cracker Bread, crunchy whole wheat crackers with sesame seeds.

Your area will have additional choices, we're sure. Just read the label with those "undesirable" ingredients in mind.

SOMETHING TO DO WITH CRACKERS: CRUMBS

Aside from serving these whole grain crackers with cheese, hors d'oeuvres, salad, and soup, they should be used to make homemade cracker crumbs. No need to spend your money on packaged cracker crumbs which are made from white flour crackers (with all the undesirable ingredients therein). For speedy homemade cracker crumbs, break chemical-free whole grain crackers into the blender container and process several seconds at medium speed until finely ground. Your yield will depend on the size of the particular cracker you use.

You can prepare crumbs when you need them or make up a batch and store them in a covered container at room temperature so they're always convenient. Use for toppings and crumb crusts.

RECOMMENDATIONS

General Rule of Purchase: All ingredients on label. Look for those made with whole grain flours, honey, vegetable oils, wheat germ, and seeds.

Be on the lookout for white flour, wheat flour, synthetic enrichment, sugar, dextrose, corn syrup, hydrogenated shortening, margarine, artificial color and flavor, citric acid, yeast nutrients, and preservatives.

> EXEMPLARY BRANDS:
> Whole Wheat
> *Ak-Mak* Armenian Cracker Bread

      Allgrane Wheat Wafers
      Holgrain Wheat Crackers
      Venus Wheat Wafers

Rye
      Finn Crisp
      Ideal Flatbrod (includes wheat and barley flours)
      Kavli Crispbread
      Kings Bread Crisp Bread
      Master Old Country Hardtack
      Ralston Purina Natural (or Original) Rye Crisp
      RYVITA Crisp Ryebread
      SILJANS KNACKE Crispbread
      Wasa Ry-King

Rice
      Devonsheer Brown Rice Wafers
      Feather River Rice Cakes
      Holgrain Rice-Crackers

Matzoh
      Horowitz Bros. & Margareten Whole Wheat Matzoh
      Manishewitz 100% Whole Wheat Matzoh
      Streit's Whole Wheat Matzoh

Corn (Tacos)—these are mostly deep fried
    East—*Old El Paso* Taco Shells
      Ortega Taco Shells
    Middle—*Diablo* Tacos
      Jimenez Taco Shells; Chalupa Shells
      La Hacienda Tacos; Tostadas
      La Tiara Taco Shells
      Mexitaco Taco Shells
      Old El Paso Taco Shells
      Ortega Taco Shells
      Rodriguez Tacos; Tostadas
    West—*Little Pancho* Taco Shells; Tostada Shells
      Lynn Wilson's Taco Shells
      Macayo Taco Shells
      Old El Paso Taco Shells
      Ortega Taco Shells
      Pocos Taco Shells; Tostadas
      Rainbo Taco Shells

Cookies, Cakes, and Pastry

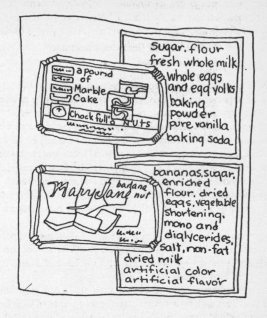

Sweets rank high when it comes to violating the laws of nature. Between the usual bleached white flour, refined sugar, artificial flavoring, preservatives, emulsifiers, and stabilizers, you have little to look forward to but one very unwholesome dessert. Unlike bread, these baked goods must let you know on the label everything that's in them.

COOKIES

Cookies made with whole grains, dried fruits, unsaturated fats, and honey could easily be marketed as a nutritious snack item. So far no major bakery has picked up on this idea so we had to supply you with some wholesome cookie recipes in the chapter "Satisfying Your Sweet Tooth—Sanely."

Some local and specialized bakeries do turn out cookies from unrefined, real ingredients. Until recently they have been confined to natural foods stores, but lately more and more brands are reaching the supermarket through the new natural foods departments. You know what to look for, so read the label. *El Molino* and *Old Stone Mill* by *Balanced Foods* are some recommended brands you're likely to encounter. The cookies taste terrific.

The Slim Pickings

There is little to choose from the general offering in the supermarket. One superior cookie exists made from organically grown whole wheat and rye flour, vegetable oil, oat flakes, raw sugar, crushed nuts, wheat germ, raisins, and honey (only a partial list of the rich ingredients) called *Famila* Biscuits (after the *Familia* Cereal) and distributed by HUG. These cookies are sold in natural foods stores as well where the price may be as much as 12¢ higher. The *Famila* cookies prove that good cookies can be mass-produced and mass-marketed. *Famila* cookies come from Switzerland and are always fresh-tasting and crisp. They not only make good eating, but you can make superb crumb crusts for pies with them.

Pepperidge Farm cookies come out better than most supermarket selections. There are no preservatives, artificial colors, or flavors added, and they do use fresh eggs and unbleached flour. Unfortunately, they also include lots of white sugar.

Scattered throughout the cookie shelf there are generally a few other packages with no artificial ingredients other than bleached white flour and refined sugar. While hardly laudable, these can help fill the cookie gap.

CAKES AND PIES

As you can see from the label of most packaged cakes and pies the story here is even worse. In addition to the refined raw ingredients and artificial flavors and color, you are likely to find:

Chemical emulsifiers (mono- and diglycerides and polyethylene derivatives). Polyethylene derivatives make great paint remover. In the human body, however, they may irritate gallstones and accelerate kidney disorders. They have been banned from breads, so why not cakes as well?

Vegetable gum is added to create a smooth texture without the use of extra costly eggs and fats; it is popular both as an extender and stabilizer in pie fillings.

Preservatives are almost always found in packaged cakes while often excluded from cookies.

Lunch-Box Stuffers

Those little cakes created especially for children's lunches are almost entirely starches, fillers, emulsifiers, and phony flavors. Although the label may have more than fifteen ingredients listed, nonfat dry milk is almost always the only one with any nutritional significance. Even the "chocolate" ones often neglect to include any real chocolate.

Adults Fare No Better

Why should they bother to add bananas to "Banana Cream Pie" when imitation banana flavoring is so much cheaper and nobody ever bothers to read the label—and we were worrying about a little white flour and refined sugar!

If you would like to try a cake that has no offenders whatsoever try *Holland* Honey Cake, Honey Fruit Cake, and Raisin Date Cake. Honey keeps these cakes moist and tender, not artificial "fresheners." *Holland* Cakes, stored in the refrigerator, make fine eating for weeks. Try serving them plain or toasted with butter, jam, cream cheese, or ice cream, and you'll have a pretty wide variety of desserts.

For a dessert that at least doesn't read like a formula from a chem manual, *Chock Full O' Nuts* cakes are all "real."

Although not exactly a cake, *Thomas'* Date Nut Bread is moist, sweet, and delicious, and made with unbleached flour and no artificial ingredients or chemicals.

If your taste runs to fruit-flavored cream pies, make them yourself. That's about the only way you'll get any real fruit flavor or cream in it. Although homemade pie crusts always taste best, *Wintsen Bros.* Oronoque Orchards Frozen Pie Crust made with unbleached flour and honey will do in a pinch.

FOOD FRIVOLITY—OR IS IT FRAUD?

Although cake and cookie manufacturers are required to give a full listing of ingredients, many of them have some cute tricks to make you think the contents are realer than they are.

•Watch out for cakes that are "buttery, chocolatey, fruity" or any other "y." According to our dictionary the suffix "y" is used to mean

305

"somewhat like; suggesting." This means the flavor may be somewhat like butter, but need not have any actual butter at all.

•Remember "cream" is spelled C-R-E-A-M, not CREME, if it's the real thing. Lots of food manufacturers like to fill their cakes with "creme" filling made from corn syrup, gelatin, mono- and diglycerides, artificial flavoring, and other such ingredients. If you're a poor speller take your dictionary to the supermarket with you . . . lots of other misspelled words are just industry's way of letting you know what they're making believe the product is.

•The word "flavor" placed after the specific source of flavor usually means the flavor not the source was added. "Cherry flavor" or "real cherry flavor" means that the product has the flavor of cherries (synthetic or real), not that it contains any cherries.

•When the label or advertisement tells you "Brand X tastes *like* fresh peanut butter," don't assume that means it includes any peanut butter (or whatever else it tastes "like"). No one says why it tastes "like" it does; maybe it's the chemical flavoring agent.

•Lots of baked goods are described as "golden," "rich," "whipped," or some other taste-tempting adjective. The manufacturer is counting on you to assume that it's golden because they use eggs (even if they don't), or rich because they use butter (even if they don't), or that the whip comes from cream (even if it doesn't). Disappoint him. Don't assume his product contains anything unless you find it on the list of ingredients.

HOME-BAKED IS NOT NECESSARILY HOMEMADE: CAKE MIXES

When you decide to surprise your family and treat them to a home-baked cake, make sure it's homemade as well. Cake mixes are even more doctored up than the ready-made cakes to make them longer-lasting and insure satisfactory results under any conditions. Take a look at the label and see for yourself.

And when you go to ice the cake, don't mask it with chemicals. If you bother to read a packaged frosting label here is what you're likely to discover:

sugar, shortening (with freshness preserver), dextrose, cocoa processed with alkali, corn syrup solids, wheat and cornstarch, nonfat milk, diglycerides, artificial and natural flavor, salt, polysorbate 60, and artificial color.

If you don't want to take the trouble to make a frosting from scratch (and you'll find some simple recipes in all cookbooks and some especially healthy ones in the chapter "Satisfying Your Sweet Tooth —Sanely" of this book), just top the cake with fresh fruit and real whipped cream or yogurt with jam, fresh fruit puree, or honey.

RECOMMENDATIONS

General Rule of Purchase: Select those made with whole wheat flour, rye flour, oat flakes, honey, molasses, nuts, fresh and dried fruit, and fresh dairy products. Those made with unbleached flour are second choice.

Watch particularly for artificial coloring, artificial flavoring, preservatives, vegetable gums, mono- and diglycerides, and polyethylene derivatives as well.

While some of the items below do contain white flour and sugar, they are among the few choices on the market that do not contain any of the artificial ingredients cited above.

EXEMPLARY BRANDS:
Cookies
Archway Old Fashioned Molasses; Sugared Molasses
Au Naturelle Cookies
Busy Bee Sugar Honey Grahams
Flavor Kist Oatmeal Cookies
HUG Familia Biscuits
Huntley Palmer Wheat Meal Cookies
Keebler Old Fashioned Oatmeal
Nabisco Jeremy Potter Natural Cookies
Nabisco National Arrowroot Biscuits; Graham Crackers; Cinnamon Treats; Raisin Fruit Biscuits
Natsco or *Tohato Harvest* Natural Sesame Cookies with Honey

Peak Freans Natural Orange, Lemon, Lime and Coffee Flavoured Yogurt Wafers

Pepperidge Farm, particularly the Kitchen Hearth varieties; Oatmeal Raisin; Irish Oatmeal; Cinnamon Sugar (made with whole wheat flour)

Pogens Spirits; Oatmeal; Raspberry; Ginger Snaps; Chocolate Chip; Sugar; Florentine; Toffee Lace; Chocolate Bows

Pride of The Farm Honey and Peanut Butter; Honey and Date; Honey and Oatmeal; Honey and Carob; Honey and Sesame Cookies

Saralan Carob Cream Sandwich; Granola Cream Sandwich; Raisin and Nut Nuggets; Carob Fudge Cookies

Sunshine Golden Fruit

Susan's Giant Oatmeal Raisin; Chocolate Chip; Carob Chip

Cakes

Barbara's Fruit and Nut Muffin; Carob Brownies; Carob Macaroons; Coconut Macaroons; Butter and Nut Cookies; Carrot Cakes (all individual cakes)

Bayberry Farms Carrot Cake

Bubbles Carrot Cake Cupcakes

Chock Full O' Nuts Cakes

Holland Honey; Honey Fruit; Raisin Date

Pride of The Farm Granola; Cinnamon Crumb; Filled Carob Brownie; Raspberry Crumb; Strawberry Filled; Apricot Filled; Raisin Apple (all individual cakes)

Pride of The Farm Honey Cake

Thomas' Date Nut Bread

Pastry

Wintsen Bros. Oronoque Orchards Frozen Pie Crust

Ice Cream

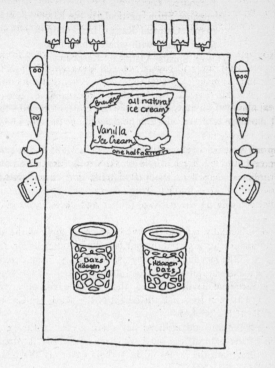

Guess what these are:

carrageenan, furcelleran, agar-agar, alcin, calcium sulfate, gelatin, gum karaya, locust bean gum, oat gum, gum tragacanth, mono- and diglycerides, polysorbate 65 and 80, sodium carboxymethylcellulose, propylene glycol alginate, microcrystalline cellulose, dioctyl sodium sulfosuccinate, sodium citrate, disodium phosphate, tetrasodium pyrophosphate, sodium hexametaphosphate, calcium carbonate, magnesium carbonate, calcium oxide and hydroxide, magnesium oxide and hydroxide*

*Just a few of the 60+ chemical additives that might be inside your favorite container of ice cream.

Rememoer the old children's song, "I scream, you scream, we all scream for ice cream"? Well, if you want your ice cream to be the real thing you'd better start screaming, or at least talking loudly, so someone does something about the frozen dessert they package and call ice cream.

If you've ever had real old-fashioned ice cream, turned from rich cream, real fruit, and salt-packed ice, you know something different is being done to make ice cream these days. What that something is, is about sixty different additives which simulate real flavor, real color, and add phony creaminess, texture, prevent crystal formation during storage, and do whatever else can be done to cut the cost of adding real rich ingredients.

The dairy ingredient alone can be as varied as whole or dried cream, butter or butter oil, fresh whole or skim milk, dry milk powder, buttermilk, condensed or evaporated milk, and cheese whey. Ice cream is one of three products which does not have to list the use of artificial coloring on the package (butter and cheese are the other two).

There is actually no way to know which, if any, of the many optional ingredients are used in your favorite brand or flavor. If you are aware of the labeling requirements, however, you can determine the presence of natural and artificial flavors.

•If no artificial flavor is added, the specific flavor only will be written in letters at least half the height of the words Ice Cream, as in "vanilla ICE CREAM."

•If both natural and artificial flavor are present with a greater percent of the natural, the label will have the word "flavored" in letters at least half the height of the specific flavor, as "VANILLA-flavored ICE CREAM."

•If there is more artificial flavor than natural flavor, the label will say "artificially flavored" or "artificial VANILLA ICE CREAM."

•If an artificial flavor other than the main flavor is used, somewhere on the label it will say "artificial flavor added," but it might not tell you what flavor.

Basically then, if you see the word "flavored" on the container, some amount of artificial flavoring has been added.

French Ice Cream

If a product is called "French Ice Cream," that means there is a greater percentage of egg solids.

310

Ice Milk

The story for ice milk is pretty much the same as ice cream, only the percentage of milk fat is lower. The label will say if it is artificially colored.

Because it has a lower fat content, many weight-conscious people replace ice cream on the menu with ice milk. But, although it has "half the fat of regular ice cream," as one brand advertises, it does not have half the calories. To compensate for the reduced butterfat, extra sugar and chemicals are included to bring the taste and texture up to par. This additional sweetening creates a product higher in carbohydrate and only slightly lower in calories than regular ice cream—about 40 calories less per halfcup serving.

Sherbet

Fruit sherbet may contain the same additives as ice cream, only it must state the presence of both artificial color and flavor on the label. Again, the amount of milk fat and solid is less than in ice cream, and the acid content is higher.

Ices

Water ices are exactly like sherbet but water takes the place of a dairy product.

WHAT TO BUY

It's difficult to give buying advice when it comes to frozen desserts since there are so many variables permitted and so many different brand names. Any way you look at it, though, even the best brands have a high fat and sugar content, so don't go too far in pushing ice cream as a nutritious dessert. Several ice cream manufacturers are experimenting with honey rather than sugar-sweetened ice cream and the use of carob, a chocolate substitute, instead of chocolate syrup. Keep an eye out for them.

In the summary at the end of this chapter are some of the companies reputed to use only the "finest ingredients" in their ice cream, which is to say cream or whole milk, real fruit and other natural flavors, no artificial coloring agents and no chemical emulsifiers or fillers.

Remember, the more far-out the flavor, the more unreal it's bound to be . . . there is no such thing as "natural" bubble gum.

HOMEMADE FROZEN DESSERTS

If you and your family are especially fond of frozen desserts (Don't panic! We wouldn't even begin to suggest you make your own ice cream!), there are some simple, nutritious desserts that are similar in nature but cut down on calories, animal fat, sugar intake, and have no hidden ingredients.

FROZEN FRUITED YOGURT

Frozen Fruited Yogurt is easily made by pureeing unflavored yogurt, fruit, and honey in the blender and then freezing the mixture. For each pint of yogurt use 1 banana or 1 orange or ½ cup of diced fresh fruit or ½ cup of diced dried fruit which has been softened in warm water, and 2 to 4 table-spoons of honey, depending on the sweetness of the fruit. Start with the smaller amount of honey; blend and taste. Transfer the mixture to a plastic container suitable for freezing, cover, and allow to harden in the freezer. This will take about 30 minutes. For a creamier product, whip the frozen yogurt in an electric mixer and let it harden again. *Yield:* about 1 pint per pint of yogurt.

ITALIAN HONEY GELATO

A low-calorie Italian Gelato can also be made quite simply and inexpensively from nonfat dry milk, gelatin, and egg whites. Each ½-cup serving contributes only 70 calories. Here is a recipe for a honey-sweetened version:
1 envelope (1 tablespoon) unflavored gelatin
½ cup nonfat dry milk powder
2 cups skimmed milk
½ cup honey
2 teaspoons lemon juice
2 egg whites
Mix together gelatin and dry milk powder in saucepan. Stir in milk. Place over low heat, stirring constantly until gelatin dissolves, 5 to 8 minutes. Remove from heat; stir in honey and lemon juice. Pour into freezer tray or shallow pan and freeze until firm. Turn into chilled bowl and add egg white.

Beat at high speed of electric mixer until mixture is smooth and fluffy. Return to freezer tray and freeze. *Yield*: about 5½ cups; 10 servings.

FRUIT ICES

If fruit ices are more your style you can create some delicious fresh fruit-flavored ones by filling your ice cube tray with orange juice, apple juice, or grape juice, and freezing the cubes until firm. To make them easy to handle you may want to insert a small wooden skewer or lollipop stick into each cube when it is almost firm.

RECOMMENDATIONS

General Rule of Purchase: No ingredients on label of ice cream, and few required for other frozen desserts. If the word "Flavored" appears on the label, this is your clue that artificial flavoring has been added (see details in text). Ice milk, sherbet, and water ices must indicate artificial coloring; ice cream may not. The brands listed here are the least tainted, no artificial coloring or flavoring, no fillers, but still plenty of sugar.

EXEMPLARY BRANDS
 East—*Breyers*
  Haagen-Dazs (particularly carob and honey)
  Louis Sherry All Natural
  Meadow Gold Old Fashioned
  Truly Nature's Own
  Waldbaum's All Natural
 Middle—*Breyers*
  Haagen-Dazs (particularly carob and honey)
  Meadow Gold Old Fashioned
 West—*Brockmeyer's* Natural
  Golden Temple Natural Honey Ice Cream
  Haagen-Dazs (particularly carob and honey)
  Lucerne Country Pure Vanilla Honey
  Sara Lee Old Fashioned

Puddings and Gelatin Dishes

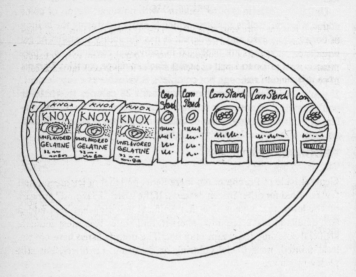

The popularity of gelatin desserts in this country needs no documentation; rarely has a food product been able to change our language as effectively as "Jell-O." Today the word "Jell-O" is invariably used to mean gelatin desserts no matter what the brand. One of the most successful advertising campaigns, however, masks one of this country's worst processed food items.

Do you have any idea what those dessert powders are made of? They're about 85 percent sugar and 10 percent gelatin plus factory-made flavorings, colors, and acid—all those things we're trying to avoid.

What did people do before these dessert mixes came in a box? Before J-E-L-L-O? Why, they made their own puddings and gelatin desserts from fresh fruit and vegetable juices, fresh dairy products, and pure unflavored gelatin. One of Nikki's first jobs included developing recipes for unflavored gelatin, a product she had never even heard of, having grown up in this age of prepared gelatin desserts. To her surprise she discovered that the amount of time and work involved in preparing fresh-flavored dishes using unflavored gelatin was almost identical to reconstituting the packaged gelatin dessert mixes.

Unflavored gelatin is pure "gelatin" with no sugar, flavor, or color added. Gelatin itself is a protein which is extracted during the boiling of bones, then dried and powdered. It has the ability to stiffen or gel liquids. Most brands are packaged in individual envelopes each pre-measured to gel up to 1 pint of liquid. Each envelope contains 7 grams of protein, which although not complete, is valuable as a supplement. If you're counting calories 1 envelope adds 28 calories to whatever you're making. If not pre-measured, 1 tablespoon will be the equivalent of 1 envelope. Any brand of unflavored gelatin is acceptable and we have seen *Knox* Unflavored Gelatine in every supermarket.

YOUR OWN GELL-O

The secret of all gelatin dishes is learning to make the basic gelatin mixture, a simple combination of gelatin plus liquid. From here you can go on to create sweet or savory salads, whips, chiffons, and mousses.

To prepare a simple gel for 4:

1. Sprinkle 1 envelope (1 tablespoon) of gelatin evenly over ½ cup of cold liquid in a small saucepan to soften. This liquid can be any fruit juice (but if it's pineapple it must be the canned type), vegetable juice, or broth. It can even be water.
2. The gelatin granules absorb the cold liquid and swell, making it easy for them to dissolve. Now place the saucepan with the softened gelatin over low heat and stir constantly until gelatin dissolves, about 2 to 3 minutes.
3. Remove from heat and stir in an additional 1¼ cups of the liquid and ¼ cup raw sugar if you're making a sweet gel. (For a sweet gell-o some form of sweetening is necessary, but at least you can eliminate the highly refined type and keep it to a minimum.)
4. Pour mixture into a bowl or 4 small dessert dishes and chill until firm. Like all packaged gelatin dishes this will take 2 to 4 hours.

If you want to add diced fruits or vegetables to your gel, chill the mixture until it is slightly thickened (the consistency of unbeaten egg whites), then fold in up to ½ cup of solid ingredients and return to the refrigerator until firm.

Gelatin Whips

A whip is simply a gelatin dessert that is beaten until light, fluffy, and double the original volume. To prepare a whip, chill the gelatin until it is partially set, then beat with an electric or rotary beater until it is frothy. Pour into dishes and chill until firm.

Mousse

A mousse is no more than the clear basic gel with whipped cream folded into the partially set mixture. An Orange Mousse, for instance, can be made by chilling the basic gel made with orange juice to the consistency of unbeaten egg white, whipping 1 cup of heavy cream, and folding it into the partially set orange mixture. If you like, you can mix in some diced strawberries or other fresh fruit just before you fold in the whipped cream. Turn the entire mixture into a bowl or dessert dishes and chill until firm.

Chiffon Pies

A chiffon is only a bit more complicated and involves the addition of eggs. This is how simply you could whip up a Banana Chiffon Pie.

BANANA CHIFFON PIE

1 envelope (1 tablespoon) unflavored gelatin
½ cup cold water
Pinch of salt
4 eggs, separated
1 cup mashed banana
2 tablespoons lemon juice
½ cup honey
½ cup heavy cream, whipped

Sprinkle gelatin on water in top of double boiler to soften. Add salt and egg yolks; mix well. Place over boiling water and cook, stirring constantly, until gelatin dissolves and mixture thickens slightly, about 3 to 5 minutes. Remove from heat; stir in banana and lemon juice. Chill until mixture mounds slightly when dropped from a spoon, about 20 minutes. Beat egg whites until stiff, but not dry. Gradually add honey and beat until peaks form. Fold in gelatin mixture, then whipped cream. Turn into your favorite baked pie crust—a crumb crust or nut crust is recommended—and chill until firm. If desired, garnish with more whipped cream and fresh berries.

Blend and Gel

Gelatin dishes can be prepared instantaneously in the blender. In this manner any chopping, whipping, or other work that would normally be done by hand can be passed on to the blender. This quick relish mold will show you how it's done:

CRANBERRY RELISH MOLD

2 envelopes (2 tablespoons) unflavored gelatin
½ cup cold water
½ cup boiling water
½ cup honey
¾ cup raw sugar
½ orange, seeded and cut in pieces
3 cups cranberries

Sprinkle gelatin over cold water in blender container; allow to stand while assembling other ingredients. Add boiling water; cover and process at low speed until gelatin dissolves. If gelatin granules cling to container, use a rubber spatula to push them into the mixture. When gelatin is dissolved, add honey, sugar, and orange; process at high speed until orange is finely chopped. Stop blender and add cranberries. Cover and process until cranberries are finely chopped. Turn into a 4-cup mold or individual molds. Chill until firm. Unmold to serve. *Yield*: 8 servings.

One Essential Reminder

The one thing to be sure and remember when you add fruit flavors to gelatin is that pineapple juice and chunks must be canned or otherwise cooked before adding to the gelatin. Fresh and frozen pineapple contain an enzyme which prevents gelatin from gelling.

PUDDINGS

Puddings are no mystery either. With a box of cornstarch or pearls of tapioca, both sold in your supermarket, you can make some pretty nutritious desserts without the chemicals included in the prepared pudding mixes. These do take more time than the instant mixes, but the richness of your puddings (and the delight of family and friends) will make it all worthwhile.

Cornstarch Pudding

Cornstarch acts as a thickening agent when cooked with liquids. By cooking it with milk and sweetening and flavoring the mixture to taste, you can control what goes into your pudding.

The cost and calories can be minimized if you start with nonfat dry milk. Try reconstituting the milk in a blender or a jar with a good cover and shake it until it's nice and foamy; your pudding will have an especially delicate texture.

When making cornstarch pudding keep the heat as low as possible to prevent scorching or curdling. A double boiler works best.

MAPLE PUDDING

Combine 2½ tablespoons of cornstarch, 2 cups of water, 6 tablespoons of nonfat dry milk powder (or amount recommended for reconstituting 2 cups of milk in brand you have selected) and ¼ cup of maple syrup in blender or jar. Cover tightly and shake until dry ingredients are dissolved and mixture is foamy. Cook over low heat, stirring frequently, until mixture thickens slightly and just begins to boil. Place over boiling water or turn heat *as low as possible*, cover and let cook 5 minutes. Pour into 4 small dishes and let cool to room temperature. Do not stir. When cool, chill in refrigerator. To serve, garnish with chopped nuts or fresh shredded coconut.

Tapioca Pudding

Methods for cooking with tapioca vary with the kind and it is best to follow the directions on the box you buy. Whole pearls of tapioca require soaking before you use them, often up to twelve hours. Cooking time is about one hour for most tapioca puddings. For anyone willing to make the time investment, this turns out a fine dessert.

Baked Pudding

Finally, less work and more nutritious than any of these is an old-fashioned baked custard.

MOLASSES CUSTARD

3 eggs
¼ cup molasses
¼ teaspoon salt

1 teaspoon pure vanilla extract
2 cups milk, scalded

Beat eggs lightly; add molasses, salt, and vanilla. Stir in scalded milk. Pour into six 5-ounce custard cups; place in shallow pan. Pour hot water into the pan to a depth of 1 inch. Bake in a 325° oven 40 to 45 minutes, until a knife inserted 1 inch from the edge comes out clean (the soft center sets as it stands). Serve at room temperature or chilled.

If you plan to unmold the custard, place a teaspoon or two of molasses in the bottom of each custard cup before the custard mixture is poured in. When unmolded you will have a molasses glaze on top. *Yield*: 6 servings.

RECOMMENDATIONS

General Rule of Purchase: Purchase the raw materials and prepare fresh puddings. Unflavored gelatin, cornstarch, and whole tapioca pearls provide the basis for them; buy freely.

Foodless Foods

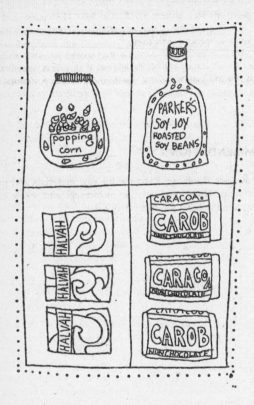

There is hardly anyone who doesn't like to snack. And why shouldn't you succumb to the alluring tastes of oversweet candy bars and highly seasoned chips?

But, these treats are not without their costs. Besides the numerous chemicals that are used in commercial snack foods there is the possibly more damaging high content of refined sugar. Those that are free of sugar contain reprehensible amounts of salt. It is a rare "treat" indeed that bears any resemblance to food. Take, for example, one of the latest additions to the list which is being billed as "a balanced nutrition between meals food" for "when you can't sit down to a well-balanced meal." This is the list of ingredients:

Corn syrup, partially hydrogenated vegetable oil (with freshness preserver), sodium caseinate, cocoa, and chocolate (processed with alkali), water, glycerine, nonfat dry milk powder, modified food starch, vegetable monoglycerides, calcium phosphate, salt, magnesium oxide, citric acid, vitamin C, iron orthophosphate, vitamin E acetate, niacinamide, vitamin A palmitate, vitamin B_6 hydrochloride, vitamin B_2, vitamin B_1 mononitrate, potassium iodide, folacin, vitamin D_2, B_{12}, and artificial flavor.

It would be a waste of time to list all the different items found in the typical candy aisle. With the few exceptions listed below, there is nothing worth your attention.

At the very least, the foods you choose for snacking should not add potentially harmful substances to your system, and without much effort they can add some good things as well. The best favor you can do for yourself is to stock your kitchen with nuts, dried fruit, fresh fruit, crackers and cheese, and some of the snack foods suggested here, so you'll never have to give in to the ersatz offerings. Strangely enough, after sampling some of the flavor-rich "real" foods that exist as alternatives, you're likely to discover your old favorites are no longer as enjoyable as you once thought they were.

POPCORN

Old-fashioned popping corn, not to be applauded for its nutritional contribution, is certainly very tasty and at least quite harmless. Bags and tins of dried corn kernels are sold everywhere, ready to be taken home and popped. Save your money and skip the kind that comes packed ready-to-pop. These "poppers" contain hardened (saturated) oils, and artificial flavoring creates the illusion in those that are "butter-flavored." You will get exactly the same results if you heat 1 to 2 tablespoons of butter or oil in a large saucepan or skillet, add the dried corn kernels, cover tightly, and shake over high heat until the popping stops. The popped corn is now ready to be salted, coated with melted butter if you wish, or sweetened with a sauce of warmed molasses or honey.

SOYBEANS: THE GREATEST SNACK ON EARTH

Let's move on to some healthier snack items. You will find a variety of roasted soy products being introduced to most supermarkets. These are soybeans which have been oven-roasted, sometimes salted, and in some cases flavored with garlic or onion. Different people prefer different brands according to taste, but these are all recommended: *Soy Ahoy*, roasted, unsalted soy nuts; *Flavor Tree Pernuts*, plain or seasoned; *Parker's* Soy Joys. Soybeans are so rich in nutrients they can be used as the basis of a meal (See "Beans, Beans, Beans"); roasted as a snack, they are outstanding.

Flavor Tree also makes a variety of "chips," tiny crackers just right for munchers. The choices are onion, cheddar, sesame, and rice chips.

CHOCOLATE

All brands of chocolate contain sugar, emulsifiers, and vanillin, an artificial vanilla flavor. They also contain caffeine, an inherent part of the cocoa bean.

There is a chocolate substitute called carob, which you should at least try; if it can be found in your supermarket it will be located in the natural foods section. Carob is made from a plant sometimes called St. John's Bread: it tastes amazingly like chocolate and is used to create carob bars and a powdered drink much like cocoa. Carob is quite good, even in the opinion of a chocolate lover.

If you do use chocolate, particularly for baking, choose *Hershey's* Baking Chocolate or *Baker's* Unsweetened Baking Chocolate. *Baker's* says right on the label, "no ingredients other than chocolate."

TWO MORE, WITH RESERVATIONS

There are two other candy items sold generally in the supermarket that we will suggest, with reservations. One is halvah, a Mid-Eastern confection made from ground sesame seeds and shaped into a bar or large block from which a hunk is cut. It can be bought plain, marbled with chocolate, or studded with pistachio nuts.

The other is "sesame snaps," or "sesame crunch," flat, crisp crackerlike nuggets and bars of sesame seeds compressed in a sweet syrup.

The reservation for both comes from the huge amount of sugar used to create them, but as sesame seeds are very good for you, and no chemical emulsifiers, stabilizers, fresheners, etc., are included in either, these rank way above other popular candies.

THE REST, THE BEST

When it comes right down to it, the best snack foods you can buy are nuts, seeds, and dried fruits. These fill you up and satisfy your craving for either something savory or something sweet. At the same time they make significant contributions to your diet.

For other candies that will tempt you, but not harm you, see the simple homemade suggestions in the chapter "Satisfying Your Sweet Tooth—Sanely."

MAKING YOUR OWN POTATO CHIPS

Just for fun, you might want to try some homemade potato chips one day—totally free of preservatives and grease from overheated oils, salted to taste, and with some of the nutritional contribution a real potato can make:

REAL POTATO CHIPS

Peel potatoes and cut in half crosswise to give you two flat surfaces. Using a potato peeler, cut paper-thin slices from the flat surface until the entire potato is sliced. Spread slices out on an oiled cookie sheet. Brush the top surface of the potatoes with oil and bake in a 450° oven 8 to 10 minutes, until brown. Place the chips in a brown paper bag with ¼ teaspoon of salt per potato and shake to season. Vary the flavor with chili powder, garlic, onion, or seasonings of your choice. Store in an airtight container to preserve freshness.

RECOMMENDATIONS

General Rule of Purchase: The one essential rule is to keep your purchase of "empty calorie" foods to a bare minimum. Most foods designed for snacking are highly sugared, or highly salted and deep fried. Thus, although some snack foods do not contain any additives, they still cannot be thought of as whole foods.

EXEMPLARY BRANDS

Snacks (mixed nuts and fruits)
Au Naturelle Snacks
Balance of Nature Raisin Snack Mix; Fruit-Nut Snack Mix; Date Snack Mix
Nature Kist Nutrimix; Nutrisnak
Woodfield Farms Power Snacks

Nuts
Fishers Toasted Sunflower Seeds
Flavor Tree Pernuts
Laura Scudders' Dry Roasted Sea Salted Soyas
Nature Nut Mix
Parker's Pepita Nuts; Soy Joys
Planter's Soy Nuts
Soy Ahoy Roasted Soybeans
United Roasters Golden Soyas (unsalted, sea salted and barbeque)

Sweet Treats
Baker's Unsweetened Baking Chocolate
Barbara's Famous Peanut Butter Crunch, Sesame Crunch; Indecently Delicious Fudge Carob
Flavor Tree Caro-sel Carob Covered Pernuts; Carob Covered Raisins
Hershey's Baking Chocolate
Joyva Sesame Crunch
Sahadi Dry Roasted Sesame Crunch

Savories
Barbara's 100 Whole Wheat Pretzels; Whole Wheat Sesame Sticks
Flavor Tree Sesame and Bran Sticks; Onion, Cheddar, Sesame and Rice Chips
plain popping corn

Supply Meets Demand:
The Natural Foods Department

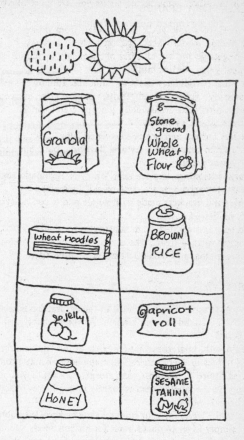

Many of you may now be greeted with the option of doing some of your shopping in a new section in the supermarket—the natural foods department. One outgrowth of the increasing concern with nutrition and whole foods is that many stores have begun buying items previously found only in natural foods stores. When you can't find what you're looking for on the regular supermarket shelf, chances are it will be stocked in this section. Although the products carried vary with the store, some of the goods you are most likely to find include:

•A variety of whole grain flours, often from organically grown grain, including whole wheat, rye, buckwheat, and soy.

•Pure vegetable and nut oils, free of chemicals, including safflower, corn, wheat germ, and walnut.

•Raw nuts, particularly cashews, almonds, sunflower seeds.

•Organically grown dried fruits, particularly apricots, figs, monukka raisins, and occasionally pineapple and banana.

•Brown rice and soybeans.

•Pure nut butters and honey-sweetened jams.

•Whole grain cereals with natural flavoring, both hot and cold.

•Raw wheat germ.

•Natural seasonings like sea salt, "raw" or turbinado sugar, brewer's yeast, tamari soy sauce, sesame salt (gomasio).

•Cookies and crackers made with whole grains and no synthetics.

•Pure, unfiltered honey.

•Herb teas and roasted grain substitutes for coffee.

•An assortment of treats, like carob, soy nuts, and "chips" made with whole grains, and baked instead of deep-fat fried.

BUY FREELY?

Just because something is situated in the natural foods section can you assume it is suited for your kitchen? As you probably suspect, our answer is NO.

To begin with, misrepresentation exists in the "natural foods" industry as it does in every other. The manufacturer may promote his product as "pure," "natural," and "organic," but if you read the ingredients on the label instead of merely taking his word for it, you may find this is not so.

Secondly, the buyer for your store may not be knowledgeable in this area, but simply eager to do a service for his customers. He may rely on the word of a salesman, often without realizing that the product he is offering is a sham.

Does your store manager distinguish between "natural foods" and "diet foods," or does he lump them together under the category "health foods"? Those foods manufactured with the diet market in mind are frequently the most chemicalized—such items as diet jams, salt substitutes, low-calorie salad dressings, artificially sweetened fruits and beverages, diet candies. Make sure you don't pick these off the shelf under the assumption they are whole foods. Almost the only foods that "diet departments" offer in common with whole foods is their selection of crackers, and even all of these do not qualify.

Gourmet Foods and Natural Foods

"Gourmet foods" often find their way onto the shelf alongside "natural foods". The fancy label and high price might lead you to assume these products are better than the average supermarket fare, while in reality they contain the same refined sugars and flours, artificial coloring and flavoring, undesirable oils and preservatives. The reason most of them are "gourmet" is that the demand for them is limited.

WHAT TO BUY

The major difference between the whole foods offered on the regular supermarket shelf and the whole foods in the natural foods department should be that those reserved for the special section should be organic as well as whole. Check the label to find out if the ingredients are "organically grown." If not, a similar whole food, free of chemicals, offered on its usual shelf will be every bit as good and will probably cost you less.

Ecology at Home: Basic Training

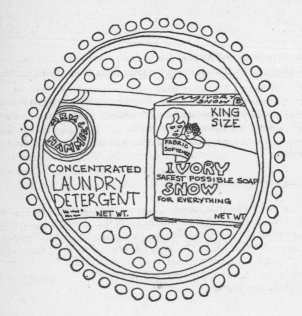

There are many people who visualize the earth as a sort of spaceship. They see the earth hurtling through space with the population as the crew and all its resources as supplies. This simplification enables them (and us) to easily analyze some of earth's contemporary problems, for we can step back and see our world in perspective.

Unlike mechanical spaceships that have limited stores, our spaceship Earth has the ability to regenerate its own supplies—indefinitely. Every day new supplies are created, in the form of freshly grown crops and newly born livestock, naturally purified air and water, and even new members of the crew. As you can see, present-day spaceships have re-created some of these processes in their ability to reuse and recycle water and air.

Recently man has realized that some of the mechanisms on our spaceship are starting to malfunction. The cause, ironically, is the crew itself. The crew (all of us) has been taking the machinery for granted and we are actually throwing monkey-wrenches into it. For example, by using too much power we consume our fuel supply faster than it can regenerate itself. The use of certain chemicals, like those often found in our modern "washday miracles," may actually destroy some of nature's systems that give us fresh water, air, and food. Can you imagine an astronaut doing the same thing to his life-supporting apparatus?

It is important to remember that whenever something is produced, a fuel is consumed. Eventually the product will be returned to nature to disintegrate and become fertilizer or fuel through the recycling machinery of our spaceship. This fuel can then be used to produce something else. In other words, nothing is lost. When a nonbiodegradable product like plastic is manufactured, however, the fuel is used but the plastic cannot be returned to the soil. Nature's cycle is ended— forever.

If we continue to use materials that are incapable of returning to their basic state (biodegradable), eventually we will have mounds of nondegradable garbage and diminished natural resources. Plastic, Styrofoam, glass, and aluminum are prime examples of materials that last virtually forever and could literally bury us.

We must all learn to be good members of the crew. Basic training isn't hard, and in the long run it is more satisfying, less expensive, and maybe will even save the earth.

This chapter will deal with the most basic training. We will try to show you some of the minimal steps you can take to make things run better.

GENERAL PRINCIPLES

Reuse and Recycle

Your basic rule should be to avoid all nondegradable items such as plastic, glass, coated paper (plastic coating prevents disintegration), and aluminum. It is difficult to totally eliminate the use of these items. What you can do is understand that *these products must be used sparingly,* and when used, reused and recycled.

Returnable bottles are preferred over the disposable kind and should always be returned. Plastic bags, jars, aluminum foil, and even waxed paper can be reused many times. Dirty plastic bags can be washed and hung to dry or used for wet garbage or cleaning the kitty litter.

When reuse is no longer possible, these items should be recycled (taken to a local recycling center) along with your aluminum or steel cans and paper. Some countries recycle as much as 45 percent of their paper; we recycle only 10 to 20 percent.

Avoid Products with Excessive Packaging

Packaging does nothing more than make a product more marketable. It does not enhance the value of the product, although it does enhance the cost. An aerosol can accounts for as much as 16 percent of the price of the item and is not biodegradable. Does the product also come in a mechanical spray? If so, then purchase that version; it will probably be less expensive and the container will be reusable and recyclable (ever try to reuse an aerosol can?).

Does one supermarket use plastic meat trays and another compressed paper? Patronize the one with the recyclable paper trays. If you buy something with unnecessary packaging send it back to the manufacturer or leave it in the store for them to figure out what to do with (like the *cellophane* that wrapped the *box* that housed the *bottle* the shampoo came in).

Use the Real Thing Whenever Possible

Cloth napkins are nicer and cheaper than paper ones. Adopt the European custom and give everyone his own napkin ring so the napkins can be used for several days. Use rags instead of paper towels. Get a set of inexpensive plastic dinnerware for use on a picnic or at the beach. They will outlast you. There is no excuse for using paper plates and cups in the home—having a kitchen includes the responsibility of washing dishes. Minimize the use of supermarket paper bags (they come from trees, you know) and bring your own shopping bag as the Europeans do.

HOUSEHOLD PRODUCTS

The following is an outline of some recommended household items which will minimize pollution, with suggestions for their use.

Cleaning Substances

Laundry: Originally we were going to list laundry products in order of acceptability. As our research progressed, however, we found that this would be impossible. There are so many products on the market today claiming to be ecologically sound and so many different standards for judging whether a product is really safe that we decided to recommend the one product that can be recommended without hesitation: pure soap.

Soap would have been our first choice anyway. There is nothing that can match the basic cleaning power and safety of plain soap. People were getting along fine with soap until that washday miracle made us want our wash "whiter than white." Despite all the fancy products that have been coming out since the 1940s, *Ivory, Duz,* and *Lux* have continued to sell plenty of powdered laundry soap. You use it too.

LAUNDERING WITH SOAP

1. Do not use too much. Use a measuring cup and experiment until you find the minimum amount necessary.
2. For extra cleaning power, use soap with ½ cup of washing soda. It is advisable, especially in hard-water areas, to rinse first with ¼ to ⅓ cup of washing soda to eliminate the detergent ingrained from previous washings, or a curd may form. The U.S. Department of Agriculture recommends using 1 to 1½ cups of white vinegar to eliminate the curd.

Other Laundry Products: Phosphates are chemicals that were first used in Tide and eventually became the major ingredient in most laundry detergents. Although a great cleaning aid, phosphates are now being blamed for causing serious damage to our water supply.

Phosphates are really only needed in hard-water areas. If you use anything other than soap, check the box and find a product that has no or low phosphates. You should also stay away from any product that lists NTA, enzymes, or arsenic. All have been shown to be personal and ecological hazards.

Remember, the term "biodegradable" is a shuck, since all detergents have been biodegradable since 1965. It still does not mean harmful chemicals and potential polluters are not included in the box.

As with soap, make sure you follow directions and use the minimal amount necessary.

Laundry Boosters and Presoaks: Most presoaks are very high in phosphates and should generally be avoided. Presoaking with *anything,* by the way, will help your wash. The following have no phosphates:

> *Arm & Hammer* Washing Soda
> *Borateem*
> *Addit*
> *Brion*

Water Softeners: If you really need your water softened, look into the mechanical softeners. *Calgon* Water Softener is low in phosphates.

Whiteners: Most bleaches are acceptable.

Starch: Use vegetable starch. It comes in liquid and solid form, is very inexpensive, and does not come in wasteful aerosol cans.

Liquid Hand Soaps: Most liquid soaps designed for hand-washing are very low in phosphates. Use them for washing dishes, lingerie, and other delicate items. The following have no phosphates:.

> *Dove*   *Lux*
> *Fels*   *Swan*
> *Ivory*   *Sweetheart*
> *Joy*   *Trend*

All-Purpose Cleaner: Your best bets are the old standards, pure soap and water, ammonia and water, baking soda and water, and washing soda and water solutions. All are good for cleaning almost anything except aluminum which they may discolor. If you prefer prepared products, the following are recommended as low in phosphates:

> *Bon-Ami* (the only nonchlorinated cleanser)
> *Kirkman's* Borax Soap
> Kosher Soap
> *Pinesol*
> *Whistle*

Dishwasher Aids: Dishwashers use an enormous amount of water and high-phosphate detergents. If you have one, use it as little as possible and *only* with a full load. Try hand-drying and avoid the expensive and toxic "rinse aids." For best results:

1. Experiment to find the minimum amount of soap needed.

2. Use the correct formula for your area. The leading dishwashing detergents are especially prepared for different waters and come in soft, medium, and hard. Ask your grocer.

These are the lowest in phosphates:

Electrasol
Finnish

Personal Soap: The best is again the simplest: pure soap like *Ivory*. Deodorant soaps have antibacterial agents and perfumes that can irritate the skin.

Paper Products and "Modest Proposal"

Paper should always be used sparingly and, when possible, reused and recycled. Use handkerchiefs instead of tissues. Save disposable diapers for traveling. Look for items that use recycled paper like *Hudson* products.

There are many environmental areas that even the experts are unsure about. One is dyed paper products, such as tissues, paper towels, and toilet paper. Some time ago many people believed that the dyes in the products were a matter of environmental concern—today they are unsure.

We have a modest proposal. It is that we go on using white paper products only. You will still have an attractive home even if the paper towels, napkins, toilet paper, and tissues don't match the decor. Let it be a sign of your concern.

A Special Problem: PVC

Polyvinyl chloride (PVC) is used to make clear, nonrigid, glasslike plastic, the type that shampoos, hand lotions, mouthwashes, cooking oils, and hair tonics come in. When burned in incinerators, PVC gives off corrosive gases which are capable of severely damaging the air-cleaning devices in the incinerator. If excessive quantities are burned, damage to buildings may also result. In this case it is better to buy products in glass containers or *nonclear* plastic bottles.

Pesticides

There are many pesticides like DDT that are harmful to you, your family, and your pets. Many of them don't even do the job. Never use DDT, chlordane, lindane, mercury, lead, arsenic, dieldrin, endrin, aldrin, toxaphene, or heptahlor compounds.

The following are considered safe:

Household Insects: Dri-Die, Drione, diatomaceous earth. Also products containing malathion or diazonin

Household and Garden Pests: Products containing pyrethrum, rotenone (poisonous to fish), ryania, sabadilla (poisonous to bees).

If unsuccessful with these, try pyrethrium-based sprays:

Raid

D-Con

Hot-Shot

Hargate

WARNING: Always follow directions. Remember, any product that says "Danger," "Warning," or "Poison" is toxic and should not be used in the home. Never dispose of pesticides in the sewage system.

Special Cleaning Solutions

In most situations soapy water and arm power can replace the more potent chemical compounds which are extremely powerful and extremely toxic.

Window Washings: One tablespoon of ammonia and one quart of water in your own squirt bottle. Try polishing your windows with old newspapers.

Household Cleaning: A solution of 2 tablespoons baking soda in 1 quart warm water cleans almost anything.

Household Odors: Try fresh flowers, incense, *Air-Wick,* or pomander balls. Pomander balls are a traditional sachet, particularly effective in closets and small, enclosed areas. Children enjoy making them and giving them as inexpensive gifts. This is the "recipe."

POMANDER BALLS

For each ball, select a large, firm orange. Stick whole cloves into the peel of the orange until completely covered with cloves. Insertion will be easier if the holes have been made with the prongs of a fork or a very sharp pencil point. When completely covered, roll the balls in a mixture of equal parts of orrisroot and ground cinnamon. Use about 1½ tablespoons of combined spices per orange. Pat in as much of the spices as will adhere to the orange and wrap in tissue paper. As pomander dries and shrinks, its fragrance develops. Remove from paper, shake off any loose powder, and it's ready to use. To hang, attach a piece of ribbon.

You can also cut down on household odors if you stop smoking. (As if you need a reason not to smoke, you might be interested to know that there are no pesticide tolerance tests for tobacco. In 1971 the amount of DDT in tobacco was twelve times that of 1957.)

Heavy Stains: Treat with a solution of 2 tablespoons of washing soda diluted in 1 cup of lukewarm water.

Dirty Diapers: Presoak in baking soda and water.

Fruit and Wine Stains: Apply corn starch or talcum powder immediately. Soak in milk before washing.

Grease Stains: Fresh grease spots can be treated with cornstarch or talcum powder. Pour boiling water or baking soda on stains before washing.

Ink Stains: Blot up carefully and apply cornstarch or talcum powder. Soak in milk.

Bloodstains: Soak in cold water.

Scalded Pots: You can eliminate scrubbing and using harsh cleaning products by boiling an acidic agent like vinegar or tomato juice in the pot if it is aluminum, or by boiling a basic solution of 2 teaspoons baking soda and 1 quart water in utensils made of iron, tin, enamel or glass.

Oven Cleaning: Loosen baked-on dirt by placing a small dish of ammonia inside a closed oven for several hours. Clean with a mild ammonia solution or soap and water regularly and heavy grease accumulation will not occur.

Tarnished Brass and Copper: Sprinkle with salt and a little vinegar or lemon juice; rub, rinse and dry.

Clogged Drains: Pour scalding water down kitchen sink daily to prevent clogging. When drains become sluggish dissolve 1 pound washing soda in 3 gallons of boiling water and pour through drain. Commercial lye preparations can cause permanent damage to porcelain, eat through clothing and can seriously burn your skin.

ECOLOGICAL ABOMINATIONS

1. *Styrofoam products,* especially disposable ones. ZERO biodegradable.

2. *Disposable diapers.* Diaper that kid. These disposables are heavy users of paper and plastics, cannot be flushed down the toilet, should not be thrown in the garbage uncleaned (because of the health hazard), and appear to be running second behind soft drink cans as highway litter.

3. *Plastic cups and utensils.* Some plastic cups are even called "reusable—disposable," so you can have it both ways. Unless they are

made of sturdy plastic and you mean to reuse them, they should be avoided.

4. *Disposable toilet bowl cleaners.* A brush from the hardware store will last a long time and will save paper and money.

5. *Pre-moistened towels.* Use soap and water.

A Short Primer on Food Labels

HERCULO

FLAKES

Nutritive Values

Nutrient	In 1oz.
Vitamin A	33%*
Vitamin D	33%
Vitamin C	33%
Niacin	33%
Thiamine (B_1)	33%
Riboflavin (B_2)	33%
Iron	7%
Phosphorus	1%
Calcium	0%
Vitamin B_6	0.6%mg
Vitamin B_{12}	1.6%mg
Magnesium	2.0mg

Typical Nutritional Composition In 1oz.

Protein	2.1gm
Fat	0.3gm
Carbohydrates	24.2gm
Calories	108

Ingredients

milled corn, sugar salt and malt flavoring with vitamins A+D in vegetable oil, sodium ascorbate, niacinamide thiamine (B_1) riboflavin (B_2) Pyridoxine (B_6) vitamin B_{12} and iron phospate added

BHA and BHT to preserve freshness

*% of R.D.A.

The Federal Code not only sets forth a guideline for what goes into food products, it also outlines those details that must be given on the package label. Like most of the food laws, these regulations hold back valuable information from the consumer.

As the Code is interpreted today, it often works to the disadvantage of the consumer where food labeling is concerned. It does not demand of industry such vital facts as freshness of the contents and expected life span, weight of the contents minus the water, or means by which the food was grown, held during storage, or otherwise handled; it does not require any display of inspection for cleanliness of the product or the processing plant; it does not call for any information on storing or using the product; it does not necessitate specific naming of many additives and where it does it often permits such vague references as spices, flavoring, coloring, vegetable oil, and emulsifiers—meaningless terms, especially to people with allergies and other health problems.

We are not informed as to how much of the contents is real and how much is chemical additive. The Code also exempts those products given a standard of identity from disclosing their basic ingredients.

There should be one basic rule for all food labels: *Complete disclosure on the label of all information which could in any way aid the consumer in buying and handling the item.*

Although this chapter does not solve the problem of inaccurate and insufficient labeling, it will tell you what the government has decided you have a right to know thus far, and how to take advantage of this information.

HOW TO READ A FOOD LABEL

In order to evaluate the processed, packaged goods in your supermarket you should learn to decipher the label. Every requirement must be satisfied in English, even on imported products. In accordance with the federal law, you will find:

1. The name of the product.
2. The variety, style, and packing medium in conjunction with the name. For instance, "sliced" beets, "creamed" corn, peaches packed in "heavy syrup."
3. The net quantity. This is the total amount (liquid included) *in* the container, expressed in ounces. For foods generally sold by weight

the measurement for the whole unit and remaining ounces is given as well, as in "40 ounces (2 pounds, 8 ounces)." For foods generally measured by volume (liquids), the volume will be expressed in whole units and remaining ounces as well, as "10 ounces (1 pint, 2 ounces)."

4. The name, address (which means city and state) and zip code of the manufacturer, packer, or distributor. If you have any questions, comments, or complaints about the product this is where to send your letter.

5. A list of special dietary properties if significant, such as "salt-free," "artificially sweetened," "enriched," etc.

6. Some indication if the product differs from government specifications, in which case the label will read "imitation" or "Below Standard of Quality."

7. A list of ingredients in descending order of predominance. This is where it gets a bit tricky. As we have said, certain products have a definition created by the federal government which sets forth mandatory and optional ingredients for the product. In these products all of the mandatory ingredients must be present in the specified amount. Because you are technically free to look up this standard of identity by consulting the appropriate legal documents (Title 21, Code of Federal Regulations) they do not have to be on the label. Certain optional ingredients, though, must appear on the package. Illogically, other optional ingredients can be included without being listed.

   Just so you aren't misled by any labels that say nothing, or say some things but may not be complete, here are the foods which *do not* have to list all ingredients:

cocoa products	processed cheeses
flour	frozen desserts
macaroni and noodle products	food flavorings
white bread and rolls	salad dressing
enriched bread and rolls	canned fruit and fruit juices
milk bread and rolls	fruit pies
raisin bread and rolls	fruit butters
whole wheat bread and rolls	jellies and preserves
milk and cream	nonalcoholic beverages
natural cheeses	canned vegetables

8. Any food which does not have a standard of identity must list all ingredients used. Although the specific name of most ingredients

Cheesecake
Ingredients:
Sugar, wheat &
graham flour,
dried cheese,
hydrogenated
coconut and soy
bean oil, dried
buttermilk,
modified tapioca
starch, sodium
phosphate, sod-
ium silico alum-
inate, invert
sugar syrup,
salt, sodium
caseinate,
polyalyceroI
ester of fatty
acids, leavening,
artificial and
natural flavor,
BHA and BHT

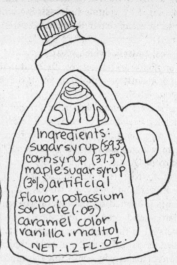

Ingredients:
Sugarsyrup (59.3),
cornsyrup (37.5%),
maplesugarsyrup
(3%) artificial
flavor, potassium
sorbate (.05),
caramel color,
vanilla, maltol
NET. 12 FL. OZ.

2 Packs NOODLE SOUP MIX
Contains: Egg noodles, salt,
whey, starch, vegetable shortening, monosodium glutamate,
onion powder, hydrolyzed
vegetable protein, flavorings,
dehydrated parsley, disodium
inosinate

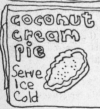

coconut
cream
pie

Serve
Ice
Cold

Ingredients: water, sugar, shortening,
corn syrup, coconut, whey solids,
corn sugar, food starch modified,
sodium caseinate, whole milk solids,
mono and diglycerides, polysorbate
60, hydroxypropyl cellulose,
monosodium phosphate, quar
gum, lectin, artificial color

must be given, exceptions include "spice," "flavor," "color," and "vegetable oil," which can be stated in those general terms.

9. Whenever any artificial flavor, color, or preservatives are used, they must be stated as such on the label. With the exception of butter, cheese, and ice cream, which for some strange reason do not have to mention artificial color, this holds true for foods which have a standard of identity as well as those which do not.

10. Any ingredient which itself contains optional ingredients must list them, for example, "vegetable shortening with freshness preserver."

11. If any food item is made from a blend of an expensive ingredient and a less expensive ingredient, and less than 20 percent of the expensive ingredient is used, the percent of this ingredient must be given. Therefore, a pancake syrup that contained less than 20 percent maple syrup combined with corn syrup would have to say just how much maple syrup there really was.

Some additives always exempt from labeling include fumigants applied to the product during storage, defoaming agents added during production, and anticaking agents added to the product along with the salt.

A LABEL THAT SPEAKS FOR ITSELF

The following list of ingredients is quoted from the label of a popular "toaster Danish." We feel it is especially complete as far as revealing its contents is concerned. Certainly if every label were this honest, you could make more informed choices.

bleached wheat flour, shortening, sugar, corn syrup, invert sugar syrup (derived from natural sugar), blueberries, glycerine (retains moistness), dried apple powder, precooked cornmeal, precooked corn starch, mono- and diglycerides and soybean lecithin (emulsifiers for uniform dispersion of shortening), salt, baking powder, aritficial flavor, citric acid (for tartness), wheat starch, potassium sorbate (a preservative), sodium bisulfite (controls texture), artificial color, propylene glycol and BHA (a preservative).

NUTRITIONAL LABELING

The latest step toward enrichment of food labels is the FDA's guidelines for nutritional labeling. Compliance with the regulations is voluntary, under the theory that competition will coerce all food companies to remodel their labels. In time we shall see.

Foods making nutritional claims, including references to protein, fat, calories, vitamins, minerals, dieting, etc., or foods that are "fortified" or "enriched" are subject to mandatory nutritional labeling.

The voluntary labeling rules affect all foods except fresh bakery goods, raw fruits and vegetables, and unprocessed dairy products. Although standardized products are not subject to the usual labeling requirements, if any "enrichment" is added, they too must comply with the federal regulations for nutritional labeling.

The rulings call for labels to include: serving size, servings per container, calorie content, protein content, carbohydrate content, fat content (including the amount of saturated and unsaturated fatty acids and cholesterol only if the processor desires) and percentage of U.S. Recommended Daily Allowances for protein, vitamin A, thiamine, riboflavin, niacin, vitamin C, calcium, and iron in each serving. The listing of other vitamins and minerals is optional.

The United States Recommended Daily Allowances (US-RDA) are derived from the Recommended Dietary Allowances set up by the National Academy of Sciences (NAS-RDA). They are designed to maintain good health in all healthy persons living in the United States. Although nutrient needs vary with age and sex, the values expressed on the label will be figured in terms of the highest recommendation of the National Academy of Sciences for males and non-pregnant females above age four for all nutrients except calcium and phosphorus (which vary widely depending on age) and biotin, pantothenic acid, copper and zinc (for which no previous recommendations exist). Formerly the percentage of protein, vitamins and minerals on a food label was expressed in relation to minumum daily requirement (MDR), or the amount of a nutrient necessary to prevent deficiency symptoms.

How Nutrition Labels Can Be Useful

Nutritional labeling is actually of greater value to the consumer of processed foods than to you who are now purchasing whole foods. With the use of whole foods it is easy to include sufficient fruits and vegetables, milk and milk products, grains, nuts, beans, eggs, meat, fish and poultry in your daily meals to meet your needs. Because the recipes for prepared foods are so complex, it is almost impossible to determine what is being offered in terms of food value unless it is printed on the package. The nutritional information on the label helps you to determine where to place these foods in the dietary scheme of things.

By becoming a label reader you can begin to compare foods and see which ones are important sources of key nutrients. Unfortunately, many consumers are not now conscious enough of food values to use nutritional labeling to its fullest advantage. With prolonged exposure to this information perhaps the awareness will come; in the meantime nutritional labeling should make food manufacturers more accountable to the consumer.

Why Nutrition Labels May Prove Harmful

There are certain drawbacks to nutritional labeling. According to current regulations there is no provision for labeling the percentages of ingredients in the food. We may find food companies, feeling pressure to "out-nutrition" competitors, relying on synthetic enrichment since they are not compelled to list the actual amount of each ingredient in their product. "Fun foods" thus enriched might enjoy increased consumption, taking the place of more sound, economic purchases. Highly chemicalized convenience meals will be enriched to bring them up to nutritional standards. The result is that our already highly processed food supply will become even more synthetic. Without knowing the percent of each ingredient, all the nutrition may be in the form of synthetic substitutes, as we have already witnessed in the case of dry cereal enrichment. Consequently, a formula diet for humans, not unlike experimental animal feeding, may come into being; a diet that not only lacks sufficient research common to the use of most chemical additives, but which may mean meat and vegetable prices for inexpensive, chemical substitutes.

We can only speculate as to why food manufacturers and the FDA are so willing to list nutrients and at the same time refuse to divulge the actual percent of meat, vegetables and other valuable ingredients, and the amount of water, starch, sugar, fat, filler and synthetics of little worth. Is their silence due to this likely trend of excessive chemical enrichment and economic trickery?

VOLUNTARY DISCLOSURE

Some companies give you some extra information on the label to help you make your choice. This is basically advertising. Aside from the descriptive phrases like "old-fashioned," "home-style," "creamy rich," and "juicy sweet," which tell you absolutely nothing, you may find a picture of the product, the size of the product (like "colossal" olives), the degree of maturity of the product (like "baby" peas), the color ("green" lima beans), and the number of cups or servings within. Some brands give a grade, like Fancy or Grade A. The grade is not mandatory, but if it is given in a USDA official seal it must meet government specifications. Details regarding food grades are included in the discussion of appropriate food items.

OTHER LABELING INFORMATION

In some states certain foods must have the date of processing, packaging, or last possible sale date on them. These will be explained further in the next chapter.

Although the label does not tell you as much as it possibly could or should, take advantage of what it does offer and make yourself familiar with the product you are buying. When you don't find what you want to know, write to the manufacturer and ask. If they don't reply (as often happened to our inquiries), you can suspect they have something to hide.

Interpreting Food-Dating Codes: Blind Dates

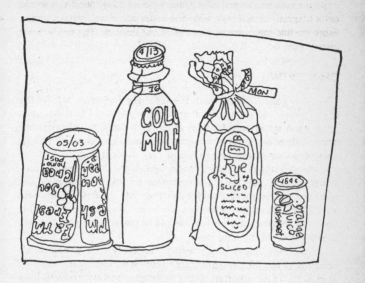

When we began writing this book we were very anxious to let people in on the secrets of supermarket food coding. If you take time to investigate you will find that almost every food item on your grocer's shelf is coded with a set of numbers and/or letters which is the manufacturer's way of conveying information concerning the freshness of the product. What a wonderful thing, we thought, if everyone could interpret these mysterious digits and know when the product was manufactured. Or is it when the product should no longer be sold? Or used? Well, that's just the problem; we discovered as we went about researching these codes that everybody's numbers, or letters, referred to something else.

As it turns out, the code changes from item to item, and store to store. In most cases the manufacturer determines whether the code corresponds to the date of manufacture, or the pull date (last day it should be sold), or the expiration date (the last day it should be eaten). Other characters are added to the code which have nothing to do with freshness at all, but refer to the plant, the vat number, or the packer. Furthermore, the codes change frequently.

By the time we jumped off the merry-go-round we decided it would be best simply to tell you what the codes are about, what you can expect to find, and how you can go about deciphering them in your own store.

OPEN DATING

Food dating, as it turns out, is not for the consumer, but for the manufacturer and the retailer as an inventory device. The codes allow for stock rotation so that older products are distributed first; they enable companies to remove overage products from the shelf (which doesn't always mean they will) and they make it possible to trace consumer complaints. Dating that is understandable to you the consumer is rare at this time. The manufacturer and the retailer do not want you to read these dates for fear that only the freshest products would be sold and the older ones left on the shelf to spoil. The cost of all this spoilage, they contend, would be passed on to you, through higher prices, in the long run.

On the other hand "open dating," or easily read dating on all products, is not the guarantee many think it is. Time is not the only or even the most important factor in judging quality. You still have no assurance the package has not been opened, since some customers like to sniff at products before buying them; opening starts product decay and renders the date meaningless. You have no guarantee a product hasn't been rewrapped in the morning to make it look like a new shipment. Also, there is no way of knowing if the food was stored properly, improper storage being more destructive of nutrients and more likely to cause spoilage in many foods than the time factor.

Despite these drawbacks, open dating is a step in the right direction toward truth in buying, and many stores have initiated open dating on their own brands. Certain cities and states have laws calling for clear marking on certain perishables, like milk and bread, indicating the last day of sale. Local consumer agencies or government offices can provide you with additional information along these lines.

DECODING

The most effective way you have of learning what the code in your supermarket means is to ask the employees or the manager. Many stores have prepared leaflets which explain the procedure. All have a master code for their own use in interpreting the numbers placed on the package by suppliers. Ask to see it.

Don't attempt to interpret the code on your own without a lead of some sort. Many of the codes are as simple as a four-digit number with the first two indicating the month, the second two the day, so that 1019 would mean October 19. By the same token, another manufacturer might use a four-digit code in which the first number indicates the year, and the last three the day, as in 2032, in which the 2 refers to 1972 and the 032 the 32nd day of the year, or February 1. Even if you have broken the code you'll have to determine if this is the date of production or the last day of sale.

In most cases, nationally distributed items show the date of manufacture. In locally sold items, where the salesmen do the policing, the date of removal from the shelf is more common so the trucker can spot it for easy removal. The food may still be good for several days past this date to allow for normal home storage.

When it comes to fresh fruits and vegetables your eye will be the best guide. But for other products, such as meat, fish, poultry, eggs, bread, and dairy products, you should have some idea of what the numbers mean. Of course if you don't buy many canned and packaged prepared foods, then you won't have to concern yourself with their age.

Baked Goods

Most bread and baked goods remain on the shelf for forty-eight hours, after which they are removed or marked down. Many of the richer whole grain products made with honey or molasses, which improve keeping quality, are designed to remain longer. Many of these companies are on the side of the consumer and indicate clearly on the package the last day of recommended purchase. For the others, the code appears at one end of the package and is often accompanied by a color-coded tie twist so the trucker can spot it easily when he makes his rounds. Pick out your favorite breads and ask the store manager or deliveryman what those funny numbers mean. Then you'll know for all future purchases.

Dairy Products

In some cities the health code requires milk to have a pull date stamped on the top of the carton which states: "Not to be sold after midnight of." If date of pasteurization is indicated, sale should be within sixty-six hours of this time (about three days). This leaves adequate time for home storage, which should be only two to three days after pull date. If neither of these dates is marked, buy at your own risk, and if the milk smells the least bit suspicious, return it for another. Most stores are quite obliging in this matter. The same goes for cream.

Other dairy products, like yogurt, cottage cheese, and sour cream, usually have a date on the top or bottom of the container. Use common sense here. If you interpret the date as some time in the near future, this is the pull date. If the date is already past, it is probably the date of manufacture (although if your store has a slow turnover it could just as easily be an outdated item). Inquire, and if you get no helpful information, make another selection (of product or supermarket). Don't buy any of these products more than two weeks after the manufacturing date. Some distributors are beginning to clearly mark the length of time you can expect the product to remain fresh. *Dannon* yogurts provide a model for other food companies to follow.

The end sticker on a package of butter holds the code for this item. It is usually very long, since part of the number may be the government certification that the butter meets the grade indicated on the label. One common way of marking butter is to reserve four numbers for the date the butter is cut (sliced from the large brick and packaged). How long that is from the date of manufacture is anyone's guess. From this date the holding time can be from one to two months, and one retailer remarked that most butter is frozen for at least six months before it ever reaches the display shelf. So much for butter; we're as bewildered as you. Your best bet is to buy sweet, unsalted butter. Salt is a good cover-up for off-flavors, while rancidity is hard to disguise in sweet butter.

Eggs

While eggs do not have to carry a pull date, any eggs graded by the USDA as Grade AA or Grade A must state clearly when the last day of sale is. Grade AA eggs are supposed to be tightly controlled and should be fresh when you get them. Policing of Grade A eggs is up to the store. The pull date of eggs must be less than ten days from packing and they must be packed within six days of shipment, allowing them at the most sixteen days in the store . . . which is too much if you intend to keep them another two weeks at home. Buy eggs with the most time left you can find, and assume they are already a week old when they get to the display shelf. If they are not in a refrigerated showcase, consider them well past their time and look for a store that handles their eggs properly.

Meat, Fish, Poultry

Stores generally package their own meat, so there are no general truths here, although meat and fish and poultry are about the most perishable items you can buy. Here "pull date" is less effective than "cutting date," since the store might consider three days a fine shelf-life for meat, while you may be thinking more in terms of one or two days. Since ground meat has a shorter shelf-life than others, the marking on a fresh-looking package of ground beef can be of some help in finding a clue if your butcher is less than cooperative. Most markets grind beef at least twice daily, so when you find a package you believe is fresh, you can assume it is marked with that day's code. Other meats similarly marked should, therefore, be fresh that day too. If a letter is used to indicate the day, count back the letters on other meat packages and maybe you'll have some idea of how long they've been there. If a package has more letters than most or an X on the wrapping, it is usually an indication that it has been rewrapped, which means it's less fresh than you'd like to purchase.

Any precooked meat or fish product should be consumed within two to three days of preparation, regardless of what the wrapper tells you. Cooked breaded fish sticks dated for sale up to two weeks from the day you find them in the store (something we observed in a local supermarket) are a sign of an irresponsible merchant.

Frozen Foods

Frozen products, if properly frozen, can remain on the shelf for several months—and most do. Remember though, if this is the case, don't plan on keeping them for another several months or you'll be greatly disappointed in the quality you receive. If an item is not properly frozen—and many aren't—it will be of lesser quality the moment you buy it. Some indications of improper freezing are soft-ness or pliability; stickiness on the surface of the package; a large accumulation of ice crystals; package discoloration from leaking con-tents; or large cartons of frozen goods waiting in the aisles to be unpacked.

Part 2

In Your Kitchen

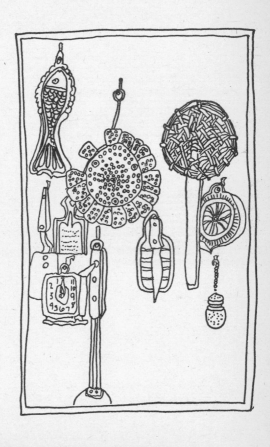

Breakfast:
Unseating the Sugar-Frosted Fortified Fakes

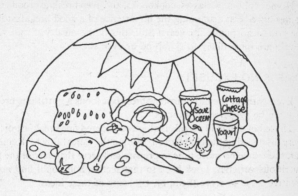

Some of the most depressing foods are those created and marketed for the American breakfast table. Despite the importance of the early morning meal, the products that are promoted as breakfast foods are primarily sugar and starch, like dry cereals, instant breakfasts, muffin mixes, and pop tarts. You'll probably welcome some ideas about now as to what you can serve instead.

WHY IS BREAKFAST IMPORTANT?

Think about your body for a minute. While you were asleep, your system was still busy at work, digesting your food, pumping blood, and keeping your respiratory system going. By the time you awaken, your system has been without food for eight hours or more. You can hardly expect it to carry you through the morning at an increased pace without some sort of inducement. That inducement must come in the form of food, or fuel for the system. A high carbohydrate (sugar and starch) breakfast may provide that necessary energy, but sugar burns through the system rapidly and within an hour your body will be nagging for more. When your body needs more fuel it lets you know in subtle ways—you become bored, your mind wanders, your eyes and head begin to ache. How many children do you know who lose patience in class and find it difficult to absorb what is being said?

Often it's because they haven't had a good breakfast. That edginess you feel before lunch is not the anticipation of a work break, but your body calling for replenishment.

Home economics classes, cookbooks, and even breakfast food companies have been drumming the importance of a good breakfast into the American public for years. Still, this is the meal you and your family are most likely to skimp on or even skip.

TIME IS NO EXCUSE!

Even without the aid of instant breakfast foods a nutritious breakfast can be prepared in minutes.

Those hot and cold cereals that are considered fine breakfast dishes were discussed in the chapters on "Filling the Cereal Bowl." Remember, these take no more time to prepare and serve than any of the less nutritious varieties. Look back to that section and you'll find many creative ways to serve them; or, try some of these ideas.

INSTANT BREAKFAST DRINKS

Instant breakfast drinks don't have to come out of a package. They can be made just as easily from the fresh, natural ingredients in your refrigerator and kitchen cabinet. If your family doesn't have time or appetite for a full breakfast, serve them one of these.

DATE NUT NOG

For each serving: Grind ¼ cup of almonds to a powder in the blender. Add 3 pitted dates, ¾ cup of milk, and blend until smooth.

TOMATO WHIP

Blend at high speed of blender until thoroughly mixed:
¾ cup tomato juice
1 egg
⅛ teaspoon pepper sauce
⅛ teaspoon salt
2 tablespoons nonfat dry milk powder
Serve at once. *Yield:* 1 serving.

SUNSHINE BREAKFAST

¾ cup orange juice
1 small carrot, sliced
½ banana
1 egg
1/3 cup nonfat dry milk powder
1 teaspoon honey

Pour orange juice into blender container, add carrot, and process at high speed until carrot is liquefied. Add remaining ingredients, cover and process until smooth, about 10 seconds. *Yield:* 2 cups or 2 servings.

BREAKFAST SUNDAES

Another breakfast dish that's no work for "the cook" and can be varied daily to prevent breakfast boredom works like an ice cream sundae and centers around yogurt (for protein), nuts (for protein and minerals), and fresh and dried fruits (for vitamins and minerals). To get this together:

1. Place your storage containers of nuts (walnuts, raw cashews, almonds, sunflower seeds, pumpkin seeds) and dried fruits (raisins, dates, apricots, figs) on the kitchen table.
2. Give each person a container or bowl of plain, unflavored yogurt.
3. Bring out a plate of fresh fruits.
4. Now let everyone make their own "Breakfast Sundaes."

Let the season determine what the fresh fruits will be. In the winter, offer bananas, pears, and apple wedges and plenty of raisins and dates. As spring rolls around, you can add strawberries, then melons, peaches, apricots, grapes, and gradually more and more fresh fruits, cutting back on the dried until the fresh supply becomes sparse again.

Always include some walnuts and sunflower seeds to vary the texture. If you like, you can add a topping of toasted wheat germ, dry cereal, or "wet nuts" made by combining honey or maple syrup with chopped walnuts and peanuts.

You can vary your sundae with cottage cheese served along with or instead of the yogurt.

BREAKFAST FROM THE TOASTER

Pop-up breakfasts are extremely popular with adults because they're quick, and with children because they're fun. It's a lot less costly and a lot more healthy to make a couple of pieces of whole grain toast (which is exceptionally flavorful) and offer them with any of these toppings:

• Peanut butter, alone or with sliced bananas, raisins, jam, honey, and a sprinkling of wheat germ.

• Cottage cheese or ricotta cheese mixed with chopped walnuts and dates.

• Butter, honey, and cinnamon.

• Sliced cheese, especially good when melted onto the toast.

• Cold sliced meat or fish.

• For Orange Pecan Swirls, trim the crust from the bread, toast on one side, butter the untoasted side and coat with a mixture of 1 teaspoon of honey, 1 teaspoon of thawed, undiluted frozen orange juice concentrate, and 2 teaspoons of chopped pecans. Broil until topping is bubbly and lightly browned.

Serve these as open-faced sandwiches; that way you get more filling for less bread. If you like, you can do the same things with crackers.

QUICK BREADS

Biscuits, muffins, and coffee cakes are not a breakfast by themselves, but eaten with eggs, cereal, or cheese they can be valuable breakfast foods. A standard recipe for muffins and biscuits will turn out nine to twelve at one time. Make one or two batches so that you can serve some fresh and freeze the rest to use during the next few weeks. It is best to freeze each muffin separately, or pre-slice coffee cakes and freeze in individual servings. This way you can place the foil-wrapped packages in a 350° oven when you wake up and in fifteen minutes, by the time you're ready to eat, you'll have a hot bread waiting to be devoured.

All of these are easy to fix and freeze well.

CINNAMON–APPLE COFFEE CAKE

1 cup minus 1 tablespoon whole wheat flour
1½ teaspoons baking powder

¼ teaspoon salt
1½ teaspoons cinnamon
½ cup raw sugar
1 egg
Milk
½ cup safflower oil
1 apple, peeled and thinly sliced

Mix dry ingredients. Break egg into a measuring cup, beat lightly and add milk to measure ½ cup. Using a knife or pastry blender cut oil into dry mixture until uniformly blended. Reserve 2 tablespoons of this mixture and add egg mixture to remaining dry ingredients. Stir only until moistened.

Spread batter into an oiled 8-inch square baking pan. Arrange apple slices on top and sprinkle with reserved flour mixture. Sprinkle with additional cinnamon. Bake in a 375° oven 20 to 25 minutes, until lightly browned.

WHOLE WHEAT RAISIN MUFFINS

2 cups minus 2 tablespoons whole wheat flour
½ teaspoon salt
3 teaspoons baking powder
3 tablespoons oil
1 egg
1 cup milk
¼ cup honey
¼ cup raisins

Combine dry ingredients. Beat together oil, egg, milk, and honey, and add to dry ingredients. Stir only enough to moisten. Fold in raisins (or other chopped dried fruit). Spoon into oiled muffin cups, filling them 2/3 full. Bake in a 400° oven 15 to 20 minutes. *Yield:* about 9 muffins.

ONION CORNBREAD

1 tablespoon butter
1 tablespoon oil
¾ cup cornmeal
1 egg
1/3 cup chopped onion
½ teaspoon baking soda
1 teaspoon salt
A pinch of pepper
1½ cups unflavored yogurt

(continued)

357

Combine butter and oil in a 9-inch baking dish or 1-quart casserole and place in a preheated (425°) oven to melt. Mix together remaining ingredients and pour into hot baking dish. Bake in a 425° oven 30 minutes, until just set. Serve warm or at room temperature.

SKILLET MAIN DISHES

Pancakes

Pancakes are a special treat for breakfast. If you have time in the morning you can serve a fresh stack of pancakes. A recipe using whole wheat flour appears in the chapter "Sifting Out the Flour." For a quick pancake breakfast you can freeze cooked pancakes by placing a sheet of foil or waxed paper between each, then wrapping the entire package in freezer paper or foil. At breakfast time remove as many pancakes from the pile as you need and pop them in the toaster to restore them. Pancakes can be stored in the freezer in this way for three to four months.

To vary your pancake batter, replace half the flour with an equal amount of cornmeal or buckwheat flour.

Quick Blintz

Blintzes are a Russian specialty. The true cheese blintz is made by filling a paper-thin pancake with a sweetened cheese filling and frying the bundle in hot butter until it's golden. It is much easier to fashion a Quick Blintz in this way:

For each blintz:

1. Trim any tough crust from a slice of whole grain bread.
2. Roll with a rolling pin to flatten.
3. Make an aisle of 1 tablespoon of cottage cheese along the center. Add a few raisins and drizzle with 1 teaspoon of honey. Sprinkle on ⅛ teaspoon of cinnamon.
4. Bring side edges of bread together in center, to cover filling.
5. Dip briefly in milk on both sides.
6. Fry in hot butter until browned on both sides, about 1 minute per side.

Serve blintz with a dollop of sour cream or unflavored yogurt.

Fried Mush

Fried mush may not be a very appealing name, but crisply fried slices of cornmeal (which is what "mush" really is), topped with butter and honey or maple syrup, make a beautiful breakfast. If you plan to serve it, you can do all the preparation the day before. Cold mush can be stored in the refrigerator for several days.

FRIED MUSH

Cook cornmeal (or any hot cereal) following your usual method until thick. Pour the cereal into a loaf pan or shallow baking dish and chill until firm. Just before serving, slice the chilled cereal and fry each piece in hot oil or butter in a skillet until crisp and golden on both sides. Serve piping hot with more butter, if desired, and your favorite topping.

EGGS

Serving eggs for breakfast isn't a new idea to anyone. What you should keep in mind is that you don't have to turn on the stove to serve an egg dish for breakfast. We always keep a supply of hard-cooked eggs in the refrigerator. This way we have a meal ready when we don't feel like cooking. Sliced egg on toast is a delicious morning meal and one you can enhance with cheese, leftover meat, or turn into egg salad. Some particularly nice ways to fix egg salad include:

1. Combine chopped egg, mayonnaise, salt, and chopped fresh mushrooms.
2. Combine chopped egg, salt, and sesame seeds; moisten with unflavored yogurt.
3. Add crunch to the salad with diced green pepper, celery, walnuts, and for hardy souls, onion.
4. Toss a tablespoon of wheat germ into any of the above.

When you do make scrambled eggs or omelets, add a few spoonfuls of cottage cheese or yogurt to the pan and the eggs will be lighter, tenderer, and of higher food value. Some wheat germ beaten in will go completely unnoticed, but will add valuable vitamins.

MISCELLANEOUS BREAKFAST IDEAS

There is no rule that says breakfast must be limited to cereal, eggs, and bread. Nikki had a friend who made a practice of eating lettuce and tomato sandwiches for breakfast. When Nikki was a child, her mother often gave her a bowl of soup in the morning. Cold rice pudding (made with brown rice, of course), leftover soup (pureed in the blender), cold fish, and poultry are all good for breakfast.

Recipes for elaborate breakfast dishes are available in all cookbooks if you're willing to spend a little time in the kitchen. The most elaborate breakfast we know, though, is practically work-free and extremely impressive. We call it "The Kibbutz Meal" because it is the daily fare (in the morning and the evening) on every kibbutz in Israel.

THE KIBBUTZ MEAL

Place on the table:

tomatoes	sea salt and pepper
cucumbers	sour cream
green peppers	yogurt
radishes	cottage cheese
scallions	hard-cooked eggs
kohlrabi	herring
olives, black and green	sardines
carrots	tahina, butter
cabbage	honey
parsley, dill	assorted breads and crackers
oil, lemon, vinegar	a pot of coffee, tea, and a pitcher of
garlic	milk

Let everyone choose what they like, cut as they like, and flavor as they like. Do not peel anything—just place a large bowl in the center of the table and let everyone toss their egg shells, vegetable peel, etc., into it.

Homemade Soups

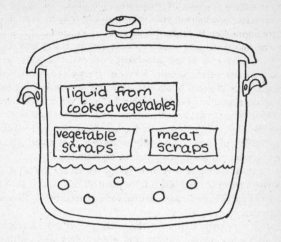

When it's cold and rainy out, make up a big pot of soup to fill the house, and later cold bodies, with warmth and comfort. Likewise, on hot summer days feast on iced soups to revive your spirits.

With the dearth of unchemicalized soups on the market it's reassuring to know that the work and time involved in making homemade soups are minimal. Soup-making is also the best way we know to make a little bit of food seem like a lot. By using odds and ends of grains, vegetables, and meat we can save money, often wasted nutrients, and cut down on garbage as well.

Since we had very little redeeming to tell you about prepared soups, this chapter is a lesson in basic creative soup-making. When you've finished, you'll never have to rely on a can for soup again.

STOCK-MAKING

The simplest of all soups is the stock or clear soup, also known as broth, bouillon, or consommé. This is the soup that often provides the liquid for other soups, sauces, and gravies. As is, it makes a delicate appetizer, low-calorie appetite-depressant, or hot beverage.

This is the soup that really takes advantage of "leftovers" like vegetable peelings, leaves, tough stems, meat bones, and the liquid left from cooking vegetables. In preparation for stock-making, set aside three closable containers in your refrigerator or freezer, depending on how soon you plan to make the soup.

In one container save your vegetable scraps: celery and scallion tops, tough broccoli stems, asparagus bottoms, pea pods, parsley stems, vegetable peelings, outer leaves of greens, overripe tomatoes, discarded ends of green beans, and even leftover cooked vegetables.

In another, save any liquid which is left after you cook vegetables. This liquid is rich in flavor and nutrients and enriches your stock. The liquid from broccoli, cabbage, and other strong-flavored vegetables should be left out since these will overpower your stock, although these vegetables in small amounts can be included.

In the third container save meat scraps which are too small to be otherwise consumed, and bones from poultry, beef, and veal. Again, lamb and ham are too strong-flavored for a general broth. Save these for flavoring bean soups.

When you're ready to prepare the stock, get out those storage bins along with a few onions, carrots, and whole celery stalks with tops.

STOCK-MAKING

Crack or saw up the bones as much as possible and place in a deep pot along with the meat scraps. Add liquid from cooked vegetables and/or water to cover by about 2 inches. Bring to boil, cover, and cook over low heat several hours to extract the flavor. Then add some freshly chopped onions, carrots, and celery, and the saved vegetable scraps. Chop all the vegetables coarsely to expose the most surface to the liquid and extract the most flavor. Again, use strong-flavored vegetables with discretion so they don't overpower your broth. For additional flavor you can add a clove or two of garlic, a bay leaf, and a bouquet of fresh herbs—parsley, dill, basil, thyme. If fresh herbs aren't available, add dried, allowing about 2 teaspoons per quart of broth. If necessary, add more water, then cover and cook gently 1 hour (or longer for more flavor). The less water you use, the stronger the flavor; the longer it cooks the richer it will be. Just before it's done, add sea salt and pepper to taste.

When the stock is finished, very little flavor or vitamins will be left in the meat or vegetables. Strain them out. You can then refrigerate the stock. When the stock is completely cooled, the fat will rise to the top and you can skim it off.

You now have a clear soup ready to serve as is, or you can add some pasta and cook until tender for a simple consommé. You can store the stock in the refrigerator several days, or freeze it in pint containers for future use.

Vegetarian Stock

By the way, a delicious vegetarian stock can be made in only one hour if you skip the simmering of the bones and begin at the point where the vegetables are added. Use just enough liquid to cover the vegetables, and when finished add 2 tablespoons of oil for each quart of soup for extra richness.

Chicken Soup

Another popular broth which doesn't have to come from a can is chicken soup. Use this homemade broth wherever a recipe calls for chicken broth or bouillon. As for the chicken you've used, dice it for a delicious salad or casserole base.

CHICKEN SOUP

1 chicken, whole or cut up
1 quart water
1 onion, sliced
1 carrot, diced
4 celery tops
2 bay leaves
2 teaspoons salt
½ teaspoon whole peppercorns

Put the chicken in a kettle, add water and remaining ingredients. Bring to boil, then cover tightly. Reduce heat and simmer 45 minutes. Remove from heat, strain broth and refrigerate both the chicken and the broth immediately. When the chicken is cool you can remove the meat from the bones. *Yield:* about 1 quart chicken broth (and about 2½ cups diced cooked chicken).

CHUNK SOUPS

A chunk soup is very much like a stew in a thick or thin broth. Chunks of vegetables, beans, grains, and meat all add texture and taste to this soup, which is otherwise prepared very much like the simple clear soups. Here, however, you will want to begin with fresh vegetables and eliminate the scraps, since nothing will be thrown away in the end.

All vegetables are welcome in the chunk soup pot. Fresh beans, corn, and asparagus in the summer, and don't forget cauliflower, sweet potatoes, and red cabbage in the winter.

CHUNK SOUP

Start this soup in vegetable broth or the liquid reserved from cooking vegetables if you can; otherwise use plain water. Make sure you have a tomato or two (save your soft tomatoes for soup) to sieve into the kettle. Begin all chunk soups by heating 1 or 2 tablespoons of oil or butter in the soup pot, then sauté a chopped onion or leek in the oil until tender and transparent. From here on, it's just like the clear soup; add lots of freshly chopped vegetables, a large soup bone or small pieces of meat if you wish, herbs (and always a bay leaf), cover with liquid, and bring to boil. Reduce heat, cover, and cook gently until all vegetables are tender (about 45 minutes to 1 hour), and if you've included meat, until the meat is cooked. When the vegetables are barely tender add a few tablespoons of rice, barley, cracked wheat, or pasta, and continue to cook until the grain is tender. This will take 15 minutes to 1 hour, depending on the grain you've added. The grain will absorb some of the liquid and your soup will thicken, much like a stew. You can add more liquid at any time to thin it, using stock, water, or tomato juice.

When adding green leafy vegetables like spinach, cabbage, lettuce, etc., to chunk soups, wait until the last ten minutes to do so. These vegetables cook very quickly and longer cooking destroys their delicate flavor. If you have any leftover grains on hand, add these instead of raw grains for convenience. They will take only ten minutes to reheat.

This Mushroom and Kasha Soup will demonstrate how easily a chunk soup can be made.

MUSHROOM AND KASHA SOUP

Heat 2 tablespoons of oil in large soup pot. Add 1 large sliced onion and a handful of diced mushrooms and sauté until the onion is limp and transparent. Add 5 cups of water or stock, 1 carrot thinly sliced, 1 sieved tomato, 1 bay leaf, and 1 tablespoon soy sauce. Bring to boil, reduce heat, and simmer 20 minutes. Add ¼ cup of raw kasha (buckwheat groats) and 1 cup shredded cabbage; replace cover and simmer 15 minutes, until grain is tender. Season with 1 tablespoon of salt and ½ teaspoon of pepper. *Yield:* 1 quart soup; 4 servings.

Bean-Based Chunk Soups

For a chunk soup made with dried beans, begin with the beans.

Soak them overnight or by the quick-soak method (see directions in the chapter "Beans, Beans, Beans") in 1½ to 2 times the usual amount of water, or 4½ cups of water per cup of beans. Bring to boil, then reduce heat, cover, and cook very gently, just as you would in normal bean cookery, for 1 hour. At the end of the hour add an assortment of fresh chopped vegetables (and don't forget that sieved tomato), herbs, a bone or pieces of meat if desired, and continue to simmer gently until the beans and vegetables are fork tender, about 1 hour longer. Add salt and pepper to taste, about 2 teaspoons of salt and ¼ teaspoon of pepper for each quart of liquid.

In making bean soup you can add many vegetables, as you would for a straight vegetable soup, or simply add lots of fresh garlic and onion. Lentil and split-pea soup are made the same way, except you can skip the soaking and the first hour of cooking and simply combine the beans, vegetables, and meat, and cook them together for about an hour.

Additional flavoring for chunk soups can come from a tablespoon or two of wine, vinegar, or lemon juice stirred in at the end. Meat can be added or excluded in any recipe. If you leave out the meat and desire a richer flavor add 2 tablespoons of oil and 1 tablespoon of soy sauce or powdered brewer's yeast per quart of soup.

To get you started with bean-based chunk soups, try this one.

MARIA'S WHITE BEAN SOUP

1 pound white beans
8 cups water
2 onions, diced
4 carrots, sliced in rounds
1 cup celery tops, chopped
2 tomatoes, sieved
2 sprigs parsley
½ cup olive oil

(continued)

2 teaspoons salt
¼ teaspoon pepper

Soak beans in water overnight, or bring to boil, remove from heat, and let soak 1 hour. Cook the beans in the soaking liquid in a covered pot 1 hour. Add the onions, carrots, celery tops, sieved tomatoes, parsley, and oil. Cover and cook gently 1 hour longer, until beans and vegetables are tender. Season with salt and pepper. *Yield:* 6 servings.

PUREES

A puree is nothing more than a chunk soup which has been forced through a sieve or processed in the blender. The resulting potage can be thick and smooth or have small pieces of vegetables or grain left for texture. By introducing leftover chunk soup to the blender you can completely change it into a new soup for another day.

This Black Bean Soup demonstrates the technique especially well, for it is prepared just like a chunk bean soup and then half is pureed.

BLACK BEAN SOUP

1 cup black beans
3½ cups water
1 bay leaf
1 clove garlic, crushed
1 small onion, chopped
½ green pepper, chopped
1 teaspoon oregano
.2 tablespoons wine vinegar
2 teaspoons salt
½ teaspoon hot pepper sauce

Soak beans in water overnight or bring to boil, remove from heat, and let soak 1 hour. Add bay leaf, garlic, and onion, and cook 1½ hours in a covered saucepan. Add remaining ingredients, cover, and cook 1 hour longer, until beans are tender. Puree half the beans, return to pot, and reheat, adding up to ½ cup more water to thin the soup. Serve with brown rice and raw, chopped onion. *Yield:* 4 servings.

Purees are also popular in warm weather, served iced. Potato, broccoli, avocado, beets, even fruits are all common bases for these chilled soups. Instead of resorting to a can, take twenty-five minutes and prepare this Vichyssoise yourself from scratch. Serve it hot in the winter, icy cold in the heat.

VICHYSSOISE

2 tablespoons butter
1 leek, sliced
1 small onion, chopped
2 medium potatoes (2 cups peeled, diced)
3 cups water or broth or vegetable cooking liquid
1 teaspoon salt
¼ teaspoon pepper
½ cup half-and-half (or cream for a really rich soup)

Melt butter; sauté leek and onion in hot butter until limp, about 5 minutes. Add potatoes, water or broth, salt and pepper, and bring to boil. Reduce heat, cover and cook over low heat 20 minutes, until potato is tender. Puree in blender or food mill and chill. Just before serving stir in half-and-half and adjust seasonings to taste. Garnish with fresh chopped parsley or watercress. Serve very cold. *Yield:* 4 appetizer servings.

Purees can be garnished with homemade croutons. Use stale brown bread or leave a few slices of fresh bread exposed to the air to dry. If time is short, dry the bread in a slow oven (250°). When bread is very dry, cut or break into cubes.

CREAM SOUPS

A delicate homemade cream soup is one of the easiest and quickest soups you can make. Any vegetable alone, or in combination, can be used. Squash, carrots, peas, asparagus, or spinach all work beautifully. This is another way to use up the less desirable parts of the vegetable, like tough broccoli stems.

Each cup of soup calls for ¼ to ½ cup of vegetable puree, depending on whether you want to emphasize the soup or the vegetable. To prepare the vegetable, cook it in just enough water to keep from sticking, until tender enough to mash or puree in the blender. The time will vary with the vegetable, but twenty minutes will be the maximum. Leftover cooked vegetables can be pureed instead.

The basic pattern for cream soups is always the same.

CREAM OF VEGETABLE SOUP

1 cup pureed vegetable
1 tablespoon oil or melted butter
1 tablespoon cornstarch
2½ cups milk, or 1½ cups milk and 1 cup liquid from cooked vegetables
½ teaspoon salt
¼ teaspoon pepper
Additional seasoning as desired

Heat the butter or oil and stir in cornstarch to form a smooth paste. Gradually stir in liquid and cook until mixture thickens and just reaches boiling. (This is a thin white sauce; fresh milk or reconstituted dry milk can be used.) Remove from heat, season, and gradually add pureed vegetable, stirring until smooth. Just before serving reheat, but *do not boil. Yield:* 4 servings.

Seasonings for All Cream Soups

The seasoning you use will add life to your soup (and this is true for all soups, not just the cream soups), and here you can be really creative. The following suggestions will set you on the right track:

CREAM OF	SEASONING
asparagus	basil, marjoram and rosemary
broccoli	nutmeg or mace
cauliflower	dill or caraway seeds
spinach	dried mustard or sesame seeds
pea	coriander
tomato	Italian seasonings or celery seed
pumpkin or winter squash	cinnamon

• For additional flavor, try sautéing a small chopped onion in the oil or butter at the start.

• Add pieces of cooked seafood or meat and vegetables to your cream soup and you have a chowder.

• For the finishing touch, garnish cream soups with toasted wheat germ or coarsely chopped peanuts or walnuts.

JELLIED SOUPS

All soups can be thickened and chilled for a refreshing jellied soup by the addition of unflavored gelatin.

All you have to do is soften 1 package of gelatin (1 tablespoon) in ½ cup of cold water (or cold soup or juice), stir over low heat for three to five minutes until gelatin dissolves, then add to remaining hot or cold soup. Chill in refrigerator until thickened, then cut into cubes or pile with a spoon into serving dishes. To speed chilling, place bowl with gelatin mixture in bowl of ice water or freezer for ten minutes. A jellied soup should be thinner than a mold, so use 1 package of gelatin (1 tablespoon) for each 2½ to 3 cups of liquid. Top jellied soups with a spoonful of yogurt or sour cream.

JELLIED BORSCHT

2 large beets
½ cup chopped fresh onion
¾ teaspoon salt
2½ cups cold water, divided
1½ teaspoons honey
1 teaspoon lemon juice
1 envelope unflavored gelatin

Wash beets, peel and chop to make about 3 cups of chopped beets. Place beets, onion, and salt in large saucepan, add 2 cups of water, and bring to boil. Reduce heat, cover and simmer 35 minutes, until beets are tender. Strain, reserving both chopped vegetables and the liquid. Add honey and lemon juice to liquid and return to saucepan. Heat to boiling. Sprinkle gelatin over remaining ½ cup of cold water to soften. Add to boiling beet liquid; stir until gelatin dissolves. Remove from heat. Chill, stirring occasionally, until slightly thickened. Reserve ½ cup of cooked beets and fold remaining beets into chilled gelatin mixture. Turn into bowl and chill until mixture forms a soft gel. To serve, spoon ½ cup of mixture into chilled soup plates. Garnish with reserved beets and sour cream or yogurt. *Yield:* 6½-cup servings.

INSTANT SOUPS

For really quick service, here are some soups that require almost no work or time before they're ready.

NO-COOK VEGETABLE BROTH

Collect the bases of carrots, celery, parsnips, and the tops and outer leaves of vegetables and greens. Dice each vegetable and combine or process separa-

(continued)

tely in the blender with just enough water to get the machine going. When finely chopped, pour the vegetables into an ice-cube tray and store in the freezer. To use, defrost cubes in a covered saucepan over low heat, or add directly to other soups and sauces for flavoring. Two cubes can replace ¼ cup of liquid in a recipe. Use to flavor the liquid for cooking grains also.

BROWN BROTH

This is a quick, flavorful appetizer soup made by sautéing 4 chopped scallions in 1 tablespoon of oil until tender, about 5 minutes, adding 2 cups of water, 2 tablespoons of soy sauce, and bringing the liquid to a boil. Reduce heat and cook briefly to let flavors blend. If you like, you can add leftover cooked grains to this soup.

TOMATO-AVOCADO SOUP

Quickly made in the blender, needs only gentle warming before serving. For 3 cups of soup combine:
½ cup water
1 cup tomato juice
1 small carrot, diced
1 stalk celery with leaves, diced
1 tomato, quartered
½ avocado
¾ teaspoon salt
¼ teaspoon basil
in blender container. Blend at high speed until smooth and heat gently to serve.

QUICK CREAM SOUP (from leftovers)

For each cup of soup combine 2 to 3 tablespoons of leftover cooked potato, brown rice, or whole wheat macaroni, 1 cup of milk, and ½ cup of cooked vegetable in blender. Process at medium speed until creamy and heat gently.

BLENDER SALAD SOUP

A spicy soup that needs no cooking at all.
2 ripe tomatoes
¼ large green pepper
¼ small onion
½ cucumber

½ clove garlic
⅛ teaspoon pepper sauce
½ teaspoon salt
1 tablespoon olive oil
4½ teaspoons wine vinegar
¼ cup ice water

Quarter tomatoes; seed and slice green pepper; peel and slice onion and cucumber; peel garlic clove. Place in blender. Add remaining ingredients, cover, and blend 3 seconds. Allow small pieces of vegetables to remain. To serve, pour into soup plates with an ice cube in the center of each. This makes 3 servings. Recipe may be doubled, but you will have to fill the blender twice to process this amount.

LAZY COOK'S SOUP

Prepare any vegetable or bean soup in twice the quantity you need. Then freeze half to use sometime in the next six months.

SOUP DINNERS

By now you are probably a master soup-maker and should begin to think really creatively about serving your family a dinner based on rich, thick, truly novel soups. The addition of hunks of whole grain bread, spread with cheese or nut butter, salad, and pudding or fruit can complete the menu. In warmer weather, plan on crackers rather than bread for a lighter meal. Any cookbook can supply you with some interesting ideas. Here are three of our favorites that you might want to begin with. To suit our preference, they are all particularly easy to make.

BREAD AND CHEESE SOUP

6 onions, thinly sliced
3 cloves garlic, minced
1 large bunch broccoli, chopped
2 tablespoons oil
4 teaspoons salt
½ teaspoon pepper
2 quarts boiling water

(continued)

½ pound whole grain bread, thinly sliced
½ pound grated Swiss cheese
½ pound grated Parmesan cheese

Sauté onion, garlic, and chopped broccoli in oil until onion is golden. Season with salt and pepper, add boiling water, cover and cook 20 minutes, until broccoli is tender.

Line bottom of a 4-quart casserole with half the bread. Sprinkle with 1½ cups of cheese, top with remaining bread, and add another 1½ cups of cheese. Pour broccoli soup into the casserole; sprinkle with remaining cheese. Brown in a 375° oven for 5 to 10 minutes. *Yield:* 4 to 6 servings.

SOPHIA'S GREEK FISH SOUP

2 pounds white fish (such as cod or flounder)
3 teaspoons salt
2 large lemons
1 medium onion, sliced
4 carrots, sliced
2 stalks celery with leaves, diced
4 potatoes, peeled and sliced
8 cups water
¼ cup olive oil
5 peppercorns
1 bay leaf
2 eggs, separated

Cut fish in large pieces, rub with 1 teaspoon of salt and the juice of 1 lemon, and let stand while you prepare soup.

Combine the vegetables, water, remaining 2 teaspoons of salt, oil, peppercorns, and bay leaf. Cook over medium heat 35 minutes, until vegetables are just tender. Remove 1 cup of the broth, add the fish and any liquid with the fish to the pot, lower heat and cook gently 15 minutes.

While fish cooks, beat the egg whites with a few drops of water until foamy. Add yolks and continue to beat until light. Slowly beat in the juice of the remaining lemon, then the reserved cup of hot broth. Stir the egg and lemon sauce into the *hot* soup just before serving. If it is necessary to reheat the soup once the egg and lemon sauce has been added, heat very gently; *do not boil* or the egg will curdle. *Yield:* 5 to 6 servings.

COLD FRUIT SOUP

2 peaches
2 plums
½ medium cantaloupe

2 oranges
1 cup yogurt
2 tablespoons honey, optional
1 cup blueberries

Dice peaches and plums; cut melon from rind and dice pulp. Combine the diced fruits and the juice from the oranges in blender c . . . . puree at high speed until liquefied. Add the yogurt and honey (if your f . . is not sweet enough) and process at low speed until smooth. Stir in blueberries and chill until serving time. *Yield:* 4 servings.

Do-It-Yourself Sauces

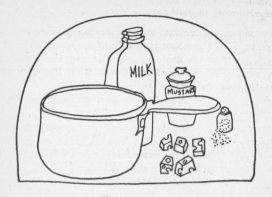

Most sauces can be made from scratch in five to ten minutes, including white sauce, cheese sauce, and gravies. Starch is the common ingredient for thickening these sauces and they are all based on the same recipe pattern. Here is a table with directions for preparing the standard sauce base:

STARCH-THICKENED SAUCES

Sauce	Fat	Cornstarch	Liquid
Thin	1 tablespoon	½ tablespoon	1 cup
Medium	1 tablespoon	1 tablespoon	1 cup
Thick	2 tablespoons	1½ tablespoons	1 cup

The normal method for preparing sauces is more complicated and more time-consuming than it need be. Try this shaker method instead:

1. Place fat (oil or butter) and most of the liquid in a saucepan and heat over a low flame until liquid warms and fat, if butter, melts.
2. Combine cornstarch and remaining liquid—about 2 tablespoons liquid per tablespoon of cornstarch—in a jar with a tight cover and shake to liquefy the cornstarch. The liquid you use must be cold.
3. Pour the starch mixture into the heated liquid and stir constantly over

.medium low heat until the sauce comes to a boil. Cook 1 minute longer to remove the starchy taste.

4. Season with ½ teaspoon of salt and ¼ teaspoon of pepper.

These sauces will provide the base for making most other sauces and gravies. The Thin Sauce is prepared for cream soups and meat gravies. The Medium Sauce is best for all-purpose sauces, cheese sauce, and creamed meat or vegetable dishes. The thick sauce is reserved for fillings.

Once you have prepared the basic Medium Sauce you can vary it like this:

Cheese Sauce: Prepare the basic Medium Sauce with milk or a milk-vegetable liquid combination. Add 1 to 1½ cups of grated cheese and stir until melted. If necessary return to low heat. Add a dash of dry mustard or nutmeg to heighten the taste.

Curry Sauce: To 1 cup of Medium Sauce made with milk add 2 teaspoons of curry powder, 1 teaspoon of lemon juice, and ⅛ teaspoon of ginger. If desired, stir in a few spoonfuls of yogurt just before serving.

Béchamel: Use ½ milk and ½ chicken stock to prepare this sauce. Season with ¼ teaspoon of thyme and 1 teaspoon of fresh minced onion. Serve over croquettes, meat loaf, chicken, or vegetables.

Meat Gravy: Gravy for roasts is prepared by the same method as other starch-thickened sauces with the liquid supplied by the juices left in the pan the meat or poultry is cooked in. Additional liquid is usually needed and this can come from wine, water, or a combination. Let the fat come from the meat drippings as well. Follow the pattern for a thin or medium sauce, depending on how thick you like your gravy. The proportions for a thin sauce are standard.

Onion Gravy: The proportions are the same here but the method varies slightly. To prepare this sauce, chop 1 large onion and sauté in 2 tablespoons of oil. While the onion cooks, add 1 teaspoon of salt and 1 teaspoon of honey for a rich glaze. When the onion is just golden, add 1 cup minus 2 tablespoons of water or broth, reserving the 2 tablespoons of cold liquid to liquefy 1 tablespoon of cornstarch. Now proceed as you would for any starch-thickened sauce. Season if you wish with 1 teaspoon of brewer's yeast or soy sauce.

White Sauce: Choose milk as the liquid and season with ½ teaspoon of herbs of your choice. Use with diced meats and vegetables for a "creamed" dish, allowing ½ cup of sauce for 1 cup or ½ pound of solid food.

Tomato Sauce

Homemade tomato sauce doesn't take much longer than the canned to prepare. This recipe produces a fast, but flavorful sauce.

HOMEMADE TOMATO SAUCE

Heat 2 tablespoons of safflower or olive oil in a large skillet or saucepan. Chop 1 large onion and 1 clove of garlic and sauté in the oil until onion is limp and transparent. Meanwhile chop ½ green pepper or 1 Italian frying pepper. Add to onion in skillet and continue cooking until pepper is softened and onion begins to turn golden. The time required so far will be about 10 minutes. Add 3 or 4 diced tomatoes to the pot, about 1 teaspoon of salt, 1 teaspoon of dried herbs, 1 teaspoon of honey, and pepper to taste, cover, turn heat down low, and cook until tomatoes melt, another 10 to 15 minutes. Adjust seasonings to taste, and your sauce is ready. You will have enough for a casserole dish for 4, or a pasta main dish for 2.

This tomato sauce may be a bit thinner than you're accustomed to. If you find this consistency doesn't suit your needs, add a tablespoon of canned tomato puree or tomato sauce to thicken it.

Meatless Main Dishes and Nutrition

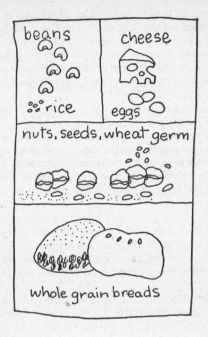

In the chapter "Meeting the Challenge of Meat" we mentioned that many people have begun using less meat in their diet. For some this means cutting out meat entirely, for others simply a reduction of present intake. Vegetarianism is not right for everyone; breaking the daily habit of meat is.

There are many reasons for the re-evaluation of "two servings of meat, fish, poultry, or eggs" daily. Here are some of the motivating forces behind the move toward low meat diets. Consider them seriously.

HEALTH FACTORS

From the standpoint of personal health many people have realized the importance of reduced meat intake. Those saturated fats we are constantly being warned about come from fats of animal origin, and nowhere do we find as much animal fat as in the meaty parts of the carcass. Cholesterol, too, is in high concentration in animal tissues. With the great war being waged against heart disease, meat is one of the first foods doctors suggest potential cardiac victims cut down on. Everyone is a potential victim.

What about the effect of some of the other meat "ingredients" on the rest of your system? The antibiotics and hormones used to raise animals destined for consumption are linked to many human disorders; these range from the increase of drug-resistant strains of bacteria and allergic reactions to drug treatment (a result of the indirect ingestion of antibodies) to cancer (traced to stilbestrol).

Even the toxicity of chemicals used on other foodstuffs creates a problem for meat eaters. Widespread use of chemicals affects the air, water, and food crops. As these potentially toxic substances travel through the food chain—from plant to animal to man—they do not depreciate, but, rather, the residue progressively accumulates to higher levels. Therefore, the lower you eat on the food chain, i.e., plant foods, the more you can control pesticide residue in your own system.

People who are so busy making sure they eat enough meat have a tendency to ignore other foods, deeming them less important. Meat may be rich in protein and B vitamins, but it's a poor source of most other vitamins. Without these catalysts your body cannot utilize the protein properly or carry on its daily functions in good health.

ECOLOGICAL FACTORS

Animal-raising is wasteful. It costs money, land, and lots of grain (potential feed for man) to raise an animal from birth to the time it is ready for slaughter. Even the USDA in the latest *Yearbook of Agriculture* admits that "if we ever chose to have a 'no meat' diet, our

HOW MUCH FAT DO YOU EAT?

Food	Total Fat	Saturated Fat[1]	Unsaturated Fat[2] linoleic acid
(1 pound)	(grams)	(grams)	(grams)
Almonds	254.9	20	49
Bacon	314	101	28
Beans			
chickpeas, dry	21.8	2	8
soybeans, dry	80.3	12	42
Beef			
hamburger	96.2	48	2
sirloin, bone in	108.4	52	2
Cheese			
Cheddar	146.1	80	4
Swiss	127.0	70	4
cottage	19.1	10	1
Chicken	13.1	5	3
Egg	45.9	15	2
Lamb			
leg, bone in	73.5	41	2
rib, bone in	137.9	77	4
Milk			
whole	16.8	9	1
part skim	9.1	5	–
Peanuts, unroasted	215.5	47	63
Pork			
fresh ham, bone in	102.6	37	9
spareribs, bone in	89.7	32	8
sausage	230.4	83	7
Salmon	70.8	22	1
Tuna, canned	31.6	10	6
Veal, rib with bone	49.0	23	1
Wheat germ, toasted	52.2	8	25

1. A saturated fat is one in which all possible locations for hydrogen atoms have been filled. Saturated fats are thought to accumulate in the cells of the heart and blood vessels, blocking the passageway and bringing about thickening and hardening of the arteries. Saturated fats may also increase the level of blood cholesterol.

2. Unsaturated fats have one or more possible sites available for hydrogen atoms. They do not contribute to bodily cholesterol and are the preferred form of fat consumption. Linoleic acid is only one of many unsaturated fats, but it is the most important. It is necessary for proper functioning of the nerves, brain, hormones, digestive system and general upkeep of the body. Linoleic acid cannot be synthesized by the body and therefore must be supplied by food. It is found primarily in fats of vegetable origin.

current production capacity would feed four or five times as many people as it does. Feeding animals to furnish us with meat is less efficient than direct use of crops for food."

ECONOMIC FACTORS

Not only is meat production wasting our nation's resources, it is doing the very same thing to many of our pocketbooks. The body needs protein, there's no doubt about that. But meat is not the only source of protein, albeit the most expensive. Eggs, cheese, and milk products (and don't forget yogurt) are capable of providing protein *equal* to that of meat at a much lower cost. Still cheaper are the equally valuable protein dishes you can make from combinations of dried peas and beans, nuts, seeds, whole grains, and other vegetable sources—those foods that are termed "incomplete" proteins. (If you don't believe it, a look at the table "Protein for Pennies" on page 122 may help change your mind.) This latter group is referred to as "incomplete" because each of these foods lacks one or more of the protein building blocks, called essential amino acids, needed by the body to carry out the functions of a high-quality protein. By combining these foods, however, you can easily supply the lacking amino acids and create a source of protein of *equal value* to the high-quality protein foods like milk, eggs, cheese, and meat.

These food combinations in your meal will create "complete" proteins:
    rice and beans
    cornmeal and beans
    rice with nuts and sesame seeds
    whole grain breads and nut butter or beans
    a variety of nuts
    or any of these foods with eggs, cheese, or milk

Remember, once your body has satisfied its need for protein, the excess, just like the excess of all food, becomes fat, and tomorrow your need for more protein will begin again. High protein consumption, common in many people who follow the home-economics-class guidelines of high levels of meat daily, is a very expensive source of calories.

AESTHETIC FACTORS

There are so many good things to eat in this world and people who build every meal around a meaty main dish miss many of them. Once you curtail your meat intake you begin to experiment and learn about new foods. You'll find dried beans are really delicious; that nuts can be shaped into a hundred new dishes. You begin eating vegetables you never dreamed existed. You discover a whole world of tastes and textures you never experienced. Our own experimentation led to Nikki's first cookbook, *Cooking What Comes Naturally* (Doubleday and Co.)

IT'S MORE THAN A MATTER OF MEAT

If you simply stop eating meat and continue to eat the empty calorie foods that characterize "the American way" you won't be doing yourself much good. Slow down when it comes to meat, but pick up on the other rich foods your supermarket has to offer, like whole grain breads and cereals, beans and nuts. Buy the least processed fruits, vegetables, and dairy products; not only are these important from an "unchemical" standpoint, but these are also the richest sources of all the essential nutrients.

Throughout this book, recipes are given stressing nonmeat foods to awaken your taste buds to the other things the "natural supermarket" has to offer. If you haven't already done so, go back through the buying guidelines and try some of the recipes we've suggested for the foods you've bought. And since we're sure you'll enjoy them, here are a few more protein-rich, meatless main dishes that will help you use a variety of the whole foods which now stock your kitchen. Some suggestions for the rest of the meal are given along with the main dish recipe in case the absence of meat throws you in the beginning. Soon you'll find it easy to build your own menus without including meat.

VEGETABLE PIE

Crust: ¾ cup rye cracker crumbs
        ½ cup wheat germ
        ½ teaspoon salt
        1 tablespoon caraway seeds
        2 tablespoons oil
Filling: 1 onion, thinly sliced
        2½ cups combined diced cauliflower and broccoli flowers
        1 cup shredded Gouda cheese
        2 eggs
        1 cup milk
        ½ teaspoon salt
        ¼ teaspoon dry mustard powder
        ¼ teaspoon pepper

Combine all crust ingredients and press into a 9-inch pie plate. Chill.

Spread onion over bottom of crust. Fill with diced vegetables. Cover with shredded cheese. Beat together eggs, milk, and seasonings, and pour over cheese and vegetables. Bake in a 375° oven 40 minutes, until brown and set. Let stand 5 minutes at room temperature, cut and serve. *Yield:* 4 servings.

Serve with marinated bean salad and sliced tomatoes.

EGGPLANT LASAGNA

2 cups tomato sauce
½ teaspoon oregano
¼ teaspoon basil
½ clove garlic
1 teaspoon salt
1 large eggplant (2 pounds), or 2 small, thinly sliced
oil
1 cup Ricotta cheese
2 tablespoons fresh parsley, chopped
3 tablespoons grated Parmesan cheese
4 ounces Mozzarella cheese, thinly sliced

1. Cook tomato sauce with oregano, basil, garlic, and salt.
2. Place eggplant on large baking sheet, brush with oil and broil about 5 minutes on each side, until lightly browned.
3. Layer ingredients in a large casserole as follows:
    Sauce
    Eggplant
    Ricotta mixed with parsley
    Parmesan

Sauce
Eggplant
Mozzarella
Sauce . . .

continuing until all ingredients are used. End with a layer of Mozzarella, and sprinkle top with Parmesan cheese.

4. Bake in 350° oven 20 to 25 minutes, until cheese is melted. *Yield:* **4** servings.

Serve with individual antipasto or salad and bread of your choice.

EGG AND VEGETABLE STEW, INDIAN STYLE

3 tablespoons oil
1 large onion, chopped
1 teaspoon ground coriander
½ teaspoon chili powder
Pinch of turmeric
1 teaspoon chopped chives
1 teaspoon parsley
1 large carrot, sliced
½ cup green beans, cut up
1 cup shredded cabbage
1 medium potato, diced
2 tablespoons tomato paste
1 teaspoon salt
1 cup boiling water
4 hard-cooked eggs, halved

Fry onion in hot oil for 5 minutes. Add ground coriander, chili powder, turmeric, chives and parsley; continue cooking for 1 minute. Put in carrot, green beans, cabbage, potato, tomato paste, salt, and boiling water. Cover and cook gently until vegetables are tender, about 30 minutes. Add halved eggs and simmer 5 minutes longer. *Yield:* 4 servings.

Serve with sliced tomatoes and cucumber with yogurt dressing and whole wheat or pita bread; stew may be served plain in shallow bowls or over brown rice.

NUT CUTLETS

4 slices whole wheat or sprouted wheat bread
Tomato juice for soaking

(continued)

2 cups mixed nuts (almonds, walnuts, sunflower seeds, raw cashews), finely
    ground
1 carrot, grated
Up to ½ cup chopped raw vegetables (onion, mushroom, zucchini, cauli-
    flower, broccoli), optional
2 teaspoons chopped parsley
½ teaspoon chili powder
1 teaspoon salt
2 eggs, lightly beaten

Soak bread in tomato juice until soft; squeeze out all the liquid and combine
with remaining ingredients. Shape into 4 large or 8 small patties. Bake on a
greased baking sheet in a 350° oven 20 to 25 minutes, or sauté in hot oil until
browned on both sides, about 10 minutes. *Yield:* 4 servings.

Serve with chutney or relish, creamed spinach or salad, and your favorite
grain.

GOURMET MEATLESS MEALS

If you've enjoyed this detour in your eating habits and want to
pursue the idea of eating more meatless meals, there are a number of
vegetarian cookbooks on the market that can set you on the right
path. In addition, foreign cookbooks can be a valuable source for
finding other suitable recipes, since with the exception of this country
and parts of western Europe, meat is considered a luxury and the
majority of people have been enjoying wonderful substitutes for ages.
Greek, Mid-Eastern, Indian, Chinese, Italian, Mexican, and South
American cuisines all have ideas you can offer to your family and
friends with pride and the assurance that they will not feel the least
bit cheated when a meat dish doesn't appear on your table.

House Dressings

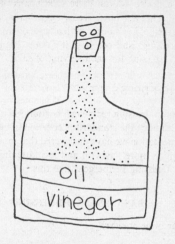

When you bypass the bottled salad dressings on the supermarket shelf you make a tremendous saving, both health- and money-wise. As we discussed in the chapter "Salad Dressing, Oil and Vinegar," there is almost nothing available in the supermarket in prepared dressings that is free of undesirable additives. On the other hand, there are many varieties of vinegar, oil, and seasonings that you can bring home for whipping up delicious salad dressings of your own. The average time commitment for a homemade dressing is a mere five minutes, and unused portions can be stored, just like bottled dressings, in the refrigerator for future salads.

The cost saving of homemade vs. prepared dressings is impressive. A 12-ounce bottle of the best wine vinegar in our supermarket sells for 45¢; a 24-ounce bottle of peanut oil for 85¢. Based on the standard 2:1 proportion of oil to vinegar in the French dressing outlined here, it costs 37¢ for 8 ounces of homemade French dressing (which includes a generous 5¢ for any additional seasonings). This is based on the *highest price* ingredients in our store. A similar dressing, purchased in the supermarket, costs 45¢ per 8-ounce jar (and that's far from the most expensive brand). Quite a difference for less than five minutes' labor!

While you're saving money, and avoiding many potential chemical dangers, you can also add an extra food bonus to simple salads by including fresh cheeses, nuts, seeds, eggs, herbs, and vegetables in your dressing recipe. Let's begin with a basic oil and vinegar dressing (or French dressing) and see how it's done. Plan on using 1 to 2 tablespoons of dressing for each serving of salad.

BASIC FRENCH DRESSING

A basic French dressing recipe can be found in almost every cookbook. You will notice the standard proportion of oil to vinegar is 3:1. In our experimentation we have discovered that more vinegar and less oil makes a much more flavorful and less fattening dressing, so our Basic French Dressing recipe goes like this.

BASIC FRENCH DRESSING

1/3 cup vinegar (wine or cider)
2/3 cup oil
½ teaspoon salt
½ teaspoon dry mustard powder
¼ teaspoon freshly ground pepper
Combine all ingredients and shake before pouring.

More often than not, we replace all or part of the vinegar with freshly squeezed lemon juice. The oil we use varies: safflower or peanut oil for general use; olive oil for Italian-style meals.

From this starting point you can add a variety of herbs and other flavoring ingredients to completely change the look and taste of your dressing. Here is a list of ideas you can employ to change Basic French Dressing to:

Garlic Dressing: Mince 1 clove of garlic and add to Basic Dressing.

Herb Dressing: To Basic Dressing, with or without garlic, add ¼ teaspoon of dried basil, thyme, or chervil, or 1 to 2 tablespoons of fresh herbs (parsley, dill). Any herb can be added or deleted to suit your taste.

Blue Cheese Dressing: Beat in 3 tablespoons of crumbled Blue cheese. To make the dressing Greek, use feta cheese instead.

Cheese Dressing: Grate 2 to 4 tablespoons of Parmesan or Swiss cheese into the dressing.

386

Creamy Dressing: Make the dressing thick and creamy by mashing a hard-cooked egg or egg yolk with the lemon juice or vinegar before adding the rest of the ingredients.

Indian Dressing: Add ½ teaspoon of curry powder and a pinch of ginger. Raisins can be added to this dressing, along with 1 teaspoon of finely chopped onion.

Italian Dressing: Make Basic Dressing with olive oil and omit the mustard. Add ¼ to ½ teaspoon of basil and oregano, 1 tablespoon of fresh parsley and 1 minced clove of garlic.

Chinese Dressing: For spinach salads, bean sprouts, or Chinese cabbage make a soy sauce dressing. Make the Basic Dressing with peanut oil and replace the vinegar with soy sauce. Add 2 tablespoons of lemon juice and season with 1 tablespoon of sesame seeds.

FRUIT SALAD DRESSING

Fruit salad dressings can be made in much the same manner as the Basic French Dressing, but this time use lemon juice to replace the vinegar. For even more flavor use the juice of a fresh lime or orange as well. Some of these suggestions can make the dressing really tasty:

Creamy Dressing: Beat 3 tablespoons of heavy cream or yogurt into the Basic Fruit Salad Dressing.

Honeyed Dressing: Add 1 to 2 tablespoons of honey and, if you like, 1 teaspoon of grated lemon, lime, or orange rind.

Mint Dressing: Add 2 tablespoons of freshly chopped mint to the Honeyed Dressing.

Nut Dressing: Chop 1/3 cup of walnuts, sunflower seeds, or raw cashews; add to Basic Fruit Salad Dressing or Honeyed Dressing.

Citrus Dressing: Highly recommended for salads which include grapefruit or orange sections and avocado wedges. Add 2 tablespoons of honey, ½ teaspoon of ginger, and 1 tablespoon of toasted sesame seeds to Basic Fruit Salad Dressing.

This is just a starting point. You have probably thought of a long list of other variations you can make on your own. Try them; it's hard to miss. Don't forget to taste as you go along.

HOMEMADE MAYONNAISE

Even with all this variety you're bound to tire of oil and vinegar dressing after a while. So slip in a mayonnaise dressing on occasion. In Europe people are appalled at the idea of buying bottled mayonnaise. If you've ever tasted the homemade kind you know why. The cost of making your own mayonnaise may be equal to the ready-made, but the flavor is far superior.

The hardest part about making your own mayonnaise is the slow addition of the oil and the simultaneous whipping of the mixture to keep it from breaking, or separating. If you have a blender, this problem is solved. It is best to have all ingredients at room temperature when you begin.

BLENDER MAYONNAISE

2 eggs
1 tablespoon lemon juice
1 teaspoon dry mustard
1 teaspoon salt
2 cups safflower oil

Combine eggs, lemon juice, mustard powder, and salt in blender container. Add ¼ cup of oil, turn blender to high speed and process, immediately adding remaining oil in a slow, steady stream through the feeder cap until completely blended. Store in refrigerator. *Yield:* 1 pint (2 cups).

A word of comfort: If your mayonnaise does separate (either during preparation or storage), you can repair it simply enough; beat an egg yolk and slowly beat in some oil until the mixture starts to thicken. Then add the broken mayonnaise gradually as if it were oil. After all the mayonnaise has been beaten in, you can add more oil if necessary to get the desired consistency. Then adjust the seasoning to taste.

Just like the other basic salad dressings, plain mayonnaise can be jazzed up for a whole line of flavorful dressings. For instance:

Green Mayonnaise: Add ¼ cup of combined chopped parsley, chives, and scallion, and for a more pungent dressing 1 tablespoon of lemon juice for each cup of mayonnaise. Delicious with fish and raw vegetables such as cauliflower, broccoli, carrot and celery sticks.

Creamy Blue Cheese Dressing: Whip together ½ cup of mayonnaise, ½ cup of Basic French Dressing, and ¼ cup of crumbled Blue cheese.

Thousand Island Dressing: Combine 1 cup of mayonnaise, ¼ cup of catsup, 1 finely chopped hard-cooked egg, 3 tablespoons of chopped onion, 3 tablespoons of finely chopped celery, and a couple of chopped olives.

Horseradish Dressing: Another seafood favorite, add ¼ cup of prepared horseradish to 1 cup of mayonnaise.

Garlic Dressing: Serve this one over leftover vegetables, cooked beans, boiled potatoes, and fish. Mash 1 to 2 cloves of garlic and blend into 1 cup of mayonnaise.

YOGURT DRESSING

Unflavored yogurt makes another excellent base for salad dressings. To flavor 1 cup of yogurt for vegetable salads, add a finely minced clove of garlic, ½ teaspoon of salt, and 2 tablespoons of grated cucumber. Vary this with additions of chopped onion, finely chopped tomato, and fresh mint. You can add bite with a tablespoon of vinegar or lemon juice.

For a fruit salad dressing, sweeten yogurt with honey to taste, figuring on 2 to 4 tablespoons per cup; use chopped dried fruits and nuts to enhance the dressing as well. Mint is nice with fruits too. To give the yogurt a fruity flavor, add a tablespoon of orange or pineapple juice.

COTTAGE CHEESE DRESSING

Cottage cheese, like yogurt, furnishes a low-calorie base for a salad dressing. A blender will help make this dressing smooth and creamy.

LOW-CALORIE COTTAGE CHEESE DRESSING

¼ cup cottage cheese
½ cup juice (tomato, orange, or pineapple)
1 tablespoon lemon juice

Puree all ingredients at medium speed in blender. This dressing can be made without the blender by pressing cottage cheese through a sieve or strainer with a wooden spoon, then thinning with the liquid ingredients.

For added flavor stir in ½ teaspoon of curry powder, or 1 tablespoon of chopped fresh herbs for vegetable salads, or ¼ teaspoon of cinnamon for fruit salads. *Yield:* 2 servings.

For vegetable salads use tomato juice as the liquid. For fruits, try orange or pineapple juices. Season as you would a Basic French or Mayonnaise Dressing.

MARINADES

For marinated salads, including cucumbers, mushrooms, artichokes, tomatoes, and bean salads, you can prepare the following marinade and let the cooked beans or raw or cooked vegetables stand in the dressing at least half an hour at room temperature before serving.

BASIC MARINADE

Beat together 3 tablespoons of wine vinegar, 2 tablespoons of oil, ½ teaspoon of salt, 3 finely chopped scallions, and any herbs desired. Pour over vegetables. *Yield:* marinade for 1 cup of beans or vegetables, or 2 servings.

A REALLY SPECIAL DRESSING

A vegetable-nut dressing is highly recommended when you're serving all-green salads—either a combination of greens or something as plain as shredded cabbage. This is our favorite.

CARROT PEANUT CREAM

10 roasted peanuts, unsalted, in the shell
1 small carrot, chopped
1 tablespoon lemon juice
2 tablespoons oil
1 teaspoon soy sauce
½ cup unflavored yogurt

Remove shells from peanuts and combine with carrot, lemon juice, oil, and soy sauce in blender container. Process at high speed until peanuts are ground and carrot is as fine as possible. Add yogurt and process at low speed until creamy. *Yield:* 2 servings.

Other additions you can experiment with in all dressings include:
- 1 tablespoon of peanut butter
- 1 tablespoon of tahina (sesame butter)
- 1 tablespoon of seeds, as celery, caraway, sesame, dill

RICHER SALADS

Before pouring on the dressing, add flavor, texture, and lots of vitamins and minerals to your salad with a garnish of:

- chopped nuts, especially peanuts, sunflower seeds, and raw cashews
- wheat germ
- bean sprouts
- grated cheese
- raisins
- grated raw beets
- orange, grapefruit, and melon sections
- odds and ends of cooked and raw vegetables (and you'll be surprised how many vegetables taste great raw, like cauliflower, broccoli, mushrooms, green beans, asparagus). Before you cook any vegetable, taste it. If it's good then save some to garnish your next salad.

SERVING HINTS

It's best to pour the dressing over the salad at serving time (unless, of course, you're making a marinated salad). This avoids wilting of greens, softening of crunchy raw vegetables, and leaching out of vitamins into the dressing. You can make your dressing well in advance, though, and store it in the refrigerator in a covered jar until it's needed. Just before pouring, shake the dressing, if it's the oil and vinegar kind, to get a good distribution of all ingredients; stir it until smooth if it's one of the creamy versions.

Satisfying Your Sweet Tooth—Sanely

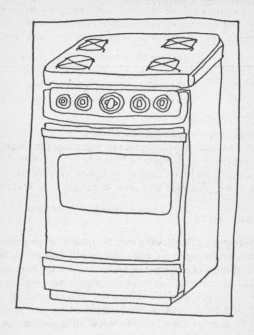

The temptation of desserts almost always outweighs the fact that most of them have negligible nutritional value and are overloaded with calories. All they may contribute to a meal is pleasure, but that's quite a lot.

Although a glance at most of the ready-made desserts available might make you think otherwise, it is very possible for a dessert to be healthy as well as delicious. Since we haven't found too much worth buying in the supermarket in this category, and since we have absolutely no desire to give up dessert, Nikki has learned to innovate. We'd like to propose some homemade desserts, made with the fine ingredients you have been able to purchase in your supermarket, as an alternative to what your store has to offer. Of course these will involve more time than it takes to open a package of cookies or a cake box, but certainly no more time than it would require to whip up the same dessert from a prepared mix.

COOKIES

When Nikki was in college there was a cook in her dormitory who baked fresh cookies every morning. Since then, she's never felt the same about store-bought cookies. Just recently we began making our own, and we were really surprised at how quickly you can turn out a couple of dozen.

How to Bake Wholesome Cookies

Cookie-making can really be an exercise in creativity. Since drop cookies are the simplest, this is the best place to begin your baking venture. This is our pattern for making delicious-tasting, nutritious, whole wheat cookies, fortified with nonfat dry milk powder.

BASIC DROP COOKIES

1 cup safflower oil
1 cup honey
1 egg
¼ cup liquid (milk or juice)
2 cups whole wheat flour
¼ teaspoon salt
4 tablespoons nonfat dry milk powder
1 teaspoon flavoring extract, optional
½ cup chopped nuts, optional
½ cup chopped dried fruits, optional

Beat together oil and honey. Beat in egg and 2 tablespoons of the liquid. Add flour, salt, and dry milk powder and stir only until smooth. Stir in remaining liquid and the optional extract, nuts, and dried fruit. Drop by rounded teaspoons onto an ungreased cookie sheet. Bake in a 325° oven 10 to 15 minutes, until lightly browned. Let cool 1 minute, transfer to a wire rack and cool completely. *Yield:* about 4½ dozen.

By playing around with flavoring ingredients you can change the basic recipe to make your favorites.

Extracts: Pure vanilla, almond, lemon, and orange extracts will impart a delicious flavor to your cookies. If you can't get hold of the unadulterated kind, you can substitute freshly grated lemon or orange rind. To do this, replace each teaspoon of extract with 1½ tablespoons of the rind. Add these along with the flour.

Spices: Your favorite spices can be used to flavor cookies. Ginger, cinnamon, and nutmeg are the most popular. When adding spices, leave out the flavoring extract. The amount of spice will vary with taste, but in general plan on ½ teaspoon of spices per cup of flour. Add the spices along with the flour.

Nuts: Pecans, walnuts, almonds, peanuts, or whatever your favorite nut is, can be added to the cookie dough for flavor and crunchiness. Plan on adding ¼ to ½ cup of chopped nuts for each cup of flour. Stir in the nuts at the end, mixing as little as possible.

Seeds: Seeds, like caraway, anise, poppy, and sesame, greatly enhance your dough. A ratio of ¼ cup seeds per cup of flour works out about right.

Fruits: Dried fruits and freshly grated coconut can be added to your dough in exactly the same manner as the nuts, again allowing ¼ to ½ cup for each cup of flour. Make sure the fruit is surrounded by batter and watch the baking time extra carefully. They burn easily and burning can really ruin a great cookie. Diced fresh fruits can enrich your cookies too. Drain the fruits well before you add them to the batter and if your recipe calls for any liquid, use a little less than usual.

Homemade "Slice and Bake Cookies"

Rolled cookies call for a few minutes more in the preparation, which we don't like to be bothered with. The same stiff dough, however, makes excellent "slice and bake" cookies. You can keep a log of this dough in the refrigerator or freezer and when friends drop in you can serve freshly baked cookies in fifteen minutes. This Spice Cookie recipe shows you how it's done. You can be just as creative with these as you were with your drop cookies by following the same guidelines for flavoring.

"SLICE AND BAKE" SPICE COOKIES

½ cup butter
2/3 cup honey
1 egg
1¾ cups whole wheat flour
2 tablespoons wheat germ

½ teaspoon cinnamon
½ teaspoon nutmeg

Beat butter and honey together until smooth and creamy. Beat in egg. Add flour and spices, and stir until smooth. Shape into 2 logs, each about 8 inches long, wrap in foil, and refrigerate or freeze until needed (at least 1 hour). When you're ready to bake, slice the dough into rounds about ¼ inch thick. Thinner slices will make a crisp cookie, thicker ones a heavier, chewier cookie. Place cookies on an ungreased baking sheet and bake in a 350° oven 10 to 12 minutes. *Yield:* about 4 dozen cookies, depending how thick you slice 'em.

Brownies, Brownies, Brownies!

No cookie repertoire is complete without a recipe for brownies, and these, made with whole wheat flour and safflower oil, are as rich and fudgy as any. If you have any left over, your friends have more willpower than ours. Hopefully they do, because these are really great chilled; after a night in the refrigerator a kind of icing forms on top.

NIKKI'S BROWNIES

Melt 2 squares (2 ounces) Baker's chocolate with ¼ cup of milk. Stir to a paste. Beat 2 eggs; beat in ½ cup of honey and 6 tablespoons of raw sugar. Beat in cooled chocolate and 1 teaspoon of vanilla extract. Stir in ½ teaspoon of salt and ½ cup of whole wheat flour. Beat in ¼ cup of safflower oil and ½ cup of broken walnuts. For cakelike brownies, bake in a greased 9-inch square baking pan in a 350° oven, 25 minutes. Use a 9 x 13-inch pan for chewy brownies. Cool in pan.

Storage

The nice part about baking cookies is you can make so many at one time. If you don't eat them all, you can keep them in the cookie jar. Cookies made with butter will keep about one week; those made with oil will keep for three months. If you like, you can store baked cookies in the freezer, where they will stay fresh up to six months. Don't store crisp and soft cookies together or your crisp ones will become soft. If this does happen, though, you can recrisp them in a 300° oven for five to ten minutes. An orange or apple placed in the cookie tin will keep your soft cookies soft.

If you'd rather have fresh-baked cookies you can store the unbaked batter in the refrigerator for about three weeks, or in the freezer up to six months.

Baking Hints

Baking cookies requires some attention. It's almost impossible to give an exact baking time because of variations in oven temperature, cookie sheets, and the dough itself. It's best to watch the first batch carefully and then allow the same amount of time for the later batches (or run a test batch of two cookies first). As soon as they are nicely browned, they're done. Wait a minute (to avoid breaking) and then lift with a spatula and let cool on a flat surface. Don't wait too long, though, or they'll stick to the cookie sheet. If this occurs, you can run the sheet quickly over a warm burner to loosen them.

If you want well-browned, evenly baked cookies, bake them on a cookie sheet. A pan with sides prevents browning. If you can't get hold of a cookie sheet, use a cake pan upside down.

Cookies with a lot of shortening are usually baked on an ungreased surface.

MAKE YOUR OWN CANDY—QUICKLY

Homemade candy-making is an activity not many people indulge in nowadays. Often it is quite laborious, time-consuming, and sticky, so we won't even begin to go into traditional candy-making.

A little bit of unconventional candy-making, however, is called for, especially when you consider the fact that candy and other similar snack items are laden with chemicals, while homemade candy can be very nourishing. Here are some recipes worth your attention; it will take you far less time to prepare any of these than it would to run down to the corner store to buy a candy bar.

This is the ideal candy for children. Not only is it made with wholesome ingredients, but kids can prepare the logs themselves. No cooking is involved.

PEANUT BUTTER LOGS

2 rounded tablespoons honey
2 rounded tablespoons peanut butter
2 to 3 rounded tablespoons nonfat dry milk powder
Chopped nuts, seeds, and dried fruits

1. Blend honey and peanut butter together with a wooden spoon.
2. Work in enough dry milk powder to make a dry, stiff paste.
3. Shape into a square ½ inch thick on a board dusted with a little milk powder.
4. Leave to set 1 hour.
5. Cut into ½-inch cubes, or shape into balls or a roll 2 inches wide.
6. Let the young cooks decorate the candy any way they wish by pressing in nuts, seeds, or diced dried fruits. Wrap and chill.

These candies can be stored in the refrigerator for snacking during the following week or two.

CITRUS NUGGETS

1 pound dried fruit
Rind of 1 orange
Orange juice
½ cup finely chopped nuts

Chop dried fruit and orange rind together until as fine as possible. Moisten with as much orange juice as needed to hold mixture together. Form into balls 1-inch in diameter. Roll in chopped nuts. *Yield:* about 2 dozen.

SNACKS

This fruit-nut mixture is packed and sold in almost every natural foods store. To make your own "Snacks" take out a large jar or bowl and fill with any combination of the following: shelled walnuts, peanuts, almonds, raw cashews, sunflower seeds, pumpkin seeds, sesame seeds, raisins, chopped dried fruit, wheat germ.

INSTANT CANDY

One of the most delicious sweet snacks we know of can be made by replacing the pit of a date with a spoonful of cream cheese. Try doing the same thing with prunes and peanut butter.

MORE LUSCIOUS DESSERTS

So much for our sweet snacking items. On to some heavy desserts! There are so many good things you can create to wind up a meal with less trouble than you imagined. All your old cookbooks can help you out with fresh baked pies, cakes, fruit dishes, and puddings. All you have to know is how to substitute the good for the bad. In any recipe that calls for all-purpose flour, unbleached flour can be used instead. In addition, you can experiment with traditional recipes by following the charts for substitution of whole grain flours, natural sweeteners, and oils offered in the chapter "Ingredient Substitution: Out with the New, In with the Old."

We are including some of our favorite desserts here in the hope that you like them as well as we do. We make them because they can be put together quickly and can easily replace the sweets we used to bring in from the outside world. Other homemade versions of some store-bought favorites appear throughout the book and can be located by consulting the index.

APPLE PUDDING

Grease a baking dish or casserole. Sprinkle with wheat germ and cover with a layer of peeled apple slices, raisins, honey, cinnamon, wheat germ . . . making at least two layers of apple. Allow 1 apple per serving and 2 teaspoons of honey per apple. The raisins and cinnamon can be added to taste. When you've used all your apples and have a top layer of wheat germ, dot with butter, cover, and bake 30 minutes in a 350° oven. Remove cover, sprinkle with additional wheat germ, cinnamon, and ½ teaspoon of raw sugar per apple. Replace cover and bake 15 minutes longer, until the pudding is a deep, rich brown. Remove cover, turn off the heat, and let pudding remain in the oven until serving time.

Serve plain or topped with cream, ice cream, or yogurt.

ITALIAN CHEESE PIE

½ cup cookie crumbs (*Familia* cookies are highly recommended)
4 tablespoons melted butter, divided
1½ cups ricotta cheese
2 eggs
6 tablespoons honey
Juice and grated rind of 1 lemon
½ teaspoon cinnamon
2 rounded tablespoons raisins, chopped

Line the bottom of a 9-inch pie pan or spring form with cookie crumbs combined with 2 tablespoons of the melted butter. Combine remaining ingredients and pour over cookie crust. Bake in a 450° oven 15 minutes, reduce heat to 325° and continue baking for 20 minutes. Cool to room temperature or chill before serving. *Yield:* 4 to 6 servings.

BANANA SPICE CAKE

¼ cup butter
½ cup honey
1 egg
1½ cups minus 2 tablespoons whole wheat flour
½ teaspoon cinnamon
¼ teaspoon nutmeg
¼ teaspoon allspice
½ teaspoon baking soda
¼ teaspoon salt
3 tablespoons yogurt
⅔ cup mashed banana (2 small bananas)

Cream butter and honey. Add egg and beat until frothy. Mix dry ingredients together and add alternately with yogurt to creamed mixture, stirring until smooth. Fold in banana. Bake in a 350° oven in a greased 8-inch square baking pan for 25 to 30 minutes, until a toothpick inserted into the center comes out clean. Cool 5 minutes in pan, then turn out onto a wire rack. When cool, frost.

MAPLE WALNUT PIE

Crust: ½ cup walnuts, chopped
¼ cup butter
3 tablespoons raw sugar
½ cup whole wheat flour

Blend chopped nuts, butter, sugar, and flour thoroughly with a fork or pastry blender. Press mixture lightly over bottom and sides of a greased 9-inch pie plate. Prick bottom with a fork. Bake in a 375° oven 10 to 12 minutes. Cool.

Filling: 2 envelopes (2 tablespoons) unflavored gelatin
⅛ teaspoon salt
3 eggs, separated
¾ cup maple syrup, divided
1½ cups milk
1 cup heavy cream

(continued)

Combine gelatin and salt in saucepan. Beat egg yolks, ½ cup of maple syrup, milk and cream together. Add to gelatin and cook until gelatin dissolves, stirring constantly. Chill until mixture is consistency of unbeaten egg whites. Beat egg whites until stiff. Beat in remaining ¼ cup of maple syrup and fold into gelatin mixture. Chill until mixture mounds when dropped from a spoon. Turn into cooled crust. Chill. If you like, garnish with walnut halves. *Yield:* 1 9-inch pie.

TOPPING IT OFF

To top off your desserts there's always homemade whipped cream. If you're conscious of calories and trying to cut down on animal fats the Lo-Cal Whipped Topping recipe given in the chapter "Milk and Its Many Forms" is almost as delicious.

If you'd rather ice your cake, try one of these.

MARSHMALLOW FROSTING

2 egg whites
¼ teaspoon salt
2 tablespoons raw sugar
½ cup honey
1 teaspoon pure vanilla extract

Beat egg whites and salt with electric beater until foamy. Add sugar gradually, continuing to beat until mixture is smooth and glossy. Beat in honey, a little at a time, until frosting forms peaks when beater is raised. Fold in vanilla. *Yield:* frosting for 2 8-inch layers.

CREAMY FRUIT FROSTING

4 ounces cream cheese
1 tablespoon honey
2 tablespoons berries mashed with 1 tablespoon milk or
2 tablespoons orange or grape juice

Beat all ingredients together with an electric or rotary mixer until smooth. Chill to stiffen, then use to frost one 8-inch or 9-inch cake.

"BUTTER CREAM" FROSTING

Cream 1 tablespoon of butter with 2 tablespoons of honey and ½ teaspoon of vanilla extract.

Beat in 1 tablespoon of milk and ½ cup of nonfat dry milk powder, adding more liquid or more powder as needed for desired consistency.

For a spice frosting add ¼ teaspoon of cinnamon and ¼ teaspoon nutmeg.

For an orange frosting use 1 tablespoon of orange juice instead of the milk and 1 teaspoon of grated orange rind instead of vanilla.

At room temperature this frosting is somewhat sticky; when chilled it hardens and is easier to eat. Frost cake while icing is still soft and refrigerate iced cake if you like. *Yield:* frosting for 1 8- or 9-inch cake.

WET NUTS

If you're a wet nuts fan, combine chopped walnuts with honey and you'll have an instant dessert topping.

DON'T FORGET FRUIT

We feel almost silly saying it, but don't forget fresh fruit makes a delicious dessert. We have found the addition of chopped dates and pecan or walnut halves makes fruit compotes something special.

FRUIT SALAD FOR A CROWD

Fill a mixing bowl or salad bowl with fresh diced fruits of the season—apples, pears, bananas, halved grapes, tangerines, and pineapple in winter; peaches, plums, cherries, berries, nectarines and more bananas in summer. Add one handful chopped dried dates and one of nut halves. Then squeeze 2 or 3 fresh oranges over all, until you have a respectable amount of juice. In winter press the juice from a pomegranate just as you would an orange and pour over the fruit salad too.

If you'd like a special sauce for your fruit mélange, let the diced fruits marinate in a mixture of ¼–½ cup of yogurt and 2–4 tablespoons of honey.

AN ADDENDUM: MORE DESSERT IDEAS

Not all desserts have to be elaborate, and not all desserts have to be sweet. Spur-of-the-moment desserts can be made simply:

•Toast a slice of whole grain bread, spread with butter and honey, and warm slightly.

•Layer fresh berries and sliced bananas on top of lightly toasted whole grain bread. Drizzle with honey or maple syrup and sprinkle with wheat germ.

•Spread a plain cookie or cracker with peanut butter and another with jam or mashed fruit. Put them together for a sandwich cookie.

•Stuff dried fruits with cheese wedges, nuts, and seeds, or roll them in freshly grated coconut.

•Stir honey, chopped fresh fruit, or fruit jam into yogurt, ricotta, or cottage cheese for a sweet fruit pudding.

•Top a whole wheat cracker with a layer of cream cheese and chopped dates.

•Go continental and serve a platter of natural cheeses and whole grain crackers for dessert.

Building a Better Baby

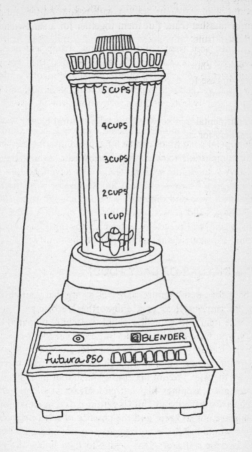

The manufacture of foods specially prepared for babies is a booming business in America. It is also a way of life for many young mothers who cannot imagine ever feeding their young ones anything else. Advertising has created the feeling that unless you feed your child prepared baby foods you may not be satisfying his/her nutritional needs. We have been sold the idea that unless your baby is a "Gerber Baby" he is not a healthy child.

Look at the facts more critically, however, and you'll find the processed, highly adulterated and overpriced baby foods are the most reprehensible aspect of the American food scene. Once you've read this section we think you'll see that this is hardly an overstatement.

All parents want their children to grow strong and healthy with sparkling eyes and a lust for life, and the food they eat plays an important part in determining that physical and mental outlook. Just like you, baby needs a rich supply of proteins, vitamins, and minerals along with carbohydrates and fats to promote growth, provide energy, and encourage proper utilization of food intake. The basic guide for feeding your child should be outlined for you by your pediatrician. He can recommend what foods can be introduced into the diet and when.

Equally important to what foods baby eats is how that food is prepared. A young child with no teeth must have food in a liquid or semiliquid form. These semiliquid foods must be smooth enough to be easily swallowed and digested, yet thick enough to be eaten from a spoon. As a child grows older, the food becomes more textured, from finely chopped pieces to larger chunks, until finally your child is enjoying the same dishes as the rest of the family.

WHAT'S IN A JAR OF BABY FOOD?

The baby food manufacturers are well aware that your child cannot handle the same meal as you, and so they've brought yet another convenience item into your household—specially prepared foods for baby. Do you have any idea what those special foods consist of?

First and foremost in most jars of baby food is water—the kind you get free from the tap. Then along with the meat or fruit or vegetables (which, by the way, are not necessarily fresh, but most likely canned or frozen) are seasonings like salt and sugar, so when *you* lick the spoon you are satisfied your child is getting a dish he can enjoy. Baby's taste buds are not so keen, and the absence of salt or sugar in those early days would hardly be noticed. After a few meals, however, your child's taste for salt and sugar begins to take hold—the reason so many children demand highly salted foods and extra sweets. A child raised on less-seasoned foods will not develop this dependency. Every jar of commercial baby food contains salt and/or sugar.

Still trying to please the parents, the manufacturers add artificial flavor and color to the foods so they seem more appealing than they really are.

Once food comes in contact with saliva it begins to soften and break down. Babies have a habit of drooling a lot, so their food often becomes soft and watery. But don't worry, the baby food manufacturers have found the solution to this problem; they've added thickeners in the form of chemicals and starch to the jar to keep the texture just as they think it should be. Because young children have difficulty digesting starch at first, they add a starch product known as modified food starch which is easier to digest. Modified food starch is treated with harsh acids. Actually baby is not too well equipped for digesting sugar either, so most manufacturers add dextrins, a highly refined form of simple sugar, to high carbohydrate dishes to help out in this area.

Here's more:

... officials of the Food and Drug Administration confirmed that, although the limit for meat and fish content of nitrate is 200 parts per million, it permitted up to 260 parts per million before seizing products as harmful.

A cancer specialist told the same subcommittee yesterday that the nitrate limit should be no more than 20 parts per million because the chemical—a curing and coloring agent—may combine in the stomach with amino acids and cause cancer.

—New York Times, March 17, 1971

Processed baby meat and meat dinners—franks, ham, bacon, luncheon meat—get treated to the same nitrites and nitrates as the frankfurters and other processed meats prepared for grown-ups. Your child shouldn't eat them and neither should you.

Then, of course, preservatives are needed to increase the life of the food.

The only thing the manufacturer doesn't skimp on is the jar—its cost to you is about a third of the price.

Still want your baby to be a "Gerber Baby"?

Special Juice for Baby

The special orange juice canned for baby is made from the same frozen concentrate you buy in your supermarket. The only difference is it's watered down, sugar is added, and so is artificial vitamin C. Compare the cost of baby orange juice (46¢ per pint) to the same quantity from the family container (21¢ per pint).

405

Young children do not need vitamin C in as large a quantity as you do, and the natural vitamin C in the orange juice, if it weren't so diluted, would surely be adequate.

Food "Fortified" for Infants

Baby cereals, too, have many questionable ingredients, like coconut oil, a highly saturated fat which has no place in your child's diet.

Those special cookies also have hydrogenated (saturated) shortening along with the highly refined flour, sugar, salt, and artificial coloring and flavoring that go into most baked treats.

To sum it all up: *Commercial baby foods are neither fresh, nor wholesome, nor properly suited to a healthy baby's needs.*

THE ANSWER

The solution, of course, is for you to prepare your child's foods. There is no reason why your baby can't share in the usual family fare as soon as your doctor recommends the introduction of new foods into his diet. With the aid of a blender, or food mill, the fresh foods you're serving to the rest of the family can become part of your baby's meals as well. This will save you the work of cooking twice, your family will reap huge savings on food bills, and when it comes time to wean your child away from baby foods and up to the family table, the job will already be done.

To show you how easy it is to make your own baby food let's see what's available in each of the basic food groups that can be easily transferred from the family pot to the baby feeder.

MILK

Milk, whether mother's or from formula, is the first food a baby gets. A breast-fed child receives all the nutrition he needs in those first few months and the decision of when to begin supplementary feeding should be left to the mother and doctor. A baby fed on formula has a greater need for iron and vitamin C. One way you can add these nutrients is to use the liquid from cooked vegetables in place of water in the formula.

CEREAL

The first food that is introduced into a baby's diet is usually cereal. Despite what baby food manufacturers think, a child should not be started on cereal until at least six months of age. By introducing cereal too early you only risk decreasing milk intake, and the refined starches fed most babies do not contribute significantly to protein, vitamin, or mineral intake. Once you do begin to serve your child cereal it should be only whole grain cereal.

You can serve baby the homemade Cream of Brown Rice cereal suggested for the rest of the family in the chapter "Filling the Cereal Bowl: Hot Cereals." If it is not quite smooth after cooking, add a little milk and process it in the blender for perfect results. There is no need to add salt to this cereal, and if a little sweetening is desired, add honey, a form of sugar much easier to digest by the very young and the very old.

Other cereals that can be made at home from the supermarket supplies include cream of cornmeal (a thin gruel of cornmeal cooked with milk which can also be thinned and smoothed if need be in the blender) and oatmeal (made specially smooth for baby by grinding the raw oats in the blender, then cooking as usual). Leftover cooked grains (brown rice, barley) can also be heated with milk and processed in the blender to a creamy consistency. Of course, any of these hot cereals can be enjoyed by other members of the family too, so cook up one big pot for everyone.

Muesli, the cold breakfast cereal imported from Switzerland, was originally developed just for feeding babies. A special box of *Familia* Swiss Baby Food is sold in the supermarket to offer a nutritious cold breakfast cereal to infants over six months. This is one prepared baby food that contains no additives or refined products.

VEGETABLES

When it comes time to serve your baby vegetables, remove a small portion from the cooked vegetables you plan to serve to the rest of the family before you add any seasoning. Combine the cooked vegetable with enough liquid to get the blender going and puree at high speed until you have reached the correct consistency The longer foods are processed, the more even-textured they become, and as your child becomes more grown up you can shorten the blending time. For infants the solid foods can be mixed with milk and processed to a very fine, semiliquid state. When your child reaches toddler stage, the liquid can be decreased and foods chopped to just the right size by switching the unit on and off repeatedly until it's just right for him to handle. Only one food at a time should be blended and introduced into his diet at a time when your child is an infant, but as his likes and dislikes become more clearly defined you can puree or chop several vegetables together for variety.

BASIC FORMULA FOR VEGETABLES

½ cup cooked vegetable pieces
2 to 4 tablespoons cooking liquid or milk

When your infant becomes a teether let him tackle a raw carrot and celery sticks while you enjoy your salad.

If you're preparing baked potatoes, save a piece for baby. Mash it right in the jacket with a little milk and he won't feel left out.

FRUITS

Fruits, the perfect sweet for baby, can be cooked gently and pureed in the cooking liquid in the same way as vegetables. Only a little liquid is needed to cook the fruit, and all of it should be used in the puree to avoid wasted vitamins. No extra sweetening is necessary.

BASIC FORMULA FOR FRUITS

½ cup cooked fruits
2 to 4 teaspoons cooking liquid or fruit juice

Both fresh and dried fruits are suited to pureeing. Soft fruits like bananas and peaches can be blended or mashed without cooking. Raw applesauce (see recipe in the chapter "Picking Fruit") is fine for baby too.

JUICE

The same fresh fruit juices you serve everyone else can be given to your young children as well. When baby is still using a bottle it may be necessary to strain the juice. Try orange, apple, and pineapple juice.

PROTEIN FOODS

Protein for your baby comes from the same sources as protein for you—meat, fish, cheese, eggs, dried beans, and whole grains. Nuts are often too difficult for a young child to swallow, although once he's eating most other food successfully ground nuts can be added.

One of the best foods for baby is egg yolks. Soft-cooked egg yolks can be served alone or blended with vegetables. As baby develops a taste for eggs they can be softly scrambled (instead of butter, use safflower oil or scramble them in the top of a double boiler set over gently boiling water), and when his system can handle it, hard-cooked egg yolks can be introduced mashed with a little milk or vegetable liquid.

Cottage cheese mixed with a little milk in the blender or pressed through a sieve can be served alone or flavored with a little orange, pineapple, or apple juice. Add 2 to 4 tablespoons of liquid to each ½ cup of cottage cheese.

The soft creamy consistency of yogurt, the ease of digestibility, and the high quality of its protein make it a perfect baby food. Serve it plain, and if your child doesn't take to it at first, try varying it with added mashed bananas, fruit puree, or a smidgen of honey. Use it in the blending of cooked vegetables for instant creamed vegetables.

All kinds of plain meats, roasted, broiled, or stewed, and fish and chicken can be mixed with broth or milk and made smooth for baby in the blender. If you plan to season the meat for your dinner before cooking, cut off a small piece for baby and cook it separately.

BASIC FORMULA FOR MEAT

½ cup cooked cubed meat
4 to 6 tablespoons broth or milk

Beans, brown rice, and barley can all be pureed before salting and served to your baby when the rest of the family enjoys these protein-rich foods for dinner.

When baby is ready for combination dinners, serve him one of these variations:

MEAT DINNER

½ cup milk
½ cup cubed cooked meat
2 tablespoons cooked vegetables
½ cup cooked brown rice or potato

CHICKEN DINNER

¼ cup chicken broth
¼ cup milk
½ cup cubed cooked chicken
2 tablespoons cooked carrot
¼ cup cooked brown rice, barley, or whole wheat spaghetti

Put all ingredients into blender container, cover, and process at high speed until smooth. If necessary heat gently in a small saucepan.

COOKIES

Cookies for baby don't have to be rich. Your child is after something to teethe on, not something to satisfy a sweet tooth. Any plain biscuit will do, but make sure there are no pieces of nuts, dried fruits, or other tiny hard foods that baby can get caught in his throat. A plain "Slice and Bake Cookie" (see "Satisfying Your Sweet Tooth—Sanely") made for older family members will be enjoyed by baby.

Instead of giving your child pretzels to teethe on, these nourishing Teething Sticks can be made and stored in a covered tin for several weeks. Try rolling some in sesame seeds before baking and serve them like bread sticks at a family meal.

TEETHING STICKS

2 cups whole wheat flour
1¼ cups milk
½ cup safflower oil
2 cups wheat germ
1 tablespoon honey

Combine all ingredients, knead until smooth, then cut dough and roll into sticks ¼ inch thick and 5 inches long. Place on oiled cookie sheet and bake in 350° oven 40 minutes, until brown and firm. *Yield:* 60 sticks.

OTHER DESSERTS

Soft puddings not only add a treat to baby's meals, but are a good source of nourishment. A baked egg custard is the ideal dessert for children of all ages. Follow the recipe for Molasses Custard in the chapter "Puddings and Gelatin Dishes."

STORING LEFTOVERS

Mini-blender containers are better than full-sized ones for making baby food. This way any extra can be refrigerated right in the jar to avoid bacteria from other utensils. Store one to two days in the refrigerator for reuse. Don't keep food longer than this, though. Baby's body is more susceptible to bacteria than yours.

MAKING BABY'S MEALS AHEAD OF TIME

You won't always be serving something that can be adapted to your baby's needs. Plan ahead for those days and prepare some of the preceding purees in quantity, then pour them into a freezer tray. When the cubes are solid, remove them from the tray and store, frozen, in a plastic bag in a zero degree freezer. When you need a meal, pull out a cube and heat it gently in a covered saucepan until thawed and warmed. One to two cubes makes an average serving.

ENHANCING YOUR CHILD'S MEALS

Everyone can stand a little extra nutrition, and it's easy to slip extra protein and B vitamins into a young child's meals when you make them at home. When you puree foods in the blender, add a spoonful of wheat germ (raw is better since it is already quite soft) or brewer's yeast. Brewer's yeast is unfortunately not available in most supermarkets and this is one instance where a trip to a natural foods store is worth the extra steps. Brewer's yeast is a dried yeast extract, originally a by-product of beer-making, but today made purposely as a food supplement. It is a rich source of B vitamins and complete protein and is often added to baby cereals by manufacturers. The powdered form is most concentrated and easiest to use. Once you've bought a jar, use it to enrich family meals too. It is rather unpleasant alone, but a tablespoon added to soups, stews, and bean dishes imparts a surprisingly nice "meaty" flavor. Pets love it too.

Wheat germ can be added unnoticed to ground meat patties and most other mixed foods to increase their food value.

All children go through a noneating phase. When your baby refuses to eat, fortify his milk instead of coaxing, coercing, and ultimately fretting.

POWER MILK

Blend together: ½ cup orange juice
½ cup milk
1 to 2 tablespoons brewer's yeast or wheat germ
1 tablespoon safflower oil
2 tablespoons dry milk powder
½ teaspoon vanilla
     or
1 teaspoon honey

THE FINALE

This is only a basic introduction to making your own baby food to give you an idea of what other mothers have done. Almost anything that can be creamed in the blender can be served to baby as long as it is not highly seasoned or fatty. Consult your pediatrician when in doubt and check your local bookstore for homemade baby food cookbooks.

When you see how easy it is to make your own baby foods, share the information with your friends.

Ingredient Substitutions:
Out with the New, In with the Old

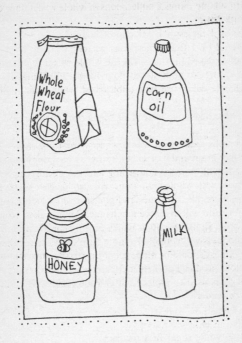

Here are some quick reference charts you can use when you're cooking to guide you in replacing the refined ingredients you encounter in your recipes with their more wholesome counterparts. Many of these substitutes are the old-fashioned pure foods your ancestors used before modern-day science and technology became involved with the food industry. Many of your finished dishes, you'll discover, will more closely resemble the rich, truly satisfying foods which constituted the American diet a hundred years ago.

IN BAKING

Flour

To replace white flour in a recipe:
- Substitute 1 cup minus 2 tablespoons of whole wheat flour for each cup of white flour.

Reduce oil by 1 tablespoon per cup of flour.

Increase liquid by 1 to 2 tablespoons per cup of flour.
- For lighter baked products, sift the whole wheat flour and return the coarse siftings to your stored flour for bread-baking.
- For delicate cakes use half unbleached white flour, half whole wheat.
- Use unbleached flour instead of regular all-purpose flour in the same proportion.

Expect breads made with whole wheat flour to be more compact with a coarser grain and a crumbly, rather than spongy consistency. These breads will be more nourishing and more satisfying.

Cakes made with whole grain flour will also have a coarser texture. Certain products, like brownies and gingerbread, which have a high liquid : flour ratio will evidence no change. Pound cakes, fruit cakes, and many other similar products which do not depend on a soft crumb for their goodness will actually be more desirable. Those cakes which demand lightness should be made according to the suggestions above.

Wheat flour produces crunchier cookies when butter is the shortening. When oil is used to replace butter your cookies will actually be softer, more tender.

Sweetening

To replace white sugar in a recipe:
- Substitute ¾ cup of honey for each cup of sugar in the recipe.

Decrease the liquid by ¼ cup for each ¾ cup of honey. If there is no liquid in the recipe add ¼ cup of flour for each ¾ cup of honey.
- For each cup of sugar specified, use ¾ to ½ cup of molasses and ¼ to ½ cup of raw sugar.

Decrease the liquid by ¼ cup for each cup of molasses.

Omit the baking powder in the recipe.

Add ½ teaspoon of baking soda for each cup of molasses.

•Use raw sugar just as you would the refined white.

•To substitute for corn syrup in a recipe, replace with an equal amount of honey.

Baked goods made with honey and molasses will stay fresh and moist longer than those made with sugar.

To make measuring easier, measure the shortening first, then measure the honey or molasses in the same measuring unit.

Shortening

•For each cup butter, vegetable shortening, or other solid shortening called for in a recipe substitute ⅞ cup of nut or vegetable oil (1 cup minus 2 tablespoons).

•For each cup of melted shortening substitute an equal amount of oil.

Cookies baked with solid shortening tend to be crunchier than those made with melted or liquid shortening. Other products do not exhibit any significant difference.

GENERAL COOKING

Flour Coatings

•Replace white flour with sifted whole wheat flour alone or combined with unbleached flour. Add 2 tablespoons wheat germ for each cup of flour.

•If desired, substitute fine ground cornmeal for white flour.

Thickening Soups and Sauces

For each tablespoon of white flour substitute one of the following:

1 tablespoon whole wheat flour
½ tablespoon cornstarch
½ tablespoon potato starch
1 tablespoon unbleached flour
1 to 2 tablespoons of peanut butter

Sweetening

When syrup is called for to sweeten soups, sauces, syrups, vegetable dishes, etc., replace sugar with an equal amount of honey or molasses.

Honey will provide a mild, mellow, sweetness. Molasses will impart a stronger, more distinctive taste. If more than ¼ cup of sweetening

415

is indicated, molasses may overpower the flavor of the dish if not specifically called for in the recipe.

Sautéing

Whenever you need to sauté or pan-fry foods oil can be used to replace an equal amount of butter, lard, or other specified shortening.

Since most oils are flavorless, you might find an additional touch of herbs and spices necessary. Olive oil and peanut oil will both give some additional flavor to the foods cooked in them, and where a butter flavor is desired (as for eggs), you might try using half butter and half oil.

USING FRESH VEGETABLES, DRIED BEANS, AND WHOLE GRAINS

Vegetables

If your recipe is based on canned vegetables and a cup measurement is given, the substitution is simple enough; just replace them with an equal amount of the fresh. When measurements are given "by the can," this information can help you:

1 pound tomatoes = 3 medium tomatoes = 1 cup pulp
When 1 can (1 pound, 3 ounces) is called for substitute 2 cups chopped tomatoes.

½ pound fresh mushrooms = 2½ cups sliced raw = 1 to 1¼ cups cooked.
When 1 can (4 ounces) is called for, substitute ⅓ pound of fresh mushrooms, sliced and sautéed.

Beans

1 pound dried beans = 2 cups raw = about 6 cups cooked.
When 1 can (1 pound) beans is called for, substitute 2 cups cooked beans or ¾ cup of dried raw beans.

Rice

Substitute brown rice measure for measure for white rice. Increase cooking time 20 minutes if cooked alone, 30 minutes when combined with other foods.

DAIRY PRODUCTS

Nonfat dry milk can be used to replace fresh, fluid milk in all cooking. Reconstitute according to package directions or add the dry powder to the other dry ingredients in your recipe and replace the milk with an equal measure of water.

1 pound cheese = about 4 cups grated.

¼ pound (1 stick) butter = ½ cup.

Future Trends

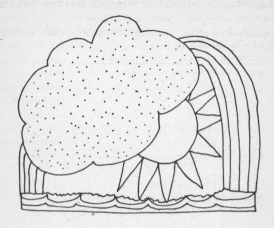

The American food scene is currently undergoing an era of nutritional concern—(what David terms the "Age of Nutrition"). In a country where there is so much wealth and affluence, the amount of hunger and malnutrition evidenced is appalling. Only a small part of serious nutritional deficiencies is the result of poverty; for the most part poor nutrition is due to misinformation or no information plus the proliferation of valueless foods on the market. Concerned citizens and government officials are at last taking note of these facts and, despite the growing selection of junk foods, progress is being made in the right direction. This new food-consciousness can be seen on both the consumer level and the decision-making level.

THE "NATURAL FOODS" MOVEMENT

Some people view the so-called Natural Foods Movement as a fad; a fly-by-night venture that should not be taken seriously. Many have called it elitist, the rich man's luxury. How foolish these folks are. Perhaps the movement began in the upper classes, with those people who have access to more information and who can afford the high prices of the natural foods store. It is not being confined to this segment of the population, however, and with the greater flow of information and books such as this one, nutritious, unpolluted foods are being made accessible to all. Perhaps some of the items recommended here are more costly than the huge loaves of white bread, large cans of fruit punch, and other low-quality foods on the market, but as soon as the people become aware of the fact that the money they are wasting on empty calorie foods will go a lot further and will provide greater enjoyment when spent on more wholesome goods, the movement will penetrate all segments of the population. Once people relearn how to prepare whole foods, they will take to them readily.

One positive step that you can look forward to seeing in more and more areas is the growth of "natural foods departments" in supermarkets. Here you will be able to purchase many unrefined, unchemicalized substitutes for the normal supermarket fare and many organically grown foods as well. As the interest continues, many of the common supermarket brands will be forced to revise their formulas too.

Some of the large universities like Yale, Harvard, and MIT have acquiesced to demands of students by including whole and organic foods in their cafeterias.

We look forward to the time when nutrition and home economics classes are not boring sessions in cookie-making, open only to women, but are interesting classes teaching young people the basics of food, nutrition, and ecology. Along this line we hope that medical schools, too, will expand their meager courses in nutrition to enable our doctors to better understand the relationship between nutrition and health.

CHANGING PRODUCTS AND SUPERMARKETS

Many manufacturers have already begun to improve their products, eliminating chemicals and introducing unrefined raw ingredients. Several bakeries have taken to using only whole grain and unbleached flours. They have eliminated many of the chemical preservatives from their bread formulas. In the last year two major East Coast companies, *Pepperidge Farm* and *Arnold,* have introduced breads made entirely from whole, high-quality ingredients. Many supermarkets are taking in baked goods made by local bakeries with the same high standards. Safeway is one of the progressive supermarket chains that is marketing its own bread based on a whole grain formula. This bread is far superior to most house brands and a sign that the message is getting across.

Granola, the rich, whole grain cold breakfast cereal that actually has nutritional value, has made its breakthrough into the supermarket, and today there is hardly a store that does not offer one or more brands of this crunchy breakfast cereal.

Wesson oil has made a move in the right direction by removing the chemical additives from some of their containers of vegetable oil. Hopefully, they will soon respond to the demand for higher quality components and remove the cottonseed oil as well.

The Florida Citrus Commission has recently agreed to cease the use of artificial coloring agents on the skins of oranges to make them more attractive. This is your chance to support these changes and encourage others to follow suit. Do not judge fresh produce based on artificially induced outward appearance. Let manufacturers know it's what's inside the product that you're concerned with.

If we were giving awards, our first would be to Esther Peterson and Giant Foods in Washington, D.C. They have proved literally that honesty is the best policy with innovations like unit pricing, open dating, and ingredient labeling of standardized products. In addition to promoting the sale of more nutritious food, they have marketed their own pure soap and have even created their own line of recycled paper products under the trade name CYCLE.

These are but a few of the positive responses the food industry has made to popular demand. If interest continues to soar and favor these changes, you can expect others to follow.

ADVERTISING DECEPTION

One way you know that something has caught on is when advertising begins to capitalize on it. This is also the time to become particularly attuned to products eager to get on the bandwagon, but unwilling to make real changes. There is nothing wrong with changing the formula of a product to meet the demands of the new food-consciousness and launching an advertising campaign to let people know about it. That is what "consumer demand" is really about.

The deception comes from the many companies who are eager to make money off the movement without truly meeting its qualifications. Beware of breads that boast "natural ingredients" but don't tell you what those ingredients are. Sure, they may use unbleached flour (which is no big deal) and no preservatives. But what about the other additives in the long list of *permissible* ingredients (which do not have to be listed) contained in the Federal Code? Don't be misled by jams implying they are better because they contain "no artificial coloring, flavoring, or preservatives" while they still depend on refined sugar. Never assume a product is "natural" or "organic" just because the manufacturer has tacked the term onto the label. "Natural" and "Organic" have many diverse meanings, and perhaps the manufacturer has chosen one quite different from yours. Foods that are "whole foods," as we have defined them, must be determined from the list of ingredients they provide, not the claims they make. In the future you will probably see more and more of this deceptive advertising. If you know how to read labels and evaluate contents you will not be a victim of this fraud. Just because one baby food manufacturer calls his product "the most natural baby food you can buy" doesn't mean it's free of undesirable additives or that a more natural baby food could not be made.

VOLUNTEERING MORE INFORMATION

State and city requirements are making more demands for adequate labeling. New York City, for instance, has passed a law requiring certain perishables, among them bread and dairy products, to clearly stamp the last day of recommended sale on the label of these products. Consult your local consumer agency or city council to learn if similar bills are proposed in your area. If so, send a letter expressing your support to the appropriate officials and, once the bill is passed, make use of this valuable information.

Because they have been shown the consumer is interested, many companies have begun to offer freshness information of their own. *Dannon* yogurt has provided a great convenience for the consumer by clearly labeling each container with the last day you can expect the contents to be usable. Where a choice exists, make an effort to purchase the brand that offers you any voluntary, helpful information for buying or using their product. In this way you will be consciously recognizing and thanking them for responding to your needs. As soon as their competitors see the results of providing better information, they too will offer a more complete label.

GOVERNMENT STEPS IN

To date, the federal government has given little tangible support to the movement toward chemical-free, nutritionally sound nourishment. They have given it some lip service, however, and perhaps with a letter to your congressman you can help push some of the proposed bills through.

Presently under consideration are bills concerning mandatory labeling of all ingredients, including those foods governed by a standard of identity (the Truth in Food Labeling Act); open dating, in order that the date itself can be deciphered and a uniform style of dating can be established; and the Honest Label Act, requiring the name and place of business of the manufacturer, packer, and distributor to appear on the label. Many manufacturers produce a product and distribute it under alternate brand names; this bill would enable you to determine if the same product was being offered under a brand and supermarket name with the only difference being the price.

The growing interest and demand for organic food has brought forth yet another proposal, a bill to amend the Federal Food, Drug and Cosmetic Act to supervise the certification of foods labeled "organic." This bill aims to define the terms "organically grown" and "organically processed" so that unethical merchants could no longer deceive the public. This bill, like the others, needs all the popular support it can get to rally the interest of other politicians.

Other ideas that need your support include labeling of drained weight, that is, how much vegetable, soup or stew is in the can once you drain off the water; handling instructions for foods which are likely sources of Salmonella poisoning; labeling of coloring agents used in fresh as well as processed foods, and labeling of biodegradability or the amount of recycled material used in the product or the packaging.

PRIVATE ENDEAVORS

While the government is tossing around proposals for the new organic food bill, Rodale Press and others are organizing organic certification programs that meet the definition of organic foods. If this undertaking succeeds, you will be able to assure yourself that the fresh produce offered in your store is indeed "organic" by the special seal it will carry.

KEEP YOUR EYES AND EARS OPEN

There are many things to watch for as the market begins to open up for whole foods. Read the labels of the products you buy and show support for any improvement a manufacturer makes through your purchases.

By learning as much as you can about your supermarket and making yourself a well-informed consumer you will encourage further improvements. In the meantime you will be making a sound investment in your own health and the health of those you feed.

A Glossary of Terms

Additives

Technically speaking, a food additive is any material, other than the basic raw ingredients required in the production of a food item, used to enhance the final product in some way. These additives can be either natural or chemical in origin. The simplest of these are in the form of natural flavoring aids such as herbs, spices, salt, and natural extractives; natural coloring from vegetable juices and extracts; fresh fruit acids; wheat germ and brewer's yeast. These are all considered "natural additives." "Chemical additives" are a bit more complex and are the result of technical alteration or fabrication done on real foods or real food extracts, for example, modified food starch or a long list of vegetable gums and related stabilizers; laboratory duplication of vitamins using synthetic ingredients; the manufacture of over 3,000 chemicals used in foods as preservatives, buffers, emulsifiers, neutralizing agents, sequestrants, stabilizers, anticaking agents, flavor enhancers, flavors, colors, and a multitude of other functions. It is these chemical additives that we refer to throughout this book.

All additives are regulated by the Food and Drug Administration, with certain restrictions as to amount and use in various foods. None are supposedly used for deceptive purposes (i.e., as a cover-up for blemishes or poor quality, or to make it look as if an ingredient has been added when it hasn't been), and they are supposedly deemed "safe under condition of its intended use." Of course deceptive use has been witnessed many times, for although legally the users of these products have not overstepped their bounds, we as consumers are constantly being suckered into thinking our foods are better than they are by all the fancy primping these additives supply. More crucial, however, is the second factor of safety.

We must consider the possibility that the chemical compound formed in the metabolic process once these additives are assimilated into the body is often more dangerous than the original chemical itself. We must take into account the fact that many of these additives destroy or inhibit natural enzymes, thereby causing disease. It is a known fact that DDT, for example, inhibits one of the enzymes in our blood.

Many chemical additives are the source of allergic reactions. Some scientists hypothesize that arteriosclerosis may be related to sensitivity to certain antibiotics ingested along with our foods.

According to the Health Research Group of Washington, D.C., Russian tests have shown that female animals fed Red Dye 2 suffered increased fetal deaths, impaired milk production, and a stillborn rate of one in seven; male animals exhibited reduced life, movement and resistance of sperm. Red Dye 2 is the most widely used food coloring in this country, present in hot dogs, sausage, soft drinks, gelatin desserts, candy, baked goods, prepared cereals, pistachio nuts, chewing gum, pet foods and many other items.

Most people feel safe in relying on the judgment of their government; it is therefore interesting to note that often additives considered safe in this country are banned from use by equally competent governments. In Great Britain the use of BHA and BHT, common preservatives in this country, is strictly forbidden.

Some food additives are listed on the label in terms of their function, such as "emulsifiers," "artificial color," "artificial flavor," "dough conditioners," etc. Others are enumerated by their more specific, technical name. Many do not appear on the label at all. To help you understand what is in the package of food you are considering, here is a list of some of the more common chemical terminologies you are likely to find on the label and the specific functions of these additives.

ADDITIVES	FUNCTION
Aluminum sulfate	firming agent
Ascorbic acid: calcium and sodium ascorbate	antioxidant
Bromates: calcium, potassium	maturing agent, dough conditioner
Brominated vegetable oil	texturizer, flavor dispersant (banned)
Butylated hydroxyanisole (BHA)	antioxidant
Butylated hydroxytoluene (BHT)	antioxidant
Caffeine	flavor
Calcium phosphate	dough conditioner
Calcium salts: acetate, chloride, citrate, diacetate, gluconate, phosphate, sulfate	emulsifier, firming agent
Carrageenan	stabilizer, emulsifier

Citrate salts: calcium, potassium, sodium	plasticizer, emulsifier, buffer
Citric acid	antioxidant, acid, flavor
Cyclamates	sweetening agent (banned)
Ethylenediaminetetraacetate (EDTA)	sequestrant
Glycerides: mono- and di-glycerides	emulsifier, defoaming
Gum tragacanth	thickener, stabilizer
Lecithin	natural emulsifier, antioxidant
Mannitol	antisticking and texturizing agent
Metaphosphates: calcium, sodium	emulsifier, sequestrant, texturizer
Methylcellulose	thickener, stabilizer
Modified food starch	thickener, texturizing agent
Monosodium glutamate (MSG)	flavor enhancer
Nitrates: sodium, potassium	color fixative
Nordihydroguaiaretic acid (NDGA)	antioxidant (banned)
Phosphates: calcium, potassium, sodium	emulsifier, texturizer, sequestrant
Phosphates: calcium acid, tricalcium, disodium, sodium acid, trisodium, sodium aluminum, sodium acid pyrophosphate	buffer
Polysorbates	emulsifier
Potassium carbonate and bicarbonate	alkali
Propionic acid, calcium propionate, sodium propionate	mold and rope inhibitor
Propylene glycol	solvent, wetting agent
Saccharin	sweetening agent
Silicates: aluminum calcium, calcium, magnesium, sodium tricalcium	anticaking agent
Sodium diacetate	mold and rope inhibitor
Sorbic acid: calcium sorbate, potassium sorbate, sodium sorbate	fungistat
Sorbitol	sequestrant, texturizing agent
Sulfur dioxide: sodium sulfite, potassium bisulfite, sodium bisulfite	antioxidant, preservative, antibrowning agent
Tocopherols	natural antioxidant
Vanillin	flavor
Vegetable gum: agar-agar, guar gum, gum karaya	thickener, stabilizer

Code of Federal Regulations: Title 21, Food and Drugs:

The Code of Federal Regulations are the federal laws which set forth the rules established for the Food and Drug Administration and include the Federal Food, Drug, and Cosmetic Act and the Fair Packaging and Labeling Act. In regard to foods, these regulations encompass a definition of certain food items (also known as the standard of identity) which names mandatory and optional ingredients to be used in preparing these foods and prohibits the inclusion of any other ingredients; provide guidelines for package labeling; and set standards for quality and container fill. Because the details of these regulations are published in the Code, those foods which are standardized are exempt from certain labeling requirements under the assumption that anyone wishing to know the formula is free to consult the text. In this book the Code is alternately referred to as the "Federal Food Code" or, when in reference to a specific food, simply the "standard of identity" or the "standard."

Food and Drug Administration

The Food and Drug Administration is a subsidiary of the Department of Health, Education, and Welfare, responsible for the promulgation of federal food regulations and the testing and authorization of food additives.

GRAS List

In addition to those substances the government defines as additives, there is a list of additional items that are "Generally Regarded as Safe" which are not considered legally as additives. Essentially they differ only in that much less restriction is placed on their use; only the "amount used must not exceed that reasonably required to achieve the desired effect" or, if not used to accomplish any effect, must be "reduced to the lowest reasonable point." While the government feels an "additive" must be used with certain limitations, those items on the GRAS list can be used with little restraint.

Although the laws have taken them out of the definition of additives, these chemical substances fall into the technical definition of additives and many of them compose the list of preservatives, colorants, buffers, emulsifiers, etc.

The story of how the GRAS list was arrived at is quite fascinating. In 1958 when the Food, Drug, and Cosmetic Act placed more stringent restrictions on food additives, the Food and Drug Administration realized that it would be impossible to test all those chemicals being added to foods at the time. So they composed a list of the most widely used ones and sent it around to 900 "experts" of their choice. Only 355 of the "experts" responded, and only 194 concurred with the list or had no negative comments to offer. Despite this, the GRAS list came into being and since then has been expanded, based on manufacturers' petitions. Although most of the items that found their way onto the GRAS list did so because the FDA felt they had withstood the test of time, many of them have since been reviewed and either banned entirely or given interim status. Some of those most recently removed from the list include:

- NDGA (an antioxidant formerly used in meats, butter, and other shortening, cake mixes, and soft drinks), which is not mentioned in this book since its use was banned long enough ago so that it is no longer found in foods.

- Many coal-tar dyes, popular in the 1940s, which, after more recent review, were found to be carcinogenic (cancer-causing) and removed from use.

- MSG
- Cyclamates
- Glycine and glycine salts

Natural Foods

Often the term "natural" is used to refer to those foods we characterize as "whole foods"; many interpret the term "natural" to mean "organic" as well. "Natural foods" are always free of chemicals in their production; those located in the "natural foods department" of the supermarket may be organic as well.

The "natural foods store," referred to alternately in common discourse as the "health foods store," is a store devoted to the sale of organic foods, whole foods, and foods suited to special dietary needs.

Because the term "natural foods" is used interchangeably with "health foods" in some circles, many "natural foods" departments and stores also include special "diet foods," made with sugar and salt substitutes and by no means additive-free. It is wise not to assume a product is untainted just because it is sold in the natural foods section of your store.

Organic Foods

Organic foods are foods grown without pesticides, in soil untreated with artificial fertilizers, but whose mineral content is enhanced by the addition of natural mineral fertilizers; these foods have not been treated with hormones, antibiotics, or processed with preservatives or synthetics of any kind.

Processed Foods

Foods that are manufactured in some way—that are refined, cooked, and combined with other food ingredients—are considered "processed." Although chemicals needn't be included in the process, they frequently are, and the amount of handling is usually sufficient to cause nutritional losses.

Processed foods are the antithesis of "whole foods" and those people who term whole foods "natural foods" should really be calling processed foods, the bulk of the American food supply, "unnatural foods."

Standard of Identity

The legal definition of certain food items which states those ingredients required and those permitted (see Code of Federal Regulations).

United States Department of Agriculture

This government agency is concerned with the production of food at the most basic level, that is, the growing of crops and the raising of animals. Known familiarly as the USDA, this is the authority responsible for federal inspection and grading of foods.

Whole Foods

Whole foods, the focal point of this book, are foods offered for sale free of chemical additives, colorants, or artificial flavoring, left in the whole, unrefined state, or processed as little as possible to render them suitable for eating. These foods are not necessarily organic, that is, grown without chemicals or pesticides, but in some cases may be.

Bibliography

All About Tuna, Tuna Research Foundation, Terminal Island, California, 1972.

Bourjaily, Vance, "Rich America's Poor Meat," *Harpers,* March, 1972.

Burns, Marjorie, and Helen Gifft, *Fish and Shellfish,* Cornell Extension Bulletin 1069, Ithaca, N.Y., August, 1965.

Burr, Horace K., PhD, and R. Paul Ellion, MS, "Quality and Safety in Frozen Foods," Council on Foods and Nutrition, AMA, Chicago, October, 1960.

Cheese from Denmark, Danish Cheese Export Board, Aarhus, Denmark.

Code of Federal Regulations (CFR), Title 21, Parts 1–119, Food and Drugs, U.S. Government Printing Office, Washington, D.C.

Composition of Foods, USDA Handbook No. 8, Washington, D.C., 1969.

Consumer Food News, Agriculture and Marketing Service, USDA, N.Y. (weekly newsletter).

Consumer Reports, Consumers Union, Mt. Vernon, N.Y. (monthly magazine).

Consumers Bulletin (now known as *Consumers Research* Magazine), Consumers Research, Inc., Washington, N.J. (monthly magazine).

Council on Food and Nutrition Policy Statements, AMA, Chicago, Ill.:

  "Composition of Certain Margarines," 1962.

  "General Policy on Addition of Specific Nutrients to Foods," December, 1961.

  "Safe Use of Chemicals in Foods," November, 1961.

Downey, Irene, *Keep the Quality in the Food You Buy,* Home Economics Extension Leaflet 19, Ithaca, N.Y., August, 1965.

Dunn, Mildred, and Helen Gifft, *Cheese: Buy It, Eat It, Enjoy It,* Cornell Extension Bulletin 1020, May, 1965.

Evaluation of Food Additives, Food and Agricultural Organization of the United Nations, Rome, 1971.

"Facts for Meat Managers: What You Should Know About New

Zealand Spring Lamb," New Zealand Lamb Council.

FDA Consumer, Food and Drug Administration, Superintendent of Documents, Washington, D.C. (monthly magazine).

Federal and State Standards for Composition of Milk Products, Agricultural Handbook No. 51, USDA Consumer Marketing Service, Washington, D.C., 1971.

Food and Home News Notes, USDA, Office of Information, Washington, D.C. (weekly newsletter).

Food and Nutrition, Section. Consumer Bulletin Annual, Consumers Research, Inc., Washington, N.J., 1972.

Frank, Helen Gunderson, and Egbert R. Ferguson Jr., *Food Standards and Definitions in the U.S.,* New York Academic Press, N.Y., 1963.

"Guide to Average Monthly Availability of Fresh Fruits and Vegetables," United Fresh Fruit and Vegetable Association, Washington, D.C., 1969.

Herber, Lewis, *Our Synthetic Environment,* Knopf, N.Y., 1962.

Hunter, Beatrice Trum, *Consumer Beware,* Simon & Schuster, N.Y., 1970.

"It's on the Label," National Canners Association, Washington, D.C.

Jacobson, Michael, *Eater's Digest,* Doubleday & Co., N.Y., 1972.

Judge, Jean F., "Freshness Codes," Grand Union Company.

Keene, Paul, "The Story of Oils," Walnut Acres, Penns Creek, Pa.

Kiernat, Barbara H., Jo Ann Johnson, and A. J. Siedler, *A Summary of the Nutrient Content of Meat,* American Meat Institute Foundation, Bulletin No. 57, Chicago, Ill., July, 1964.

Kileen, Jacqueline, *Ecology at Home,* 101 Productions, San Francisco, Cal., 1971.

Klippstein, Ruth, *The Versatile Egg,* Cornell Extension Bulletin No. 915, Ithaca, N.Y., 1963.

Knight, Granville F., MD, "What Are Pesticides Doing to Human Beings," American Nutrition Society, Los Angeles, Cal., 1952.

McIntosh, Edna Mae, *Foods for Baby and Mealtime Psychology,* Gerber Baby Products Company, Fremont, Michigan, 1963.

"Milk Information Sheet," National Dairy Council, Chicago, Ill., 1964.

"Newer Knowledge of Cheese," National Dairy Council, Chicago, Ill., 1967.

Organic Gardening and Farming, Rodale Press, Emmaus, Pa. (monthly magazine).

Rodale, J. I., and Staff, *The Complete Book of Food and Nutrition,* Rodale Press, Emmaus, Pa., 1971.

Rohe, Fred, "The Sugar Story," Los Angeles, Cal.

"Sickeningly Sweet: The Morbid Facts About Sugar," *Moneysworth,* N.Y., December 11, 1972.

The Story of Cereal Grains, General Mills, Minneapolis, Minn., 1944.

Swatek, Paul, *Users Guide to the Protection of the Environment,* A Friends of the Earth/Ballantine Books, N.Y., 1970.

Turner, James, *The Chemical Feast,* Grossman, N.Y., 1970.

United States Department of Agriculture, *Food for Us All: The Yearbook of Agriculture,* U.S. Government Printing Office, Washington, D.C., 1969.

United States Department of Agriculture, Home and Garden Bulletins No:

    103, "Eggs in Family Meals," October, 1973

    112, "Cheese in Family Meals," June, 1972

    118, "Beef and Veal in Family Meals," September, 1970

    124, "Lamb in Family Meals," February, 1971

    125, "Fruits in Family Meals," September, 1970

    127, "Milk in Family Meals," November, 1967

    150, "Cereals and Pasta in Family Meals," October, 1968

    160, "Pork in Family Meals," March, 1969

    176, "Nuts in Family Meals," May, 1970

    177, "How to Buy Dry Beans, Peas and Lentils," June, 1977

    193, "How to Buy Cheese," September, 1971

    198, "How to Buy Potatoes," February 1972

    201, "How to Buy Dairy Products," August, 1972

    208, "Soybeans in Family Meals," June, 1974

U.S. Standards for Grades of Butter, Agricultural Marketing Service, Dairy Division, USDA, Washington, D.C., 1960.

[U.S.] Standards for Meat and Poultry Products, USDA, Washington, D.C., March, 1972.

Urrows, Grace M., *Food Preservation by Irradiation,* U.S. Atomic Energy Commission, Oak Ridge, Tenn., 1968.

Vaughn, Reese, PhD, and George Steward, PhD, "Antibiotics as Food Preservatives," Council on Foods and Nutrition, AMA, Chicago, Ill., November, 1960.

Whole Grains . . . and Their Importance in the National Nutrition Program, Ralston Purina Co., St. Louis, Mo., 1942.

ADDITIONAL READING MATERIAL.

Allaby, Michael, and Floyd Allen, *Robots Behind the Wheel,* Rodale Press, Emmaus, Pa., 1974.

Coffin, Lewis A., *The Grandmother Conspiracy: Good Nutrition for the Growing Child,* Capra Press, 1974.

Composition of Foods, Agricultural Handbook No. 456, USDA.

Davis, Adelle, *Let's Eat Right to Keep Fit,* Signet, New York, 1970.

Davis, Adelle, *Let's Have Healthy Children,* Signet, New York, 1972.

Dietary Allowances Committee, Food and Nutrition Board, *Recommended Dietary Allowances,* 8th edition, National Academy of Sciences, Washington, D.C., 1974.

Feingold, Ben, M.D., *Why Your Child Is Hyperactive,* Random House, New York (co-published by Bookworks), 1974.

Goldbeck, Nikki and David, *The Dieter's Companion,* McGraw Hill, New York, 1976.

Hall, Ross Hume, PhD, *Food for Naught/The Decline in Nutrition,* Vintage Books, New York, 1976.

Hightower, Jim, *Eat Your Heart Out,* Quadrangle Books, New York, 1975.

Hunter, Beatrice Trum, *The Mirage of Safety,* Scribners, New York, 1976.

Jacobson, Michael, *Nutrition Scoreboard,* Avon, New York, 1975.

Lappe, Frances Moore, *Diet for a Small Planet,* revised edition, Ballantine Books, New York, 1975.

Lerza, Catherine and Michael Jacobson, *Food for People, Not for Profit,* Ballantine Books, New York 1975.

Pimental and Hard, "Food Production and the Energy Crisis," *Science Magazine,* No. 2, 1973.

Robbins, William, *The American Food Scandal,* William Morrow & Co., New York, 1974.

Solomon, Goody, *The Radical Consumer's Handbook,* Ballantine Books, New York, 1972.

Szykitka, Walter, *Public Works/A Handbook of Self-Reliant Living,* Links Books, New York, 1974.

Tannahill, Reay, *Food in History,* Stein & Day, New York, 1973.

The Committee on Nutritional Misinformation, "Vegetarian Diets," National Academy of Sciences, Washington, D.C., 1974.

Verrett, Jacqueline and Jean Carper, *Eating May Be Hazardous to Your Health,* Simon and Schuster, New York, 1974.

In addition, we recommend you read the publications prepared by The Food Project of Center for Science in the Public Interest, located at 1779 Church St., N.W., Washington, D.C., which include:

Creative Food Experiences for Children

Energy and Food

Food Scoreboard (an adaptation of Nutrition Scoreboard for 9 to 12-year-olds)

Food: Where Nutrition, Politics and Culture Meet; an activity book for teachers

How Sodium Nitrite Can Affect Your Health

Nutrition Action (a monthly magazine)

White Paper on Infant Feeding Practices

SOME COOKBOOKS TO GUIDE YOU ALONG:

Anderson, Lynn, *The Rainbow Farms Cookbook,* Colophon Books/Harper & Row, New York, 1974.

Brown, Edward Espe, *The Tassajara Bread Book,* Shambala, Berkeley, Cal., 1970.

Brown, Edward Espe, *Tassajara Cooking,* Shambala, Berkeley, Cal., 1973.

Kinderlehrer, Jane, *Confessions of a Sneaky Organic Cook,* Signet, New York, 1972.

Goldbeck, Nikki, and David, *The Good Breakfast Book,* Links Books, New York, 1976.

Hewitt, Jean, *The New York Times Natural Foods Cookbook,* Avon, New York, 1972.

Hunter, Beatrice Trum, *The Natural Foods Cookbook,* Simon and Schuster, New York, 1961.

Hunter, Beatrice Trum, *The Natural Foods Primer,* Fireside Books, New York, 1973.

Hurd, Frank J., and Rosalie, *Ten Talents,* College Press, Chisholm, Minn., 1968.

Lo, Kenneth H. C., *Chinese Vegetarian Cooking,* Pantheon Books, New York, 1974.

Richmond, Sonya, *International Vegetarian Cookery.*

Pipault, Christine, *Children Gastronomic,* Crown, New York, 1968.

Rombauer, Irma S., and Marion R. Becker, *Joy of Cooking,* Signet,

New York, 1974.
Thomas, Anna, *The Vegetarian Epicure,* Vintage, New York, 1972.
Standard, Stella, *Our Daily Bread,* Lancer, New York, 1970.

General Index

Recipe Index